Fifth Edition

Review Questions and Answers for Veterinary Technicians

Heather Prendergast, RVT, CVPM
President
Synergie Consulting
Las Cruces, New Mexico

ELSEVIER

ELSEVIER

3251 Riverport Lane
St. Louis, Missouri 63043

Notices

Knowledge and best practice in this field are constantly changing. As new research and experience broaden our understanding, changes in research methods, professional practices, or medical treatment may become necessary.

Practitioners and researchers must always rely on their own experience and knowledge in evaluating and using any information, methods, compounds, or experiments described herein. In using such information or methods they should be mindful of their own safety and the safety of others, including parties for whom they have a professional responsibility.

With respect to any drug or pharmaceutical products identified, readers are advised to check the most current information provided (i) on procedures featured or (ii) by the manufacturer of each product to be administered, to verify the recommended dose or formula, the method and duration of administration, and contraindications. It is the responsibility of practitioners, relying on their own experience and knowledge of their patients, to make diagnoses, to determine dosages and the best treatment for each individual patient, and to take all appropriate safety precautions.

To the fullest extent of the law, neither the Publisher nor the authors, contributors, or editors, assume any liability for any injury and/or damage to persons or property as a matter of products' liability, negligence or otherwise, or from any use or operation of any methods, products, instructions, or ideas contained in the material herein.

Library of Congress Cataloging-in-Publication Data

Names: Prendergast, Heather, editor.
Title: Review questions and answers for veterinary technicians / [edited by]
    Heather Prendergast.
Description: Fifth edition. | St. Louis, Missouri : Elsevier, [2017] |
    Preceded by: Review questions and answers for veterinary technicians /
    [edited by] Thomas Colville. 4th ed. 2010.
Identifiers: LCCN 2015044880 | ISBN 9780323316958 (pbk. : alk. paper)
Subjects: | MESH: Animal Technicians—Examination Questions.
Classification: LCC SF774.4 | NLM SF 774.4 | DDC 636.089/076—dc23 LC record available at
http://lccn.loc.gov/2015044880

Senior Vice President and Director: Loren Wilson
Content Strategist: Brandi Graham
Content Development Manager: Ellen Wurm-Cutter
Associate Content Development Specialist: Erin Garner
Publishing Services Manager: Jeffrey Patterson
Senior Project Manager: Tracey Schriefer
Designer: Margaret Reid

Printed in the United States of America

Last digit is the print number: 9   8   7   6   5   4

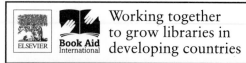
Working together
to grow libraries in
developing countries

www.elsevier.com • www.bookaid.org

Ed Carlson, CVT, VTS (Nutrition)
Technician Learning and Development Manager
IVG Hospitals, Inc.
VetBloom
Woburn, Massachusetts

Mary Ellen Goldberg, BS, LVT, CVT, SRA, CCRA
Veterinary Medical Technologist
Surgical Research Anesthetist
Instructor of Anesthesia and Pain Management
VetMedTeam, LLC
Saint Petersburg, Florida;
Certified Canine Rehabilitation Assistant
Canine Rehabilitation Institute
Boynton Beach, Florida

Brooke Lockridge, RDMS
Lead Veterinary Assistant, Nursing
Jornada Veterinary Clinic
Las Cruces, New Mexico

Tasha McNerney, BS, CVT
Anesthesia and Surgical Technician
Rau Animal Hospital
Glenside, Pennsylvania

Jody Nugent-Deal, RVT, VTS (Anesthesia, Clinical Practice—Exotic Companion Animal)
Small Animal Anesthesia and Surgery Supervisor
William R. Pritchard Veterinary Medical Teaching Hospital
University of California Davis
Davis, California

Jeanne Perrone, CVT, VTS (Dentistry)
Dentistry Instructor and Trainer
VT Dental Training
Plant City, Florida

Rachel V. Poulin, RVT, VTS (SAIM)
Internal Medicine Supervisor
Coral Springs Animal Hospital
Coral Springs, Florida

Brandy Tabor, BS, CVT, VTS (ECC)
Senior Emergency/Critical Care Technician
Animal Emergency and Specialty Center
Parker, Colorado

Marianne Tear, MS, LVT
Program Director, Veterinary Technology Program
Baker College of Clinton Township
Clinton Township, Michigan

Kenichiro Yagi, BS, RVT, VTS (ECC, SAIM)
ICU Manager, Blood Bank Manager
Adobe Animal Hospital
Los Altos, California

To my mother
~the wind beneath my wings~
who has guided and given me inspiration, motivation, and empowerment.
You have been a truly amazing woman.
I miss you dearly.

Preface

New editions of books are often more similar to previous editions than different. This fifth edition of *Review Questions and Answers for Veterinary Technicians,* however, departs significantly from previous editions in both form and content.

The content of the book is arranged to allow intuitive review for the Veterinary Technician National Examination (VTNE). The main subject areas in the ***VTNE Review*** section represent the "domains" of the VTNE that were in effect when this was written. The subjects included in the ***Foundation Knowledge Review*** section represent general knowledge that is included in all of the VTNE domains.

The 5000 questions in this book resulted from a process that began with a rigorous review of each of the questions from the fourth edition. To meet the criteria for inclusion in this edition, each question, answer, and rationale had to reflect accurate, contemporary, entry-level veterinary technology knowledge. More than 4500 of the questions, answers, and explanations are completely new, and about 500 were significantly revised.

The questions in *Review Questions and Answers for Veterinary Technicians* test factual knowledge, reasoning skills, and clinical judgment. To the best of our knowledge, none of the questions in this book have come directly from any current or previous credentialing examination. When properly used, however, the questions can help identify an individual's strengths and weaknesses in various subject areas.

Heather Prendergast, RVT, CVPM

This book is the result of the hard work of a veterinary technician team. I am honored to work with these skilled professionals, all of whom teach or work in practice.

I am grateful for the hard work and dedication given by: Kara Burns, MS, MEd, LVT, VTS (Nutrition), VTS-H (Internal Medicine, Dentistry); Ed Carlson, CVT, VTS (Nutrition); Jody Nugent-Deal, RVT, VTS (Anesthesia, Clinical Practice—Exotic Companion Animal); Mary Ellen Goldberg, BS, LVT, CVT, SRA, CCRA; Brooke Lockridge, RDMS; Tasha McNerney, BS, CVT; Jeanne Perrone, CVT, VTS (Dentistry); Rachel V. Poulin, RVT, VTS (SAIM); Brandy Tabor, BS, CVT, VTS (ECC); Marianne Tear, MS, LVT; and Kenichiro Yagi, BS, RVT, VTS (ECC, SAIM). Without their skills and knowledge, the revision would not have been possible.

Last, and certainly not least, this book would not have been possible without the support from Clint. Hats off to an awesome man who can hold down the fort while I continue to pursue my dream, and carry out an awesome career, and still have welcome arms every time I come home from another trip. I love you.

Credentialing of Veterinary Technicians

In most states and Canadian provinces, individuals who wish to work as veterinary technicians must demonstrate their knowledge and competence by completing a credentialing process that is administered by an appropriate regulatory agency. Successful completion of this credentialing process generally confers the title of Licensed Veterinary Technician (LVT), Certified Veterinary Technician (CVT), or Registered Veterinary Technician (RVT) on the individual, depending on the terminology used in each state.

Nearly all states and provinces that regulate the veterinary technology profession use the Veterinary Technician National Examination (VTNE) as the main component of their credentialing process, although some jurisdictions have additional requirements. Candidates should contact the appropriate regulatory agency in the state or province in which they desire credentialing to obtain information on processes, requirements, and deadlines. Contact information can be found on the website of the American Association of Veterinary State Boards (AAVSB) at http://www.aavsb.org.

The VTNE is offered by the AAVSB under a contractual agreement with the Professional Examination Service (PES). It is designed to evaluate essential job-related knowledge at the entry level, and it consists of 150 multiple-choice questions and 20 pilot questions in primary subject areas called "domains." The current VTNE domains are:
- Pharmacy and Pharmacology
- Surgical Nursing
- Dentistry
- Laboratory Procedures
- Animal Care and Nursing
- Diagnostic Imaging
- Anesthesia
- Emergency Medicine and Critical Care
- Pain Management and Analgesia

After a student passes the VTNE in a state or province, the examination score can be transferred to other states or provinces. Information on this process is also available on the AAVSB website.

Review Questions and Answers for Veterinary Technicians, Fifth Edition, covers every major aspect of veterinary technology. It contains 5000 questions and answers. An accompanying Evolve website contains all of the book's content in practice and exam modes, as well as rationales and source information. A 170-question practice test can be taken in the simulated exam mode. The questions are divided by section for the study mode. In exam mode, questions are organized according to VTNE domains of practice and pulled according to percentages comparable to the actual VTNE format.

The subjects covered in the **Foundation Knowledge Review** section represent general knowledge that is included in all of the VTNE domains. They are:

- Anatomy and Physiology
- Hospital Management
- Medical Calculations
- Terminology

The foundation subjects are particularly important because questions in the second section, **VTNE Review**, are built on the foundational knowledge in the first section. It may be helpful to complete the **Foundation Knowledge Review** section before beginning the **VTNE Review** section.

The VTNE Review section covers subjects related to the VTNE domains that were in effect when this edition was written. The subjects are:

- Pharmacology
- Surgical Nursing
- Dentistry
- Laboratory Procedures
- Animal Nursing
- Diagnostic Imaging
- Anesthesia
- Emergency and Critical Care
- Pain Management and Analgesia
- Exotic Animals

The primary intent of this book is to help students and graduate veterinary technicians prepare for examinations— either in academic programs or for credentialing purposes. Before beginning a section, the student should review textbooks and course notes pertaining to that subject area, and then approach each section as though it were an actual examination.

- *Carefully read each question.* Look for key words such as "most," "best," "least," "always," "never," and "except." Consider only the facts presented in the question. Do not make assumptions and inferences that may not be true.
- *Carefully evaluate each answer choice.* Each question has only one correct answer. The other three choices are incorrect "distractors." If more than one answer choice appears to be correct, closely examine each one for clues that would eliminate it from being correct.
- *Select an answer for each question.*
- *Compare your answers with the correct answers.* The correct answers are listed in the answer key at the end of this book.
- *Identify "weak" areas.* Subject areas with many incorrect answers may indicate the need for further review.

The Evolve website is set up in two different modes to better help the student study for the VTNE.

The *practice mode* includes all of the multiple-choice questions available in the book divided by section. The student chooses the specific sections he or she wishes to study, and he or she can select any number of questions to review. The student receives instant feedback as to whether the question was answered correctly or incorrectly, along with rationales and source information.

Simulated exam mode, similar to the format of the actual VTNE exam, contains 170 questions that are selected across all sections. The exam is timed and scored. After the student completes it, the results are available for viewing. The student may then review the exam in its entirety with answers and rationales.

Table of Contents

PART ONE
Foundation of Knowledge Review

Anatomy and Physiology

Brooke Lockridge, RDMS

QUESTIONS

1. Where are striated muscles located?
   a. Stomach wall and uterus
   b. Urinary bladder and intestine
   c. Ciliary body of the eye
   d. Heart and skeletal muscles

2. Systemic circulation is under:
   a. High pressure
   b. Low pressure
   c. Partial pressure
   d. Equilibrium

3. A pregnant mare has what kind of placentation?
   a. Zonary
   b. Cotyledonary
   c. Diffuse
   d. Discoid

4. The pressure in the systemic arteries during ventricular contraction is:
   a. Diastolic blood pressure
   b. Osmotic pressure
   c. Systolic blood pressure
   d. Low pressure

5. What hormone contracts the female reproductive tract to help move spermatozoa into the oviducts?
   a. Estrogen
   b. Progesterone
   c. Prolactin
   d. Oxytocin

6. Cardiac muscle is considered a:
   a. Nonstriated involuntary muscle
   b. Striated involuntary muscle
   c. Nonstriated voluntary muscle
   d. Striated voluntary muscle

7. In what order does the impulse for depolarization travel through the heart?
   a. AV node, SA node, bundle of His, Purkinje fibers
   b. SA node, AV node, bundle of His, Purkinje fibers
   c. SA node, AV node, Purkinje fibers, bundle of His
   d. AV node, SA node, Purkinje fibers, bundle of His

8. A pregnant queen has what kind of placentation?
   a. Zonary
   b. Cotyledonary
   c. Diffuse
   d. Discoid

9. The control of color changes in the pigment cells of reptiles, fish, and amphibians is associated with which hormone?
   a. FSH
   b. LH
   c. MSH
   d. TSH

10. The wave on an electrocardiogram that is associated with the atrial wall depolarization is the:
    a. PR interval
    b. T wave
    c. QRS complex
    d. P wave

11. The SA node is located in the wall of which chamber?
    a. Left atrium
    b. Left ventricle
    c. Right atrium
    d. Right ventricle

12. The muscular sphincter located between the stomach and the duodenum is the:
    a. Pylorus
    b. Cardia
    c. Chyme
    d. Rugae

13. The type of cell responsible for the transmission of impulses through the nervous system is the:
    a. Neuroglia
    b. Schwann
    c. Neuron
    d. Oligodendrocyte

14. Dogs demonstrate what type of estrous cycle?
    a. Polyestrous
    b. Seasonally polyestrous
    c. Diestrous
    d. Monoestrous

15. What system is anatomically composed of the brain and spinal cord?
    a. Central nervous system
    b. Peripheral nervous system
    c. Parasympathetic nervous system
    d. Sympathetic nervous system

16. Functions that an animal does not have to consciously control, such as peristalsis in the intestine, are influenced by the:
    a. Somatic nervous system
    b. Central nervous system
    c. Peripheral nervous system
    d. Autonomic nervous system

17. The cranial nerves and the spinal nerves are anatomically part of what system?
    a. Central nervous system
    b. Peripheral nervous system
    c. Parasympathetic nervous system
    d. Sympathetic nervous system

18. Sensory nerves are considered:
    a. Efferent motor nerves
    b. Motor nerves
    c. Efferent nerves
    d. Afferent nerves

19. When a stimulus is strong enough to cause complete depolarization, it has reached:
    a. Threshold
    b. Repolarization
    c. Refractory period
    d. Action potential

20. What happens within the neuron that allows local anesthetics to be effective?
    a. Potassium gates open
    b. The charge within the cell becomes positive
    c. The charge within the cell becomes negative
    d. Sodium channels become blocked

21. Smooth muscles can be found in the:
    a. Heart
    b. Stomach
    c. Pelvic limb
    d. Diaphragm

22. Which muscle cells have single nuclei?
    a. Skeletal and cardiac
    b. Skeletal and smooth
    c. Smooth and cardiac
    d. Skeletal only

23. Cattle and swine display what type of estrous cycle?
    a. Polyestrous
    b. Seasonally polyestrous
    c. Diestrous
    d. Monoestrous

24. What species is an induced ovulator?
    a. Bovine
    b. Equine
    c. Canine
    d. Feline

25. In what stage of the estrous cycle does the corpus luteum develop?
    a. Proestrus
    b. Estrus
    c. Metestrus
    d. Diestrous

26. Which reaction is the result of sympathetic nervous system stimulation?
    a. Decreased heart rate
    b. Dilated pupils
    c. Increased GI activity
    d. Increased salivation

27. The hormone produced by a developing ovarian follicle is:
    a. Estrogen
    b. Progesterone
    c. Prolactin
    d. Oxytocin

28. To achieve a normal pregnancy, the blastocyst attaches to what structure?
    a. Endometrium
    b. Placenta
    c. Oviduct
    d. Cervix

29. Giving birth is known as:
    a. Parturition
    b. Gestation
    c. Lactation
    d. Estrous

30. From the estrous cycle to parturition, in what order are the following hormones released?
    a. Estrogen, oxytocin, progesterone
    b. Oxytocin, estrogen, progesterone
    c. Estrogen, progesterone, oxytocin
    d. Progesterone, estrogen, oxytocin

31. All of the following are types of chorion attachments, *except:*
    a. Diffuse
    b. Cotyledonary
    c. Zonary
    d. Polycyton

32. A pregnant bitch has what kind of placentation?
    a. Zonary
    b. Cotyledonary
    c. Diffuse
    d. Discoid

33. The canine uterus is shaped like the letter
    a. U
    b. Y
    c. J
    d. V

34. How many mammary glands are typically found on a bitch?
    a. 8–12
    b. 12–14
    c. 4–6
    d. 10–16

35. Which reaction is the result of parasympathetic nervous system stimulation?
    a. Bronchodilation
    b. Pupil dilation
    c. Decreased GI motility
    d. Decreased heart rate

36. The neurotransmitter that is most responsible for the "flight or fight" reaction is:
    a. Epinephrine
    b. Acetylcholine
    c. Dopamine
    d. Serotonin

37. In the healthy heart, the heartbeat is initiated by the:
    a. SA node
    b. Purkinje fibers
    c. Vagus nerve
    d. AV node

38. On an electrocardiogram, the T wave is most closely associated with:
    a. Atrial depolarization
    b. Atrial repolarization
    c. Ventricular depolarization
    d. Ventricular repolarization

39. On inspiration, the pressure in the thoracic cavity, as compared with ambient air pressure, is
    a. Negative
    b. Positive
    c. Same as the ambient air pressure
    d. Fluctuating

40. In the healthy awake cat, the primary stimulus within blood for respiration is:
    a. Increased CO_2
    b. Decreased O_2
    c. Increased lactic acid
    d. Increased K^+

41. An increased packed cell volume (PCV) could be indicative of:
    a. Liver disease
    b. Anemia
    c. Leukocytosis
    d. Dehydration

42. Apnea will cause:
    a. Metabolic acidosis
    b. Metabolic alkalosis
    c. Respiratory acidosis
    d. Respiratory alkalosis

43. Which of the following nutrients can be used for gluconeogenesis?
    a. Long-chain fatty acids
    b. Amino acids
    c. Vitamin C
    d. Iron

44. Cataracts result from a problem with transparency of the:
    a. Cornea
    b. Vitreous humor
    c. Lens
    d. Aqueous humor

45. Within the eye, the choroid is located between which two structures?
    a. Sclera and retina
    b. Iris and pupil
    c. Lens and cornea
    d. Optic nerve and fovea centralis

46. Which of the following are considered to be a category of lipids?
    a. Neutral fats
    b. Steroids
    c. Phospholipids
    d. All of the above

47. Which of the following processes is not a function of insulin?
    a. Increased glucose transport into muscle
    b. Lipogenesis
    c. Fatty acid synthesis
    d. Increased blood pressure

48. Which endocrine cells of the pancreatic islets produce the hormone glucagon?
    a. Alpha cells
    b. Beta cells
    c. Delta cells
    d. Somatostatin

49. Long-term use of glucocorticoids will:
    a. Increase lymphocyte production
    b. Increase plasma protein levels
    c. Suppress the immune system
    d. Decrease blood glucose levels

50. Nociceptors are important for detecting:
    a. Color
    b. Warmth
    c. Lactic acid
    d. Pain

51. The sensation of hunger falls under which general sense?
    a. Tactile sensation
    b. Pain sensation
    c. Proprioception
    d. Visceral sensation

52. The vagus nerve is cranial nerve _____.
    a. X
    b. XII
    c. V
    d. VI

53. The cranial nerves originate from the
    a. Cerebellum
    b. Spinal cord
    c. Brainstem
    d. Cerebrum

54. Glaucoma is:
    a. Decreased pressure in the posterior chamber of the eye
    b. Increased pressure in the posterior chamber of the eye
    c. Increased pressure in the anterior chamber of the eye
    d. Decreased pressure in the anterior chamber of the eye

55. Aqueous humor is formed in which chamber of the eye?
    a. Posterior chamber
    b. Anterior chamber
    c. Canal of Schlemm
    d. Cornea

56. Clients should be cautioned against sticking Q-tips in the ears of their pets because they could rupture the:
    a. Oval window
    b. Round window
    c. Cochlea
    d. Tympanic membrane

57. Which condition would be typical of hypothyroidism?
    a. Decreased water consumption
    b. Oily hair coat
    c. Very active
    d. Weight gain

58. In dairy cattle, the teats and udder are gently washed before milking to stimulate the release of one of the following, to stimulate milk letdown:
    a. Adrenalin
    b. Norepinephrine
    c. Dopamine
    d. Oxytocin

59. Which hormone helps to trigger and maintain lactation?
    a. FSH
    b. Prolactin
    c. LH
    d. TSH

60. Lymph nodes that are found medial to the caudal part of the jaw are the:
    a. Popliteal nodes
    b. Inguinal nodes
    c. Mandibular nodes
    d. Prescapular nodes

61. A pregnant rodent has what kind of placentation?
    a. Zonary
    b. Cotyledonary
    c. Diffuse
    d. Discoid

62. The neurohypophysis is an anatomic section of which of the following?
    a. Hypothalamus
    b. Adrenal gland
    c. Pancreas

63. The portal vein:
    a. Carries blood from the spleen to the heart
    b. Delivers blood to the liver
    c. Delivers blood to the kidney
    d. Carries blood from the lungs to the heart

64. To proceed from a point between the eyes to the tip of a dog's nose, you would move
    a. Rostrally
    b. Cranially
    c. Caudally
    d. Laterally

65. Typically, what percentage of an animal's body weight consists of blood?
    a. 0.1%
    b. 1%
    c. 8%
    d. 30%

66. A dog that weighs 10 kg would have approximately how much blood?
    a. 50 mL
    b. 800 mL
    c. 1.5 L
    d. 2 L

67. Which of the following dissections could be made without cutting through a bone-to-bone joint?
    a. Forelimb from the body
    b. Hind limb from the body
    c. Head from the neck
    d. Tail from the body

68. If you were to grasp your hands behind your head at the base of your skull, your hands would be over which bone of the skull?
    a. Occipital
    b. Frontal
    c. Temporal
    d. Parietal

69. The glucose absorbed from the GI tract may be stored in the liver as glycogen through a process known as what?
    a. Glycogenesis
    b. Gluconeogenesis
    c. Glycogenolysis
    d. Fatty acid synthesis

70. The process of voice production usually begins in which location?
    a. Pharynx
    b. Larynx
    c. Thorax
    d. Trachea

71. Essential nutrients can be divided into how many categories?
    a. 3
    b. 4
    c. 6
    d. 10

72. Efferent nerves carry nerve impulses:
    a. To the body from the central nervous system
    b. To the body from the spinal cord
    c. From the body to the central nervous system
    d. From one part of a limb to another part of the same limb

73. The name for the bile acid–lipid units that carry fat within the gut is:
    a. LPL
    b. Micelles
    c. VLDL
    d. Chylomicrons

74. Which type of RNA copies the information in the DNA?
    a. Messenger RNA
    b. Ribosomal RNA
    c. Copy RNA
    d. Transfer RNA

75. Bile acids are important in the digestion of:
    a. Carbohydrates
    b. Electrolytes
    c. Fats
    d. Proteins

76. Which of the following lowers blood glucose?
    a. Insulin
    b. Glucagon
    c. Epinephrine
    d. Glucocorticoids

77. Which system is considered to be the largest and most extensive organ system in the body?
    a. Integument
    b. Cardiovascular
    c. Digestive
    d. Central nervous system

78. Different nitrogen bases are found in both DNA and RNA nucleotides. Which nucleotide is only found in DNA?
    a. Adenine (A)
    b. Cytosine (C)
    c. Guanine (G)
    d. Thymine (T)

79. The P wave component of a QRS complex usually corresponds to:
    a. Atrial contraction
    b. Ventricular contraction
    c. Atrial relaxation
    d. Electrical conduction in Purkinje fibers

80. The islets of Langerhans are found in the:
    a. Spleen
    b. Pancreas
    c. Liver
    d. Kidney

81. Which of the following is the basic functional unit of the kidney?
    a. Nephron
    b. Calyces
    c. Hilus
    d. Medulla

82. The kidneys are located in which cavity?
    a. Peritoneal cavity
    b. Pelvic cavity
    c. Retroperitoneal cavity
    d. Abdominal cavity

83. Which circulatory system is under the highest pressure?
    a. Pulmonary
    b. Coronary
    c. Systemic
    d. Capillaries

84. Fat in the lymph would most likely be associated with:
    a. Micelles
    b. Chylomicrons
    c. VLDL cholesterol
    d. LDL cholesterol

85. The mesovarium ligament supports which organ?
    a. Testicles
    b. Ovaries
    c. Oviduct
    d. Uterus

86. Milk fever in dairy cows is typically treated with:
    a. IV glucose
    b. IV calcium
    c. Atropine
    d. Antibiotics

87. For an animal that had lost RBCs to a moderate hookworm infection, one would expect the capillary refill time to be:
    a. Less than 1 second
    b. Greater than 4 seconds
    c. Greater than 2 minutes
    d. Greater than 4 minutes

88. A pulse taken from the inguinal area of a dog would be from the:
    a. Femoral artery
    b. Axillary artery
    c. Popliteal artery
    d. Saphenous artery

89. What is called the "knee" in the forelimb of a horse would be called the _____ in the human.
    a. Hip joint
    b. Wrist joint
    c. Finger joint
    d. Knee joint

90. The linea alba on a standing cat is _____ to the spinal cord.
    a. Ventral
    b. Dorsal
    c. Medial
    d. Contralateral

91. Arteries have relatively thick walls, which are composed of three layers. Which layer is the outermost layer?
    a. Tunica intima
    b. Tunica adventitia
    c. Tunica media
    d. Arteries only have one layer

92. Yellow mucous membranes would suggest:
    a. Renal disease
    b. Hepatic disease
    c. Shock
    d. Dehydration

93. A capillary refill time of 2 seconds would suggest which of the following?
    a. Shock
    b. Anemia
    c. A healthy animal
    d. Dehydration

94. What is the name for the large, flat projection located lateral to the head of the femur?
    a. Lesser trochanter
    b. Greater trochanter
    c. Trochanteric fossa
    d. Tubercle

95. The femur articulates distally with the tibia, forming the:
    a. Hip joint
    b. Stifle joint
    c. Tarsal joint
    d. Shoulder joint

96. What is the term for a part closer to a point of attachment or to the trunk?
    a. Distal
    b. Lateral
    c. Proximal
    d. Superficial

97. What is the term used below the carpus for the surface directed caudally or ventrally?
    a. Plantar
    b. Sagittal
    c. Palmar
    d. Longitudinal

98. In growing bone, where does lengthening take place?
    a. Epiphyseal plate
    b. Metaphysis
    c. Diaphysis
    d. Periosteal plane

99. What layer of bone tissue is necessary for the attachment of ligaments and tendons?
    a. Periosteum
    b. Endosteum
    c. Cartilage
    d. Meniscus

100. The fibrous covering around the part of the bone NOT covered by articular cartilage is:
    a. Endosteum
    b. Ligament
    c. Tendon
    d. Periosteum

101. What two valves comprise the atrioventricular valves?
    a. Mitral valve, pulmonic valve
    b. Aortic valve, pulmonic valve
    c. Mitral valve, tricuspid valve
    d. Pulmonic valve, tricuspid valve

102. What two valves comprise the semilunar valves?
    a. Mitral valve, pulmonic valve
    b. Pulmonic valve, aortic valve
    c. Mitral valve, tricuspid valve
    d. Pulmonic valve, tricuspid valve

103. The normal dentition pattern for an adult cat is
    a. Incisor 3/3, Canine 1/1, Premolar 3/2, Molar 1/1
    b. Incisor 3/3, Canine 1/1, Premolar 4/3, Molar 2/2
    c. Incisor 2/2, Canine 1/1, Premolar 3/2, Molar 2/1
    d. Incisor 2/2, Canine 1/1, Premolar 4/4, Molar 1/1

104. In the avian species, the ventral wall of the esophagus is greatly expanded to form the:
    a. Proventriculus
    b. Crop
    c. Gizzard
    d. Duodenum

105. What is the average number of air sacs that birds have?
    a. 4
    b. 6
    c. 8
    d. 9

106. In birds, the cloaca is:
    a. An appendage suspended from the head
    b. A blind sac at the distal end of the jejunum
    c. A cleft in the hard palate
    d. A common passage for fecal, urinary, and reproductive systems

107. In the avian species, the gizzard is also referred to as the:
    a. Proventriculus
    b. Ventriculus
    c. Crop
    d. Colon

108. Which muscle is the main muscle for inspiration?
    a. Epaxial muscle
    b. Diaphragm
    c. Internal abdominal oblique
    d. Hypaxial muscles

109. The uvea consists of the iris, ciliary body, and:
   a. Neural tunic
   b. Fibrous tunic
   c. Anterior chamber
   d. Choroid

110. The front surface of the lens is in contact with which of the following?
   a. Vitreous humor
   b. Aqueous humor
   c. Retina
   d. Sclera

111. The muscular structure that separates the right and left ventricles is called the interventricular:
   a. Sternum
   b. Coronary muscle
   c. Septum
   d. Myocardium

112. The muscular layer that makes up the majority of the heart mass is the:
   a. Myocardium
   b. Endocardium
   c. Myometrium
   d. Pericardium

113. The major artery that carries blood out of the left ventricle is the:
   a. Subclavian artery
   b. Carotid artery
   c. Pulmonary artery
   d. Aorta

114. All of the following major vessels contribute to blood flowing into the cranial vena cava *except* for the:
   a. Brachiocephalic vein
   b. Thoracic duct
   c. Azygos vein
   d. Femoral vein

115. Which structure drains blood from the stomach, intestine, and pancreas and flows directly to the liver?
   a. Hepatic veins
   b. Hepatic portal vein
   c. Hepatic artery
   d. Portosystemic shunt

116. The coronary veins empty blood via the coronary sinus into the:
   a. Left atrium
   b. Right atrium
   c. Left ventricle
   d. Right ventricle

117. The pulmonary circulation is under:
   a. High pressure
   b. Low pressure
   c. Partial pressure
   d. Equilibrium

118. How many teeth does an adult dog have?
   a. 28
   b. 32
   c. 42
   d. 50

119. Which of these is not a division of the small intestine?
   a. Duodenum
   b. Ilium
   c. Ileum
   d. Jejunum

120. What abdominal organ is absent in the horse and rat?
   a. Right kidney
   b. Gallbladder
   c. Pancreas
   d. Cecum

121. What is unique about the ruminant oral cavity?
   a. Presence of a dental pad
   b. Absence of salivary glands
   c. Absence of molars
   d. Presence of needle teeth

122. What is the actual true stomach called in ruminants?
   a. Abomasum
   b. Reticulum
   c. Rumen
   d. Omasum

123. What is the most common site of feed impactions in the horse?
   a. Sternal flexure
   b. Diaphragmatic flexure
   c. Stomach
   d. Pelvic flexure

124. Food is moved along the digestive tract by the process known as
   a. Mastication
   b. Prehension
   c. Peristalsis
   d. Elimination

125. The most distal portion of the monogastric stomach is the:
   a. Fundus
   b. Antrum
   c. Cardia
   d. Pylorus

126. All of the following are cells found in the fundus and body of the stomach *except:*
    a. Parietal cells
    b. Chief cells
    c. G cells
    d. Mucous cells

127. Which of the following is not a hormone produced or released by the pituitary gland?
    a. Luteinizing hormone
    b. Oxytocin
    c. Growth hormone
    d. Calcitonin

128. Which of the following is a ductless system?
    a. Exocrine system
    b. Endocrine system
    c. Lymphatic system
    d. All of the above systems contain ducts

129. The hormone responsible for maintaining pregnancy is:
    a. Oxytocin
    b. Luteinizing hormone
    c. Estrogen
    d. Progesterone

130. The structure produced immediately after an ovarian follicle has ruptured and released its ovum is the:
    a. Corpus callosum
    b. Corpus luteum
    c. Corpus albicans
    d. Graafian follicle

131. A deficiency in antidiuretic hormone causes:
    a. Diabetes insipidus
    b. Diabetes mellitus
    c. Cushing's disease
    d. Pancreatic insufficiency

132. The kidney produces what hormone?
    a. Antidiuretic hormone
    b. Adrenocorticotropic hormone
    c. Erythropoietin
    d. Adrenal cortex hormone

133. What hormone is produced by the beta cells in the pancreas?
    a. Insulin
    b. Glucagon
    c. Glycogen
    d. Somatostatin

134. Which hormone stimulates the growth and development of the cortex of the adrenal gland and release of some of its hormones?
    a. Thyroid-stimulating hormone
    b. Adrenocorticotropic hormone
    c. Prolactin
    d. Follicle-stimulating hormone

135. The endocrine structure responsible for secreting melatonin is:
    a. Pituitary gland
    b. Spleen
    c. Thymus
    d. Pineal gland

136. The lymphatic system is not involved in:
    a. Waste material transport
    b. Protein transport
    c. Carbohydrate transport
    d. Fluid transport

137. Lymph from the digestive system is known as what?
    a. GALT
    b. Haustra
    c. Chylomicrons
    d. Chyle

138. The lymphatic structure found in the small intestines responsible for the transport of fats and fat-soluble vitamins is:
    a. Afferent lymphatic vessels
    b. Lacteals
    c. Trabeculae
    d. Spleen

139. Which of the following is a lymphatic structure?
    a. Bile duct
    b. Islets of Langerhans
    c. Thyroid
    d. Tonsil

140. What structure is not found in the brainstem?
    a. Midbrain
    b. Pons
    c. Hypothalamus
    d. Medulla oblongata

141. The point at which blood vessels, nerves, and ureters enter and leave the kidneys is known as:
    a. Medulla
    b. Hilus
    c. Cortex
    d. Pelvis

142. How much urine do horses produce a day?
    a. 10 mL/kg/day
    b. 20 mL/kg/day
    c. 40 mL/kg/day
    d. 60 mL/kg/day

143. Ruminants have what type of placentation?
    a. Cotyledonary
    b. Zonary
    c. Diffuse
    d. Discoid

144. Which of the following is a posterior pituitary hormone?
    a. Luteinizing hormone
    b. Growth hormone
    c. Oxytocin
    d. Follicle-stimulating hormone

145. Sperm cells are produced by the:
    a. Seminiferous tubule
    b. Epididymis
    c. Vas deferens
    d. Seminal vesicles

146. What domestic species lacks the bulbourethral gland, also called Cowper's gland?
    a. Equine
    b. Feline
    c. Canine
    d. Bovine

147. All of the following are induced ovulators *except:*
    a. Rabbit
    b. Rat
    c. Cat
    d. Ferret

148. The time period from the beginning of one heat cycle to the beginning of the next is called:
    a. Estrous
    b. Estrus
    c. Ovulation
    d. The mating cycle

149. What muscle is responsible for pulling the testicles closer to the body?
    a. Retractor penis muscle
    b. Cremaster muscle
    c. Kegel muscle
    d. Retractor testicle muscle

150. Not all follicles that were activated in a particular ovarian cycle fully develop and ovulate. This is known as:
    a. Ovulation
    b. Follicular atresia
    c. Graafian follicle
    d. Corpus albicans

151. What primary ovarian structure is responsible for the release of estrogen?
    a. Follicle
    b. Placenta
    c. Corpus hemorrhagicum
    d. Corpus luteum

152. What is the normal gestational period for dogs?
    a. 36 days
    b. 54 days
    c. 63 days
    d. 120 days

153. The average gestational length in the ferret is:
    a. 69 days
    b. 42 days
    c. 151 days
    d. 20 days

154. The condition known as pseudopregnancy can result from an exaggerated:
    a. Anestrus
    b. Metestrus
    c. Diestrus
    d. Proestrus

155. The thorax is normally under:
    a. Partial pressure
    b. Positive pressure
    c. Equilibrium
    d. Negative pressure

156. Skeletal muscles are:
    a. Under voluntary control
    b. Nonstriated
    c. Under involuntary control
    d. Found in the walls of hollow organs

157. The two main minerals that make up bone are:
    a. Calcium and magnesium
    b. Sodium and potassium
    c. Calcium and phosphorus
    d. Calcium and potassium

158. Basic functions of bones include all of the following *except:*
    a. Protection
    b. Storage
    c. Leverage
    d. Metabolism

159. The hormone primarily responsible for preventing hypocalcemia is:
    a. T4
    b. Parathyroid hormone
    c. Calcitonin
    d. Vitamin D

160. The bone cells responsible for the removal of bone are:
    a. Osteoclasts
    b. Osteoblasts
    c. Chondroblasts
    d. Chondroclasts

161. The periosteum:
    a. Covers joint cavities
    b. Lines the heart
    c. Lines the marrow cavity of bones
    d. Covers the outer surface of bones

162. Bones come in all of the following shapes *except:*
    a. Flat
    b. Short
    c. Regular
    d. Long

163. The shaft of the bone is also called the:
    a. Trunk
    b. Epiphysis
    c. Periosteum
    d. Diaphysis

164. An example of a short bone would be a:
    a. Vertebra
    b. Tarsal bone
    c. Scapula
    d. Patella

165. The skull bone that articulates with the first cervical vertebra is the:
    a. Parietal bone
    b. Temporal bone
    c. Occipital bone
    d. Frontal bone

166. The bones known collectively as the ossicles include all of the following *except* the:
    a. Sphenoid
    b. Malleus
    c. Stapesus
    d. Incus

167. How many cervical vertebrae does the cat have?
    a. 13
    b. 7
    c. 3
    d. 10

168. The first cervical vertebra, C1, is referred to as the:
    a. Axis
    b. Atlas
    c. Arch
    d. Auricle

169. The breastbone is the:
    a. Hyoid
    b. Septum
    c. Tubercle
    d. Sternum

170. The most caudal portion of the sternum is called the:
    a. Xiphoid
    b. Coccyx
    c. Manubrium
    d. Costal

171. Claws, hooves, and horns are made up of which type of cell?
    a. Keratinized
    b. Agglutinated
    c. Calcified
    d. Crystallized

172. Which of the following is considered a part of the external structure of the equine hoof?
    a. Digital cushion
    b. Corium
    c. Lateral cartilage
    d. Frog

173. Adult cattle have how many upper incisors?
    a. 6
    b. 4
    c. 0
    d. 5

174. The anatomic term for synovial joints is:
    a. Fibroarthroses
    b. Amphiarthroses
    c. Synarthroses
    d. Diarthroses

175. Which joint is not a synovial joint?
    a. Hinge joint
    b. Gliding joint
    c. Swinging joint
    d. Pivot joint

176. The area of the kidney where urine collection occurs before entering the ureter is known as the:
    a. Renal pelvis
    b. Hilus
    c. Cortex
    d. Medulla

177. In the kidney, the primary site of action for ADH is in the:
    a. Loop of Henle
    b. Proximal convoluted tubule
    c. Glomerulus
    d. Collecting ducts

178. The renal corpuscle is located in the:
    a. Renal pelvis
    b. Hilus
    c. Medulla
    d. Cortex

179. The renal corpuscle is composed of the:
    a. Glomerulus and Bowman's capsule
    b. Collecting ducts and proximal convoluted tubule
    c. Descending and ascending loops of Henle
    d. Collecting ducts and afferent arteriole

180. The urinary bladder is not responsible for:
    a. Urine storage
    b. Urine filtration
    c. Urine collecting
    d. Urine release

181. The trunk of an animal is defined as:
    a. The front half of the animal
    b. The back half of the animal
    c. The thorax of the animal
    d. The thorax and abdomen of the animal

182. The middle phalanx is located:
    a. Lateral to the distal phalanx
    b. Distal to the distal phalanx
    c. Medial to the distal phalanx
    d. Proximal to the distal phalanx

183. The humeroradioulnar joint is located:
    a. Lateral to the carpus
    b. Distal to the left of the carpus
    c. Medial to the carpus
    d. Proximal to the carpus

184. Which organ is the largest abdominal organ in the body?
    a. Stomach
    b. Pancreas
    c. Kidney
    d. Liver

185. The leg bone responsible for minimal support is the:
    a. Fibula
    b. Femur
    c. Tibia
    d. Humerus

186. The large muscle of the caudal aspect of the canine lower hind leg is the:
    a. Tibialis anterior
    b. Gracilis
    c. Semimembranosus
    d. Gastrocnemius

187. Which of the following is not a muscle in the abdominal group?
    a. External oblique
    b. Rectus abdominis
    c. Latissimus dorsi
    d. Internal oblique

188. How many muscle heads are in the canine triceps brachii group?
    a. 4
    b. 3
    c. 2
    d. 1

189. Fascia is described as:
    a. The facial muscular surface
    b. A tough sheet of fibrous connective tissue
    c. A broad band of muscle fiber
    d. A lacy network of connective tissue

190. The deltoid muscles allow fine movements of the:
    a. Shoulder
    b. Hip
    c. Elbow
    d. Jaw

191. Which of the following structures suspends the larynx from the skull?
    a. Pharynx
    b. Epiglottis
    c. Hyoid apparatus
    d. Mediastinum

192. The two gastric sphincters of the canine are:
    a. Rectal and cecal
    b. Cardiac and pyloric
    c. Cardiac and rectal
    d. Pyloric and rectal

193. The dorsal plane divides the:
    a. Upper and lower halves of the body
    b. Front and back halves of the body
    c. Head from the rest of the body
    d. Right and left sides of the body

194. The middle portion of the small intestine is the:
    a. Jejunum
    b. Jejunem
    c. Jajunem
    d. Jujunem

195. The _____ pleura overlays organs in the body.
    a. Parietal
    b. Viscous
    c. Partial
    d. Visceral

196. Which sinus is not considered to be a "true" sinus of the dog?
    a. Frontal sinus
    b. External nares
    c. Paranasal sinuses
    d. Maxillary sinus

197. The triangular-shaped muscle that originates from the dorsal midline and inserts on the spin of the scapula is which of the following?
    a. Latissimus dorsi
    b. Brachiocephalicus
    c. External intercostals
    d. Trapezius

198. The cardiovascular system has four components. Which of the following is not part of the system?
    a. Heart
    b. Blood circulation
    c. Blood vessels
    d. Lungs

199. The appendicular skeleton includes the:
    a. Os cordis
    b. Ribs
    c. Pelvic girdle
    d. Clavicles

200. Which animal does not have an os penis?
    a. Dog
    b. Cat
    c. Wolf
    d. Pig

201. Which statement best describes short bones?
    a. Greater size in one dimension than another
    b. Filled with spongy bone and marrow spaces
    c. Thick outer layer of compact bone
    d. Irregularly shaped bones that make up the spinal column

202. The scapula is an example of a:
    a. Long bone
    b. Short bone
    c. Flat bone
    d. Irregular bone

203. An example of an irregular bone is:
    a. Cervical vertebra 1
    b. Metacarpal 3
    c. Ulna
    d. Scapula

204. Which of the following is not a part of the axial skeleton?
    a. Cervical vertebra 3
    b. Scapula
    c. Skull
    d. Thoracic vertebra 1

205. A skull suture is an example of what type of joint?
    a. Diarthrosis
    b. Synarthrosis
    c. Amphiarthrosis
    d. Cartilaginous

206. The only true pivot joint in the body is the:
    a. Spheroidal
    b. Elbow
    c. Carpal
    d. Atlantoaxial

207. Muscles and ligaments attach to structures on bony surfaces. Which of the following is not one of these found in the forelimb?
    a. Trochanter
    b. Tuberosity
    c. Spine
    d. Epicondyle

208. Which structure will not allow blood vessels and nerves to pass through?
    a. Meatus
    b. Sinus
    c. Foramen
    d. Facet

209. The joint between the bony rib and cartilaginous portion of the rib is called the:
    a. Cartilaginous junction
    b. Chondralcartilaginous junction
    c. Costochondral junction
    d. Costicartilaginous junction

210. Dogs have how many cervical, thoracic, and lumbar vertebrae?
    a. 7, 13, 6
    b. 7, 12, 7
    c. 6, 13, 7
    d. 7, 13, 7

211. Horses have how many cervical, thoracic, and lumbar vertebrae?
    a. 7, 13, 7
    b. 7, 18, 7
    c. 6, 7, 18
    d. 7, 18, 4

212. What is the value of X in this cow's dentition chart?
    I 0/3; C 0/1; P 3/3; M X/3
    a. 4
    b. 3
    c. 2
    d. 1

213. The valves that prevent backflow of blood from the arteries to the ventricles are called the:
    a. Tricuspid
    b. Bicuspid
    c. Mitral
    d. Semilunar

214. What structures disseminate electrical impulses across the ventricles?
    a. Perkinje fibers
    b. Purkinje fibers
    c. Purkinge fibers
    d. Perkingi fibers

215. Systole is:
    a. Contraction of the atria and ventricles
    b. Relaxation of the atria and ventricles
    c. Contraction of the atria and relaxation of the ventricles
    d. Relaxation of the atria and contraction of the ventricles

216. The aorta leaves the heart from the:
    a. Left ventricle
    b. Right ventricle
    c. Left atrium
    d. Right atrium

217. Blood enters the heart from the pulmonary veins in the:
    a. Left ventricle
    b. Right ventricle
    c. Left atrium
    d. Right atrium

218. Which circulation system is under the highest pressure?
    a. Coronary circulation
    b. Systemic circulation
    c. Pulmonary circulation
    d. All of the circulatory systems are under the same pressure

219. The name of the hole between the cardiac atria that closes at birth in the mammal is:
    a. Aortic hiatus
    b. Foramen
    c. Fossa
    d. Foramen ovale

220. Which of these is not a characteristic of lymph?
    a. Tissue fluids
    b. A large number of neutrophils
    c. B cells
    d. Part of the circulatory system

221. The tricuspid valve controls the flow of blood:
    a. Into the left ventricle
    b. Out of the left ventricle
    c. Into the right ventricle
    d. Out of the right ventricle

222. The thymus:
    a. Is another name for the thyroid gland
    b. Produces cells that destroy foreign substances
    c. Is more prominent in adults than in young animals
    d. Is located in the cranial abdomen

223. The eardrum is also called the:
    a. Pinna
    b. Tympanic membrane
    c. Eustachian tubes
    d. Cochlea

224. What organ is most commonly associated with the capacity for extramedullary hematopoiesis if necessary?
    a. Spleen
    b. Pancreas
    c. Lung
    d. Prostate

225. Efferent neurons are part of what system?
    a. Motor
    b. Interneuron
    c. Sensory
    d. Extraneuron

226. Afferent neurons are part of what system?
  a. Motor
  b. Interneuron
  c. Sensory
  d. Extraneuron

227. The function of the red blood cell is to:
  a. Provide defense from foreign invaders
  b. Act as a phagocyte
  c. Carry oxygen to the tissues
  d. Respond to the need for clotting

228. What artery carries deoxygenated blood?
  a. Aorta
  b. Pulmonary
  c. Coronary
  d. Carotid

229. Albumin is found in the blood and is a type of:
  a. Lipoprotein
  b. Phospholipid
  c. Enzyme
  d. Protein

230. Albumin is produced in the:
  a. Liver
  b. Red bone marrow
  c. Lymph nodes
  d. Pancreas

231. The production of platelets is known as:
  a. Hemostasis
  b. Thrombopoiesis
  c. Homeostasis
  d. Coagulation

232. What cells are involved in antibody production?
  a. Monocytes
  b. Neutrophils
  c. Lymphocytes
  d. Basophils

233. An increase in WBCs is referred to as which of the following?
  a. Leukopenia
  b. Anemia
  c. Leukocytosis
  d. Thrombocytopenia

234. Which of the following is known as the largest gland in the body?
  a. Pancreas
  b. Thyroid
  c. Liver
  d. Spleen

235. Bile is produce by which of the following organs?
  a. Gallbladder
  b. Liver
  c. Pancreas
  d. Spleen

236. What causes the gallbladder to contract?
  a. The release of CCK
  b. The release of glucagon
  c. The production of bile
  d. The gallbladder contracts involuntarily after it is filled

237. Red blood cell production is stimulated by:
  a. Hypoxia and erythropoietin
  b. Erythropoietin and thrombocytes
  c. Fibrinogen and acetylcholine
  d. Leukocytes

238. What structure is the pacemaker of the heart?
  a. Bundle of His
  b. Purkinje fibers
  c. Atrioventricular node
  d. Sinoatrial node

239. What is meant by cardiac output?
  a. Strokes (beats) per minute
  b. Volume of blood pumped per stroke (beat)
  c. Volume of blood pumped per minute
  d. Strokes (beats) per volume

240. In the normal heart ECG, the QRS complex corresponds to what portion of the cardiac cycle?
  a. The QRS complex is the entire ECG cycle
  b. Atrial depolarization
  c. Ventricular depolarization
  d. Ventricular repolarization

241. The term for accumulation of fluid in the abdominal cavity is:
  a. Pleural effusion
  b. Ascites
  c. Abscess
  d. Pneumothorax

242. Which of the following mammals does not have a gallbladder?
  a. Dogs
  b. Cats
  c. Horses
  d. Animals cannot function without a gallbladder

243. Which organ is considered both an exocrine and endocrine organ?
   a. Small intestine
   b. Thyroid
   c. Pancreas
   d. Kidneys

244. The islets of Langerhans are associated with which organ?
   a. Pancreas
   b. Liver
   c. Kidneys
   d. Adrenal glands

245. Which cells within the pancreas produce insulin?
   a. Alpha cells
   b. Beta cells
   c. Delta cells
   d. All of the cells within the pancreas produce insulin

246. In what organ are the islets of Langerhans found?
   a. Spleen
   b. Kidneys
   c. Liver
   d. Pancreas

247. Which of the following are clinical signs of diabetes mellitus?
   a. Polyuria
   b. Polydipsia
   c. Polyphagia
   d. All of the above

248. Which body system is the most important route of waste-product removal?
   a. Respiratory system
   b. Urinary system
   c. Digestive system
   d. All of the systems are equal in importance for waste-product removal

249. Which of the following is the correct path for urine elimination?
   a. Ureter, kidneys, urethra, bladder
   b. Kidneys, urethra, bladder, ureter
   c. Kidney, ureters, bladder, urethra
   d. Urethra, bladder, ureter, kidneys

250. Which organ(s) is/are responsible for acid-base balance regulation?
   a. Lungs
   b. Kidneys
   c. Liver
   d. Spleen

251. The indented area on the medial side of the kidney is known as the:
   a. Porta hepatis
   b. Hilum
   c. Convex
   d. Cortex

252. What is the basic functional unit of the kidney?
   a. Cortex
   b. Nephron
   c. Bowman's capsule
   d. Loop of Henle

253. About how many nephrons are in each kidney of the cow?
   a. 700,000
   b. 100,000
   c. 1,000,000
   d. 4,000,000

254. In which portion of the kidney is the renal corpuscle located?
   a. Cortex
   b. Medulla
   c. Renal sinus
   d. Hilum

255. Approximately what percentage of blood, pumped by the heart, goes to the kidneys?
   a. 5%
   b. 10%
   c. 25%
   d. 60%

256. Which of the following is considered the main mechanism in which the kidneys perform waste elimination?
   a. Filtration
   b. Reabsorption
   c. Secretion
   d. All of the above

257. Which of the following hormones are responsible for urine volume regulation?
   a. ADH
   b. Aldosterone
   c. Glucagon
   d. Both a and b

258. The ureters are composed of how many layers?
   a. 1
   b. 2
   c. 3
   d. 4

259. Which of the following conditions can cause prerenal uremia?
    a. Dehydration
    b. Congestive heart failure
    c. Shock
    d. All of the above

260. Which of the following is/are considered functions of the male testes?
    a. Spermatogenesis
    b. Hormone production
    c. Urine formation
    d. Both a and b

261. Which of the following best defines the term cryptorchidism?
    a. Torsion of one or both testicles
    b. One or both testes do not fully descend into the scrotum
    c. The surgical removal of both testicles
    d. An inflammatory condition of the testis

262. A flat ribbonlike structure that lies along the surface of the testis is known as:
    a. Cremaster muscle
    b. Vas deferens
    c. Epididymis
    d. Seminiferous tubule

263. All of the following common domestic animals have a bulbourethral gland (Cowper's gland) *except:*
    a. Cat
    b. Dog
    c. Horse
    d. Cow

264. The mesosalpinx ligament within the female reproductive tract supports which of the following structures?
    a. Uterus
    b. Ovaries
    c. Oviduct
    d. Vagina

265. Which of the following species is NOT considered to be multiparous?
    a. Dogs
    b. Sows
    c. Cattle
    d. Cats

266. When an animal is said to be in a period of temporary ovarian inactivity, this is known as:
    a. Anestrus
    b. Diestrus
    c. Pseudocyesis
    d. Heat

267. During pregnancy, what provides the life-support system for the developing fetus?
    a. Ovum
    b. Uterus
    c. Amnion
    d. Placenta

268. What is the gestational period for cats?
    a. 56–69 days
    b. 271–291 days
    c. 42 days
    d. 19–20 days

269. Which of the following animals has the longest gestational period?
    a. Horses
    b. Sheep
    c. Elephants
    d. Cattle

270. Which of the following conditions does the term mastitis refer to?
    a. The production of colostrum from the mammary gland
    b. An infection of a mammary gland
    c. The mammary glands in male species only
    d. A hormone produced to allow for the production of milk

271. Which endocrine gland produces the hormone prolactin?
    a. Posterior pituitary
    b. Thyroid
    c. Anterior pituitary
    d. Ovaries

272. The testes are responsible for producing which of the following hormones?
    a. Estrogen
    b. Androgen
    c. Progestin
    d. Sex hormones

273. Which hormone is responsible for the movement of glucose into cells and its use for energy?
    a. Progestin
    b. Insulin
    c. Glucagon
    d. Calcitonin

274. Which organ is part of the endocrine system?
    a. Pancreas
    b. Kidneys
    c. Stomach
    d. All of the above

275. Which hormone is secreted by the anterior pituitary gland?
    a. Melanocyte-stimulating hormone
    b. Adrenocorticotropic hormone
    c. Prolactin
    d. Follicle-stimulating hormone

276. Which hormone is responsible for triggering and maintaining lactation?
    a. Follicle-stimulating hormone
    b. Luteinizing hormone
    c. Mineralocorticoid hormone
    d. Prolactin hormone

277. Waste excretion is a requirement for maintaining homeostasis and can be achieved through which route of excretion?
    a. Urinary system
    b. Respiratory system
    c. Digestive system
    d. All of the above are routes of waste excretion

278. The kidneys are located in which cavity?
    a. Abdominal cavity
    b. Retroperitoneal cavity
    c. Pelvic cavity
    d. Thoracic cavity

279. Which species does NOT have a smooth outer surface of the kidneys?
    a. Cats
    b. Dogs
    c. Cattle
    d. Horses

280. Which of the following is the basic functional unit of the kidneys?
    a. Cortex
    b. Nephron
    c. Medulla
    d. Renal pelvis

281. What percentage of blood pumped from the heart travels to the kidneys?
    a. 1%
    b. 10%
    c. 25%
    d. 50%

282. The kidneys perform the waste-removal function by which of the following actions?
    a. Filtration
    b. Reabsorption
    c. Secretion
    d. All of the above

283. Which hormone is responsible for regulating urine volume?
    a. Antidiuretic hormone
    b. Aldosterone
    c. Mineralocorticoid hormone
    d. Both a and b

284. Birds contain an uropygial or preen gland located on the dorsal surface at the upper base of the tail. For what is this structure responsible?
    a. It secretes an oily, fatty substance that spreads throughout the feathers to clean and waterproof them
    b. It is responsible for the mating process
    c. It is responsible for the growth of feathers
    d. It is a scent gland

285. The vane is which part of the feather?
    a. The flattened weblike part of each side of the rachis
    b. The main feather shaft
    c. The opening of the feather shaft
    d. The opening at the base of the feather

286. Flight feathers within the wings of birds are known as:
    a. Retrices
    b. Remiges
    c. Auriculars
    d. Down feathers

287. Which portion of the digestive system in birds is responsible for grinding food products?
    a. Gizzard
    b. Proventriculus
    c. Glandular stomach
    d. All of the above

288. The restrained heart rate of a small bird, approximately 25 g in body weight, is:
    a. 100–150 bpm
    b. 110–175 bpm
    c. 400–600 bpm
    d. 300–500 bpm

289. Which structure of the male reproductive system is responsible for adjusting the location of the testis based on temperature?
    a. Cremaster muscle
    b. Spermatic cord
    c. Scrotum
    d. Inguinal rings

290. Which layer of the skin is the most superficial?
    a. Dermis
    b. Epidermis
    c. Hypodermis
    d. None of these

291. Which layer of skin is composed of multiple layers of cells that are continually renewed?
    a. Dermis
    b. Epidermis
    c. Hypodermis
    d. All of the above

292. Which layer of skin contains the hair follicles, sebaceous glands, and sweat glands?
    a. Dermis
    b. Epidermis
    c. Hypodermis
    d. Both a and b

293. How many different cell shapes are found within the epithelial cells?
    a. 1
    b. 2
    c. 3
    d. 4

294. Squamous cells describe cells that contain what shape?
    a. Column shaped
    b. Square or cube shaped
    c. Flattened in shape
    d. Circular shaped

295. Epithelial cells that contain tiny hairlike projections that move foreign particles along the epithelial surface are known as:
    a. Simple columnar epithelium
    b. Ciliated epithelium
    c. Stratified epithelium
    d. Transitional epithelium

296. Which of the following connective tissues contains the highest density?
    a. Blood
    b. Cartilage
    c. Fibrous connective tissue
    d. Bone

297. Which tissue is responsible for forming bone marrow within the long bones and for the formation of the blood cells?
    a. Hemopoietic tissue
    b. Areolar tissue
    c. Cartilage
    d. Bone

298. The hormone primarily responsible for preventing hypercalcemia is:
    a. T4
    b. Parathyroid hormone
    c. Calcitonin
    d. Vitamin D

299. The mammary glands contain which type of connective tissue?
    a. Tubular single
    b. Alveolar single
    c. Tubular multiple
    d. Alveolar multiple

300. Which of the following bone tissues contain an internal meshwork of trabeculae with interconnected spaces that are filled with red bone marrow?
    a. Cancellous bone
    b. Compact bone
    c. Spongy bone
    d. Both a and c

301. What substance covers the outer surface of all types of bone?
    a. Cartilage
    b. Bone marrow
    c. Periosteum
    d. Lamellae

302. The thorax is divided into right and left sides by a connective tissue septum known as the:
    a. Mediastinum
    b. Pericardium
    c. Pulmonary pleura
    d. Sternum

303. Which cavity lies immediately caudal to the thoracic cavity?
    a. Pelvic cavity
    b. Abdominal cavity
    c. Pleural cavity
    d. None of these

304. Which types of bones contain air-filled spaces known as sinuses that reduce the weight of the bone?
    a. Sesamoid bones
    b. Pneumatic bones
    c. Splanchnic bone
    d. Irregular bones

305. Cells that are responsible for laying down new bone are known as:
    a. Osteoblasts
    b. Osteoclasts
    c. Ossification
    d. Hemopoiesis

306. What is the formation called when one bone connects to another bone by articulation?
    a. Hinge
    b. Arthrosis
    c. Cartilage
    d. Ossification

307. Which of the following joints are immovable and are connected by dense fibrous connective tissue?
    a. Fibrous joints
    b. Cartilaginous joints
    c. Synovial joints
    d. None, all joints are moveable

308. The mandibular symphysis joins which of the following bones?
    a. The two hip bones
    b. Two vertebrae within the spinal column
    c. Two halves of the mandible
    d. The occipital and parietal bones

309. Which of the following is considered a range of movement that can occur in a synovial joint?
    a. Abduction/adduction
    b. Retraction
    c. Protraction
    d. All of the above

310. Which of the following correctly describes the joint movement of circumduction?
    a. The moving body part twists on its own axis
    b. The movement of an extremity of one end of a bone in a circular pattern
    c. The animal moves the limb back toward the body
    d. The animal moves the limb cranially

311. Which of the following is a type of synovial joint?
    a. Plane/gliding
    b. Condylar
    c. Ball and socket
    d. All of the above

312. Which of the following is an example of a hinge joint?
    a. Hip
    b. Shoulder
    c. Stifle
    d. Atlantoaxial joint

313. What type of muscle contraction occurs when a muscle actually moves or shortens?
    a. Isotonic contraction
    b. Muscle tone
    c. Isometric contraction
    d. None of the above

314. Muscles that form a circular ring and serve to control the entrance or exit to a structure are known as:
    a. Muscle tone
    b. Sphincter muscles
    c. Bursa
    d. Extrinsic muscle

315. Which muscle type is responsible for moving the lips, cheeks, nostrils, eyelids, and external ears?
    a. Sphincter muscle
    b. Intrinsic muscle
    c. Extrinsic muscle
    d. Digastricus

316. Before birth, the testes begin to develop in the abdominal cavity near which organ?
    a. Stomach
    b. Kidneys
    c. Bladder
    d. Gallbladder

317. The scrotum is responsible for which of the following?
    a. Regulation of temperature
    b. Production of sperm
    c. Housing of the testes
    d. Both a and c

318. Which muscle is responsible for adjusting the testes to regulate temperature?
    a. Inguinal ring
    b. Cremaster muscle
    c. Levator ani
    d. Psoas muscle

319. Which of the following is derived from the testicular veins, surrounds the testicular artery, and are described as multiple tiny veins?
    a. Spermatic cord
    b. Pampiniform plexus
    c. Cremaster plexus
    d. Vas deferens

320. What is the storage site for sperm after they detach from the Sertoli cells?
    a. Epididymis
    b. Vas deferens
    c. Visceral vaginal tunic
    d. Pampiniform plexus

321. The thick, outer layer that surrounds the testes in the scrotum and the spermatic cord is known as the:
    a. Visceral vaginal tunic
    b. Proper vaginal tunic
    c. Parietal vaginal tunic
    d. Both a and b

322. Below the tunics, a heavy, fibrous connective tissue capsule surrounds each testis. What is this known as?
   a. Common vaginal tunic
   b. Tunica albuginea
   c. Pampiniform plexus
   d. Septa

323. Where does spermatogenesis take place?
   a. Seminiferous tubules
   b. Epididymis
   c. Spermatic cord
   d. Pampiniform plexus

324. The vas deferens is responsible for which of the following actions?
   a. To mature sperm
   b. To store sperm before ejaculation
   c. To propel spermatozoa and the fluid from the epididymis to the urethra during ejaculation
   d. To produce spermatozoa

325. The accessory reproductive glands produce alkaline fluid that contains which of the following substances?
   a. Electrolytes
   b. Prostaglandins
   c. Fructose
   d. All of the above

326. Which of the following species does NOT contain seminal vesicles?
   a. Bull
   b. Cat
   c. Dog
   d. Both b and c

327. Which of the following animals does NOT have bulbourethral glands?
   a. Dog
   b. Cat
   c. Horse
   d. Ram

328. The prostate gland completely surrounds which structure?
   a. Testis
   b. Epididymis
   c. Urethra
   d. Spermatic cord

329. Bulbourethral glands are also known as?
   a. The prostate
   b. Cowper's glands
   c. Roots
   d. Seminal glands

330. Which species contain short spines that cover the end of the glans of the penis?
   a. Horses
   b. Dogs
   c. Ruminants
   d. Cats

331. Which species contains a bone within the penis that is known as the os penis?
   a. Dogs
   b. Cats
   c. Horses
   d. Ruminants

332. What structure can cause the male dog to become stuck or "tied" to the female during breeding?
   a. Testicles
   b. Bulb of the glans
   c. Os penis
   d. None of the above

333. The anatomical plane that runs the length of the body and divides its right and left parts is known as the:
   a. Median plane
   b. Sagittal plane
   c. Dorsal plane
   d. Transverse plane

334. The thoracic cavity is considered to be in what anatomical direction from the abdomen?
   a. Caudal
   b. Cranial
   c. Dorsal
   d. Ventral

335. The duodenum exits the stomach on which side of the animal's abdomen?
   a. Left
   b. Right
   c. Cranial
   d. Caudal

336. A horse's shoulder is located in which anatomical direction to its hip?
   a. Caudal
   b. Cranial
   c. Proximal
   d. Ventral

337. The caudal end of the sternum is referred to as the:
   a. Xiphoid process
   b. Trochanter
   c. Calcaneus
   d. Cannon bone

338. The back of the hind leg distal to the tarsus is known as:
    a. Plantar
    b. Palmar
    c. Lateral
    d. Medial

339. An animal's body consists of how many main body cavities?
    a. 1
    b. 2
    c. 5
    d. 8

340. The dorsal body cavity contains which of the following structures?
    a. Brain
    b. Chest
    c. Spinal cord
    d. Both a and c

341. Which of the following body cavities is the largest?
    a. Dorsal
    b. Cranial
    c. Spinal
    d. Ventral

342. Which of the following are considered to be a major structure within the thoracic cavity?
    a. Heart
    b. Lungs
    c. Esophagus
    d. All of the above

343. All of the organs in the thoracic cavity are covered by a thin membrane known as:
    a. Thorax
    b. Pleura
    c. Peritoneum
    d. None of the above

344. The visceral layer of the peritoneum covers which organ?
    a. Digestive
    b. Urinary
    c. Reproductive
    d. All of the above

345. The animal body is made up of _____ different tissues.
    a. 1
    b. 2
    c. 4
    d. 8

346. What is the main purpose of the epithelial tissue?
    a. Provides support for the body
    b. Covers body surfaces
    c. Provides movement of structures
    d. Controls the body function

347. Which types of cells carry oxygen throughout the body?
    a. Red blood cells
    b. White blood cells
    c. Nerve cells
    d. All cells carry oxygen

348. The secreting units of sweat glands, salivary glands, and mammary glands are all composed of what type of cellular tissue?
    a. Connective tissue
    b. Muscle tissue
    c. Nervous tissue
    d. Epithelial tissue

349. Which of the following is NOT a type of muscle tissue?
    a. Cardiac
    b. Skeletal
    c. Striated
    d. Smooth

350. Smooth muscle is found in which internal organ?
    a. Urinary bladder
    b. Heart
    c. Digestive tract
    d. All of the above
    e. Both a and c

351. Which of the following is the first indication that the heart is starting to fail?
    a. Decrease in blood pressure
    b. Rise in blood pressure
    c. Decrease in cardiac output
    d. Drop in oxygen saturation

352. Which of the following elements is the component of all proteins and nucleic acids?
    a. Hydrogen
    b. Oxygen
    c. Calcium
    d. Nitrogen

353. Which element of the periodic table is required for muscle contraction, nerve impulse transmission, and blood clotting?
    a. Nitrogen
    b. Oxygen
    c. Phosphorus
    d. Calcium

354. Which of the following are considered major elements found in the body?
    a. Nitrogen
    b. Calcium
    c. Magnesium
    d. Potassium

355. Oxygen is an element that makes up approximately _____ of the body mass.
    a. 18.5%
    b. 9.5%
    c. 65%
    d. 3.3%

356. Which of the following are considered as types of chemical bonds?
    a. Covalent bonds
    b. Ionic bonds
    c. Hydrogen bonds
    d. All of the choices are considered types of chemical bonds

357. A bond that is formed when electrons are transferred from one atom to another is known as what type of bond?
    a. Covalent bond
    b. Ionic bond
    c. Hydrogen bond
    d. Triple covalent bond

358. Which type of chemical reaction occurs in the body when the simple molecules absorbed during the digestive process are joined into larger molecules needed by cells for life processes?
    a. Decomposition reaction
    b. Synthesis reaction
    c. Exchange reaction
    d. None of the above

359. Which of the following are examples of inorganic compounds?
    a. Water
    b. Acids
    c. Bases
    d. All of the above

360. Which of the following is NOT an example of an organic compound?
    a. Proteins
    b. Bases
    c. Lipids
    d. Carbohydrates

361. What are chemicals that dissolve or mix well in water called?
    a. Hydrophilic
    b. Hydrophobic
    c. Solute
    d. Solvent

362. Which of the following are considered electrolytes?
    a. Potassium
    b. Sodium
    c. Calcium
    d. All of the above

363. Which of the following levels is considered the most acidic of the pH scale?
    a. 2.5
    b. 5
    c. 7
    d. 12

364. What does "buffering the solution" refer to?
    a. Creating an acidic solution
    b. Creating an alkaline solution
    c. Creating a neutral solution with the pH close to 7
    d. None of the above

365. Which of the following is an example of a buffer?
    a. Lemons
    b. Carbonic acid
    c. Ammonia
    d. Vinegar

366. What is the pH of distilled water?
    a. 1
    b. 5
    c. 7
    d. 11

367. Which of the following is an example of a carbohydrate?
    a. Sugar
    b. Starch
    c. Cellulose
    d. All of the above

368. Monosaccharides contain how many carbon atoms in a chain?
    a. 2–5
    b. 3–7
    c. 5–10
    d. 10–15

369. A sugar with 5 carbons is known as _____ sugar.
    a. Hexose
    b. Pentose
    c. Montose
    d. Tritose

370. Of the following molecules, which is not a lipid?
    a. Ribose
    b. Triglycerides
    c. Prostaglandins
    d. Steroids

371. What is the primary function of triglycerides?
    a. Act as backbone of DNA and RNA
    b. Regulate chemical reactions, enzymes
    c. Synthesize hormones
    d. Store energy

372. Which of the following molecules are nucleic acids?
    a. DNA
    b. RNA
    c. Adenosine triphosphate
    d. All of the above

373. Prostaglandins provide all of the following functions, *except:*
    a. Regulate hormone synthesis
    b. Enhance immune system
    c. Provide inflammatory response
    d. Block the COX-2 pathway

374. When two monosaccharides are jointed together, what type of reaction occurs?
    a. Synthesis reaction
    b. Hydrolysis reaction
    c. Decomposition reaction
    d. Exchange reaction

375. When water is extracted from saccharides, it is known as:
    a. Hydrolysis
    b. Dehydration synthesis
    c. Decomposition reaction
    d. Synthesis reaction

376. Lipids are made of all of the following components *except:*
    a. Oxygen
    b. Carbon
    c. Hydrogen
    d. Calcium

377. What are lipoproteins used for within the body?
    a. Energy
    b. To transport fats within the body
    c. To regulate chemical reactions
    d. To regulate hormone synthesis

378. Which types of lipids take the form of four interlocking hydrocarbon rings?
    a. Steroids
    b. Triglycerides
    c. Prostaglandins
    d. Phospholipids

379. Cholesterol is used by which of the following organs for the creation of steroid hormones?
    a. Adrenal glands
    b. Testes
    c. Ovaries
    d. All of the above

380. Which molecule is considered the most abundant organic molecule in the body?
    a. Amino acids
    b. Lipids
    c. Proteins
    d. Prostaglandins

381. What characteristic of a protein molecule directly determines its function?
    a. Size
    b. Location
    c. Shape
    d. None, proteins all have the same function

382. All of the following are characteristics of structural proteins, *except:*
    a. Stability
    b. Water-insoluble proteins
    c. Rigidity
    d. Steroid properties

383. Functional proteins are also known as:
    a. Structural proteins
    b. Globular proteins
    c. Fibrous proteins
    d. None of the above

384. Which of the following are considered the largest molecules in the body?
    a. Lipids
    b. Proteins
    c. Nucleic acids
    d. Carbohydrates

385. Nucleic acids consist of which of the following classes?
    a. RNA
    b. DNA
    c. Ribose
    d. Both a and b

386. The molecular building blocks of nucleic acids are known as:
    a. Chromosomes
    b. Nucleotides
    c. Proteins
    d. Carbohydrates

387. All of the following are nucleotides, *except:*
    a. Adenine
    b. Guanine
    c. Thiamine
    d. Cystosine

388. Which nucleotide occurs in both DNA and RNA?
    a. Thiamine
    b. Guanine
    c. Uracil
    d. Thymine

389. Which nucleotide occurs only in DNA?
    a. Adenine
    b. Guanine
    c. Cytosine
    d. Uracil

390. The aorta originates from which structure?
    a. Right ventricle
    b. Left ventricle
    c. Left atrium
    d. Right atrium

391. Which type of blood vessel carries blood away from the heart?
    a. Veins
    b. Arteries
    c. Capillaries
    d. Vena cava

392. Which types of blood vessels contain one-way valves?
    a. Arteries
    b. Veins
    c. Capillaries
    d. Aorta

393. Which blood vessel carries CO_2-rich blood from the right ventricle of the heart to the lungs?
    a. Aorta
    b. Inferior vena cava
    c. Pulmonary vein
    d. Pulmonary artery

394. Which of the following is the first main branch of the aorta?
    a. Left subclavian artery
    b. Brachiocephalic trunk
    c. The left common carotid artery
    d. Superior mesenteric artery

395. Plasma is composed of what percentage of water?
    a. 7%
    b. 92%
    c. 1%
    d. Plasma does not contain water

396. Which blood cell is the most numerous blood cell in the body?
    a. White blood cells
    b. Plasma
    c. Red blood cells
    d. Leukocytes

397. Which protein gives erythrocytes their red color?
    a. Granulocytes
    b. Hemoglobin
    c. Fibrinogen
    d. Eosinophil

398. Blood makes up approximately what percentage of body weight?
    a. 93%
    b. 55%
    c. 45%
    d. 7%

399. All of the following are a type of white blood cell, *except:*
    a. Neutrophil
    b. Reticulocyte
    c. Lymphocyte
    d. Eosinophil

400. Which structure is composed of several C-shaped incomplete rings of hyaline cartilage?
    a. Esophagus
    b. Trachea
    c. Larynx
    d. Pharynx

401. Where does gas exchange occur in the lungs?
    a. Bronchi
    b. Alveolus
    c. Alveolar duct
    d. Larynx

402. Which of the following is true about the thoracic cavity?
    a. It contains positive pressure
    b. It contains negative pressure
    c. It does not contain any fluid
    d. It is located below the diaphragm

403. What makes up the bulk of the tooth?
    a. Enamel
    b. Crown
    c. Dentin
    d. Root

404. Which of the following are the most rostral teeth in the mouth of small animals?
    a. Canines
    b. Premolars
    c. Molars
    d. Incisors

405. Which of the following animals do not have upper incisor teeth?
    a. Dogs
    b. Cattle
    c. Cats
    d. Horses

406. What regulates the size of the opening of the esophagus into the stomach?
    a. Duodenum
    b. Pyloric sphincter
    c. Cardiac sphincter
    d. Epiglottis

407. After food leaves the stomach, it is referred to as which of the following terms?
    a. Rugae
    b. Chyme
    c. Rumen
    d. Bile

408. Which is the longest segment of the small intestines?
    a. Duodenum
    b. Ileum
    c. Jejunum
    d. Colon

409. Which is the longest segment of the large intestines?
    a. Ileum
    b. Colon
    c. Cecum
    d. Rectum

410. Which vein carries nutrient-rich blood from the intestines to the liver?
    a. Inferior vena cava
    b. Portal vein
    c. Hepatic vein
    d. Splenic vein

411. Which gland is located caudal to the diaphragm and is the largest gland in the body?
    a. Spleen
    b. Pancreas
    c. Liver
    d. Gallbladder

412. The diencephalon of the brain consists of which of the following structures?
    a. Thalamus
    b. Pons
    c. Hypothalamus
    d. Both a and b
    e. Both a and c

413. What is the largest most rostral part of the brain?
    a. Cerebellum
    b. Cerebrum
    c. Thalamus
    d. Brainstem

414. Systems of folds located within the cerebrum are known as which of the following?
    a. Gyri
    b. Sulci
    c. Meninges
    d. Arachnoid villi

415. What is considered the most primitive part of the brain?
    a. Cerebellum
    b. Cerebrum
    c. Brainstem
    d. Gray matter

416. Which portion of the spinal cord is located at the cranial end?
    a. Sacral
    b. Cervical
    c. Thoracic
    d. Lumbar

417. Spinal nerves from the sacral region carry which type of nerve fiber?
    a. Sympathetic nerve fibers
    b. Parasympathetic nerve fibers
    c. Both
    d. Neither

418. How many types of cranial nerves exist?
a. 5
b. 8
c. 10
d. 12

419. Which cranial nerve is responsible for balance and hearing?
a. Trochlear
b. Vestibulocochlear
c. Accessory
d. Optic

420. The glossopharyngeal nerve is responsible for which of the following?
a. Sensations from the head and teeth, chewing
b. Eye movement
c. Facial and scalp movement
d. Tongue movement, swallowing, salivation, and taste

421. Which of the following cranial nerves is a sensory nerve?
a. Vestibulocochlear
b. Accessory
c. Trochlear
d. Hypoglossal

422. Which of the following cranial nerves is the longest cranial nerve that innervates many organs in the body?
a. Trigeminal
b. Vestibulocochlear
c. Vagus
d. Hypoglossal

423. Visceral sensations include which of the following?
a. Heat and cold
b. Hunger and thirst
c. Odors
d. Touch and pressure

424. Which of the following is NOT considered a part of the special senses?
a. Taste
b. Hearing
c. Equilibrium
d. Proprioception

425. Which of the following is a cartilaginous funnel that collects sound waves and directs them medially into the external auditory canal?
a. Pinna
b. Eustachian tube
c. Cochlea
d. Tympanic membrane

426. Which of the following is part of the inner ear?
a. Cochlea
b. Malleus
c. Incus
d. Tympanic membrane

427. Which of the following contains receptor cells for hearing?
a. Tympanic membrane
b. Organ of Corti
c. Vestibule
d. Incus

428. The vestibular sense is responsible for:
a. Taste
b. Balance and head position
c. Vision
d. Hearing

429. The clear window on the rostral portion of the eye is known as:
a. Eyelids
b. Cornea
c. Iris
d. Sclera

430. What structure is located immediately caudal to the cornea?
a. Lens
b. Iris
c. Anterior chamber
d. Vitreous humor

431. Where are visual images formed within the eye?
a. Lens
b. Cornea
c. Vitreous humor
d. Retina

432. In which layer of the eye are the rods and cons located?
a. Cornea
b. Retina
c. Iris
d. Vitreous humor

433. What area is known as the blind spot of the eye?
a. Optic nerve
b. Optic disc
c. Rod
d. Cone

434. Which of the following is responsible for draining tears from the eye?
a. Lacrimal glands
b. Conjunctiva
c. Lacrimal puncta
d. Membrana nictitans

435. What happens to the iris of the eye in dim light?
a. The muscles relax, allowing the pupil to dilate
b. The muscles contract, allowing the pupil to constrict
c. The muscles constrict, closing the pupil
d. Nothing, light does not affect the iris of the eye

436. For what is the ciliary body within the eye responsible?
a. To change the diameter of the iris
b. To change the shape of the lens
c. To produce tears
d. To drain tears

437. Which hormones are produced by the corpus luteum and are necessary to maintain pregnancy?
a. FSH
b. LH
c. Progesterone
d. Estrogen

438. Which of the following hormones are the main hormones produced by the testicles?
a. Testosterone
b. Luteinizing hormone
c. Estrogen
d. Progesterone

439. Which of the following forms the tail of the horse?
a. The cervical vertebrae
b. The sacrum
c. The coccygeal vertebrae
d. The lumbar vertebrae

440. Which of the following bones is located immediately distal to the scapula of the horse?
a. Humerus
b. Metacarpus
c. Femur
d. Ulna

441. The carpus of the horse is located proximal to which of the following bones?
a. Humerus
b. Radius
c. Ulna
d. Metacarpus

442. Which of the following bones is located distal to the tarsal bone in the horse?
a. Femur
b. Patella
c. Metatarsal
d. Fibula

443. How many ribs does the horse have?
a. 5
b. 15
c. 18
d. 6

444. At what level of vertebrae are the withers of a horse located?
a. C1
b. C2
c. C3–C7
d. T4–T9

445. Which of the following bones is considered one of the strongest bones in the horse?
a. Humerus
b. Carpus
c. Scapula
d. Patella

446. Which of the following bones is also referred to as the cannon bone of the horse?
a. Phalanges
b. Carpus
c. Metacarpals
d. Femur

447. Which of the following joints lies between the cannon bone and the long pastern?
a. Stifle joint
b. Fetlock joint
c. Pastern joint
d. Carpal joint

448. Which of the following bones is encased in the hoof?
a. Navicular bone
b. Cannon bone
c. Pedal bone
d. Sesamoid bone

449. The glenoid cavity is located immediately proximal to which of the following bones of the horse?
a. Scapula
b. Humerus
c. Ulna
d. Cannon bone

450. The deltoid tuberosity is located on which of the following bones of the horse?
   a. Radius
   b. Ulna
   c. Humerus
   d. Scapula

451. Which bone forms the floor of the pelvis of the horse?
   a. Pubis
   b. Ischium
   c. Ilium
   d. Tuber coxae

452. Which of the following is the largest bone of the pelvis of the horse?
   a. Ischium
   b. Ilium
   c. Pubis
   d. Acetabulum

453. The interosseous space is located between which two bones on the limb of a horse?
   a. Fibula/tibia
   b. Radius/ulna
   c. Cannon bone/split bone
   d. Humerus/scapula

454. The femoral condyle is located _____ to the head of the femur in a horse.
   a. Proximal
   b. Distal
   c. Lateral
   d. Medial

455. The coxal tuber is located on which of the following bones of the horse?
   a. Talus
   b. Metatarsal
   c. Hip bone
   d. Femur

456. The calcaneus bone in a horse forms which of the following?
   a. Pastern
   b. Fetlock
   c. Point of the hock
   d. The horse does not contain a calcaneus bone, only small animals

457. The tarsus of the horse is composed of how many bones?
   a. 1
   b. 3
   c. 4
   d. 6

458. Metatarsal IV in the horse is also known as:
   a. Lateral splint bone
   b. Cannon bone
   c. Talus
   d. Hock

459. Approximately how much of the weight do the forelimbs of the horse carry?
   a. 20%
   b. 40%
   c. 60%
   d. 80%

460. Which muscle is responsible for movement of the head and neck of the horse?
   a. Rhomboideus
   b. Brachiocephalicus
   c. Splenius
   d. Deltoid

461. Where is the insertion of the sternocephalicus muscles of the horse?
   a. Mandible
   b. Humerus
   c. Spine of the scapula
   d. Proximal tibia

462. Which muscle of the horse supports the rider's weight?
   a. Pectoral
   b. Semitendinosus
   c. Longissimus dorsi
   d. Rhomboideus

463. Where is the point of origin of the pectoral muscle of horses?
   a. Scapula
   b. Pelvis
   c. Thoracic vertebrae
   d. Sternum

464. All of the following muscles of the horse extend the hock, *except:*
   a. Gastrocnemius
   b. Semimembranosus
   c. Semitendinosus
   d. Biceps femoris

465. The point of origin of which muscle of the horse is at the tuber coxae of the pelvis?
   a. Gastrocnemius
   b. Infraspinatus
   c. Latissimus dorsi
   d. Superficial gluteals

466. Which of the following muscles of the horse is responsible for extending the elbow?
    a. Infraspinatus
    b. Gastrocnemius
    c. Pectoral
    d. Triceps

467. Which of the following muscles originates behind the poll (at the base of the skull) of the horse?
    a. Trapezius
    b. Splenius
    c. Sternocephalicus
    d. Brachiocephalicus

468. Which of the following muscles insert at the distal femur and tibia of the horse?
    a. Gastrocnemius
    b. Semitendinosus
    c. Biceps femoris
    d. Semimembranosus

469. Tendons attach _____ to bone.
    a. Ligaments
    b. Muscles
    c. Blood vessels
    d. Bone

470. Which of the following tendons flexes the toe in horses?
    a. Suspensory ligament
    b. Deep digital flexor tendon
    c. Superficial digital flexor tendon
    d. Lateral digital extensor tendon

471. What is the function of cheek ligaments in horses?
    a. Support and suspend the fetlock and prevent overextension
    b. Assist in the extension of the pastern joint
    c. Prevent strain and overextension of the joint
    d. Flexes the toe

472. Which of the following allows the horse to rest and sleep in a standing position?
    a. The cheek ligaments
    b. Stay apparatus
    c. Deep digital flexor tendon
    d. Superficial digital flexor tendon

473. A protective external capsule, called the _____, surrounds the internal structures of the foot on a horse.
    a. Frog
    b. Hoof
    c. Horseshoe
    d. Sole

474. Which of the following structures of the horse's hoof allows for expansion and provides strength?
    a. Bars
    b. Frog
    c. Sole
    d. Coronet

475. How long does it take for a horn to grown down from the coronet to the tip of the toe (on the ground surface) of a horse?
    a. 1–2 months
    b. 4–5 months
    c. 9–12 months
    d. 12–24 months

476. The _____ forms the outer layer to protect the hoof and maintain moisture levels.
    a. Hoof
    b. Sole
    c. Frog
    d. Periople

477. What provides nourishment to the digital cushion and functions with the frog in the horse's foot?
    a. Sole corium
    b. Frog corium
    c. Laminar corium
    d. Perioplic corium

478. The sequence in which a horse lifts its feet from the ground is described as what?
    a. Trot
    b. Gait
    c. Gallop
    d. Canter

479. In which type of gait does the floating phase occur?
    a. Walk
    b. Trot
    c. Gallop
    d. Canter

480. During which gait are there never more than two legs on the ground at the same time?
    a. Canter
    b. Trot
    c. Walk
    d. Gallop

481. A horse's vision is primarily which type?
    a. Binocular
    b. Monocular
    c. 3D
    d. All of the above

482. Which area is the blind spot for a horse?
   a. In front of the muzzle
   b. Behind the ears
   c. Right side of face
   d. Left side of face

483. What structure in horses provides additional shading for the retina to limit the entry of light?
   a. Cornea
   b. Iris
   c. Ciliary muscle
   d. Corpora nigra

484. What is the normal heart rate for a horse at rest?
   a. 25–42 bpm
   b. 40–140 bpm
   c. 48–84 bpm
   d. 260–600 bpm

485. Which of the following forms the ventral margin of each nostril of a horse?
   a. External nares
   b. False nostril
   c. Alar fold
   d. Ethmoturbinates

486. Which sinus lies in the dorsal part of the skull medial to the orbit?
   a. Frontal sinus
   b. Two maxillary sinuses
   c. Oropharynx
   d. Nasopharynx

487. Which of the following structures suspends the larynx from the skull?
   a. Epiglottis
   b. Arytenoid cartilages
   c. Laryngopharynx
   d. Hyoid apparatus

488. Which of the following is NOT part of the lower respiratory tract?
   a. Trachea
   b. Bronchi
   c. Lungs
   d. Pharynx

489. Which animal has a cotyledonary placenta?
   a. Cat
   b. Dog
   c. Horse
   d. Sheep

490. On an electrocardiogram, the P wave is most closely associated with:
   a. Atrial depolarization
   b. Atrial repolarization
   c. Ventricular depolarization
   d. Ventricular repolarization

491. Lymph nodes found on the caudal aspect of the leg at the level of the patella are the:
   a. Popliteal nodes
   b. Inguinal nodes
   c. Mandibular nodes
   d. Prescapular nodes

492. At what age do permanent teeth begin to erupt in the horse?
   a. 1 year
   b. 2½ years
   c. 5 years
   d. 6 years

493. How many permanent teeth does the adult male horse contain (minus the wolf teeth)?
   a. 24
   b. 36
   c. 40
   d. 46

494. At what age do wolf teeth develop in the horse?
   a. Less than 12 months
   b. 18 months to 5 years
   c. 5–10 years
   d. Greater than 10 years

495. How much are the occlusal surfaces worn down every year in the horse?
   a. 1–2 mm
   b. 5–10 mm
   c. 10–20 mm
   d. None, they continuously grow and are never worn down

496. What does the term hypsodontic in the horse represent?
   a. Thick layer of enamel
   b. The lack of enamel over the occlusal surface
   c. The crown reserve
   d. Continuous growth of the teeth

497. The section between the canine teeth and the first premolar of the horse is termed:
   a. Hypsodontic
   b. Wolf teeth
   c. Diastema
   d. Infundibulum

498. What is the average length of the esophagus in the average sized horse?
    a. 1.5 inches
    b. 1.5 cm
    c. 1.5 mm
    d. 1.5 m

499. What is the volume that the adult horse's stomach can hold?
    a. 1–2 L
    b. 2–3 L
    c. 7–14 L
    d. 20–25 L

500. Food passes from the esophagus into the stomach via what structure in the horse?
    a. Pyloric sphincter
    b. Epiglottis
    c. Cardiac sphincter
    d. Duodenum

501. At what level of "fullness" does the horse's stomach empty?
    a. ¼ full
    b. ½ full
    c. ⅔ full
    d. Completely full

502. Where does digestion and absorption of food take place within the horse?
    a. Duodenum
    b. Jejunum
    c. Ileum
    d. Ileocecal junction

503. Where does the microbial digestion of cellulose take place within the horse?
    a. Ileocecal junction
    b. Large intestine
    c. Small intestine
    d. Stomach

504. All of the following are part of the small intestine, *except:*
    a. Cecum
    b. Duodenum
    c. Jejunum
    d. Ileum

505. In the average horse, how many liters of ingesta can the cecum hold?
    a. 10 L
    b. 20 L
    c. 25 L
    d. 35 L

506. In the average horse, how many liters of ingesta can the colon hold?
    a. 10 L
    b. 35 L
    c. 65 L
    d. 100 L

507. How long does food remain in the colon of the horse?
    a. 1–2 hours
    b. 5–15 hours
    c. 25–35 hours
    d. 36–65 hours

508. The left kidney of the horse lies _____ to the right kidney, is located ventral to the last rib, and is near the first two or three lumbar transverse processes.
    a. Cranial
    b. Caudal
    c. Lateral
    d. Medial

509. How many grams does the average equine kidney weigh?
    a. 100–200 g
    b. 400–600 g
    c. 800–1000 g
    d. 1000–1500 g

510. How many mL of urine does an equine patient produce per day of body weight?
    a. 10 mL/kg/day
    b. 20 mL/kg/day
    c. 45 mL/kg/day
    d. 60 mL/kg/day

511. What is the normal pH of equine urine?
    a. Less than 3 pH
    b. 3–6 pH
    c. 7–8 pH
    d. Greater than 9 pH

512. At what age do the male testicles of the horse reach their full adult size?
    a. 6 months
    b. 1 year
    c. 2 years
    d. 5 years

513. Which of the following glands is a pair of smooth-surfaced, pear-shaped glands located on either side of the male bladder, and also are considered an accessory gland for the production of seminal fluid?
    a. Bulbourethral gland
    b. Seminal vesicles
    c. Adrenal glands
    d. Thyroid glands

514. The prostate gland is responsible for which of the following?
    a. Cleans the urethra before the ejaculation of sperm
    b. Neutralizes acidity of any remaining urine before ejaculation
    c. Secretes a clear fluid
    d. All of the above

515. Where does fertilization normally occur in the horse?
    a. Testicles
    b. Ovaries
    c. Fallopian tubes
    d. Infundibulum

516. What occurs to unfertilized ova?
    a. They are expelled
    b. They are reabsorbed
    c. They remain in the fallopian tube until fertilization occurs
    d. None of the above

517. The ovaries of the mare are largely inactive until sexual maturity, which occurs at what age?
    a. 6 months
    b. 1–2 years
    c. 3–5 years
    d. 7 years

518. Which of the following terms correctly describes the mare's parity?
    a. Nulliparity
    b. Uniparous
    c. Multiparous
    d. None of these

519. What is the typical breeding season of a mare?
    a. Spring–summer
    b. Summer–fall
    c. Fall–winter
    d. Winter–spring

520. The mare is considered a/an _____ ovulator, which means she will ovulate without the stimulus of mating.
    a. Spontaneous
    b. Polyestrous
    c. Anestrous
    d. Multiparous

521. How long does the typical estrous cycle last in the mare?
    a. 5–7 days
    b. 7–14 days
    c. 17–21 days
    d. 23–31 days

522. During the estrus phase of the mare, which of the following occurs?
    a. Follicle development
    b. Ovulation
    c. Secretion of estrogen
    d. Estrus does not occur in the mare

523. How long does the diestrus phase of the mare last?
    a. 7–21 days
    b. 3–5 days
    c. 14–16 days
    d. 35 days

524. The sternum of birds is extended into a laterally flattened _____, which provides a large surface area for the attachment of the major flight muscles.
    a. Coracoid
    b. Keel
    c. Beak
    d. Quadrate

525. Many of the larger bones of the bird are filled with air that is contained in membranous sacs that connect with the respiratory system and are referred to as which type of bones?
    a. Compact
    b. Irregular
    c. Long
    d. Pneumatic

526. What division are birds missing that is normally seen between the thorax and abdomen of other animals?
    a. Lungs
    b. Diaphragm
    c. Liver
    d. Keel

527. Which of the following is responsible for the perching reflex in birds?
    a. Tibiotarsus
    b. Digital flexor tendon
    c. Craniofacial hinge
    d. Supracoracoid muscle

528. Most birds have _____ toes pointing forward.
    a. 1
    b. 2
    c. 3
    d. None

529. The pygostyle found in birds is located distal to which of the following?
    a. Sternum
    b. Coccygeal vertebrae
    c. Tibiotarsus
    d. Hallux

530. Which of the following structure is the first digit in the wing of a bird?
    a. Alula
    b. Major metacarpal
    c. Tarsometatarsus
    d. Hallux

531. Which digit of the bird carries the primary feathers?
    a. Digit 1
    b. Alula
    c. Digit 3
    d. Metacarpal

532. The central shaft of a bird's feather is also referred to as:
    a. Dentary
    b. Talon
    c. Hallux
    d. Rachis

533. As feathers mature in birds, what happens to the rachis?
    a. Fills with blood
    b. Becomes hollow
    c. Molts
    d. Nothing, it stays the same throughout life

534. Secretions from which gland keeps feathers waterproof?
    a. Alula
    b. Preen
    c. Gizzard
    d. Coracoid

535. Secondary feathers are attached to which structure in birds?
    a. Digit 1
    b. Digit 3
    c. Ulna
    d. Hallux

536. Which types of feathers cover the outermost layer of the body?
    a. Primary feathers
    b. Secondary feathers
    c. Contour feathers
    d. Filoplume feathers

537. How often do go birds go through a molting process?
    a. Once a month
    b. Every 3–6 months
    c. Once a year
    d. One time after 1 year of age

538. Which surface of the wing is longer and convex? And which surface is shorter and more concave?
    a. Ventral/dorsal
    b. Dorsal/ventral
    c. Proximal/distal
    d. Distal/proximal

539. Which side of the wing does air pass over more quickly?
    a. Dorsal
    b. Ventral
    c. Proximal
    d. Distal

540. The lift force must equal which of the following parameters for flight to occur in a bird?
    a. Size of the bird
    b. Shape of the wings
    c. Weight of the bird
    d. Gravity

541. If the angle of tilt of a bird's wing is greater than _____, then lift is reduced.
    a. 5 degrees
    b. 15 degrees
    c. 25 degrees
    d. 45 degrees

542. For a bird to land, the tail is used as a _____, and the wings are extended into a stall position.
    a. Brake
    b. Guide
    c. Thrust
    d. Perch

543. All of the following special senses of birds are well developed for survival, *except:*
    a. Sight
    b. Hearing
    c. Touch
    d. All of the above are well developed in the bird

544. What structure do birds move to view an image?
    a. Eye muscles
    b. Eyes
    c. Head
    d. Optic lobes

545. Predator birds have which type of vision?
  a. Monocular
  b. Binocular
  c. 3D
  d. None of the above

546. Which of the following structures reinforces the large circumference of the eye in birds?
  a. Cornea
  b. Sclerotic ring
  c. Optic lobe
  d. Optic nerve

547. The iris of a bird's eye is formed by which muscle, which enables the bird to control the size of the pupil voluntarily?
  a. Smooth
  b. Striated
  c. Cardiac
  d. None of these

548. The vitreous humor in the posterior chamber of the eye contains a ribbonlike structure attached to the retina, and it is known as what?
  a. Nictitating membrane
  b. Pecten
  c. Third eyelid
  d. Optic nerve

549. Which type of vision do photoreceptor cells, known as rods, provide in birds?
  a. Color vision
  b. Monocular vision
  c. Binocular vision
  d. Night vision

550. Which avian species contain ear pinnae?
  a. Eagle
  b. Parakeet
  c. Parrot
  d. None, there are no external ear pinnae in any avian species

551. Where is the columella bone located?
  a. Caudal to the clavicle
  b. Proximal to the ulna
  c. Cranial to the sternum
  d. In the ear

552. Where are the free spaces within the bird located?
  a. Thorax
  b. Abdomen
  c. Major bones
  d. Wings

553. The combined effect of air passing through the larynx and what other structure produces the characteristic sounds associated with the bird species?
  a. Glottis
  b. Syrinx
  c. Bronchi
  d. Choana

554. How many air sacs do most birds contain?
  a. 3
  b. 5
  c. 7
  d. 9

555. The 9 different air sacs within birds are responsible for all of the following, *except:*
  a. Lightening the weight of the skeleton
  b. Gaseous exchange
  c. As a reservoir for air
  d. The bellows Effect

556. During the respiration process of birds, air circulates continuously and passes through the lungs _____ times.
  a. 2
  b. 3
  c. 4
  d. 5

557. The air in the _____ air sac passes straight through the lungs and out.
  a. Cranial
  b. Thoracic
  c. Abdominal
  d. Humerus

558. How many chambers does the avian heart contain?
  a. 1
  b. 2
  c. 3
  d. 4

559. The pericardial sac covers which of the following structures within the bird?
  a. Bronchi
  b. Keel
  c. Heart
  d. Syrinx

560. There is a large blood supply to the flight muscles and wings of birds, via which artery?
  a. Pectoral artery
  b. Carotid artery
  c. Brachial artery
  d. All of the above
  e. Both a and c

561. The pudendal artery in birds is located near what other structure?
    a. Ulnar artery
    b. Pectoral artery
    c. Brachiocephalic artery
    d. Rectum

562. Which of the following arteries runs parallel to the trachea in birds?
    a. Brachial
    b. Jugular
    c. Subclavian
    d. Carotid

563. Which of the following arteries runs parallel with the radial artery in birds?
    a. Brachial
    b. Ulnar
    c. Femoral
    d. Ischiatic

564. Which artery is the femoral artery distal to in birds?
    a. Coeliac
    b. Renal
    c. Pectoral
    d. External iliac

565. Food passes down the esophagus on the right side of the neck of birds and enters what structure?
    a. Gizzard
    b. Crop
    c. Duodenum
    d. Proventriculus

566. Which structure is located distal to the cecum of birds?
    a. Gizzard
    b. Cloaca
    c. Proventriculus
    d. Crop

567. Food leaves the gizzard and enters the duodenum by which of the following structures in birds?
    a. Cloaca
    b. Pylorus
    c. Proventriculus
    d. Ileum

568. How many lobes does the pancreas of birds have?
    a. 1
    b. 2
    c. 3
    d. None, birds do not have a pancreas

569. Via what structure do ureters carry urine to the outside of the body in birds?
    a. Isthmus
    b. Vagina
    c. Cloaca
    d. Proventriculus

570. Which of the following systems attach to the cloaca in birds?
    a. Reproductive
    b. Digestive
    c. Urinary
    d. All of the above

571. In female birds during the breeding season, how often is one ovum released until the clutch is complete?
    a. Every 2 hours
    b. Every 6 hours
    c. Every 12 hours
    d. Every 24 hours

572. Which of the following structures is the largest and most glandular structure of the oviduct in birds?
    a. Infundibulum
    b. Magnum
    c. Isthmus
    d. Cloaca

573. The majority of the albumen is added to the egg as it travels down which structure in birds?
    a. Infundibulum
    b. Cloaca
    c. Magnum
    d. Isthmus

574. How long does it take for calcification of the egg to occur in birds?
    a. 1 hour
    b. 5 hours
    c. 10 hours
    d. 15 hours

575. Which structure connects the testes of birds to the cloaca?
    a. Vas deferens
    b. Magnum
    c. Infundibulum
    d. Ureters

576. Where are the testes located compared to the kidneys in birds?
    a. Lateral
    b. Distal
    c. Caudal
    d. Cranial

577. In what location are spermatozoa stored in birds?
     a. Vas deferens
     b. Seminiferous tubules
     c. Ductus deferens
     d. Cloaca

578. During mating, the phallus of male birds becomes engorged with:
     a. Blood
     b. Air
     c. Lymph
     d. Water

579. Which type of vision do rabbits have?
     a. Monocular
     b. Binocular
     c. 3D
     d. Both a and b

580. Mature female rabbits develop a large fold of skin under the chin that is known as the:
     a. Philtrum
     b. Dewlap
     c. Crepuscular
     d. None of the above

581. Where are scent glands located on the rabbit?
     a. Under the chin
     b. On either side of the perineum
     c. At the anus
     d. All of the above

582. The forelegs of rabbits have _____ toes.
     a. 2
     b. 3
     c. 4
     d. 5

583. How many cervical vertebrae do rabbits have?
     a. 7
     b. 8
     c. 13
     d. 15

584. How many thoracic vertebrae does the rabbit have?
     a. 7
     b. 12–13
     c. 4
     d. 8

585. What characteristic is true about the fibula of rabbits?
     a. It is twice the length of the tibia
     b. It is half the length of the tibia
     c. It is fused with the tibia
     d. Both b and c

586. What is the average life span of the rabbit?
     a. 3–4 years
     b. 2–3 years
     c. 6–8 years
     d. 10 years

587. What is the normal body temperature of rabbits?
     a. 36.2° C–37.5° C
     b. 38.3° C
     c. 38.3° C–39.2° C
     d. None of the above

588. What is the normal respiratory rate of rabbits?
     a. 35–60 breaths/min
     b. 40–80 breaths/min
     c. 100–250 breaths/min
     d. 90–150 breaths/min

589. What is the average heart rate of rabbits?
     a. 250–500 bpm
     b. 220 bpm
     c. 130–190 bpm
     d. 260–450 bpm

590. What is the average adult weight of rabbits?
     a. 400–600 g
     b. 50–60 g
     c. 100 g
     d. 1000–8000 g

591. What is the length of the estrous cycle in rabbits?
     a. Every 4 days
     b. Every 30–35 days
     c. Every 15–16 days
     d. Every 4–6 days

592. What is the gestational period of rabbits?
     a. 28–32 days
     b. 111 days
     c. 63 days
     d. 19–21 days

593. What is the average litter size of rabbits?
     a. 1–2
     b. 2–3
     c. 2–7
     d. 6–12

594. What is the weaning age of rabbits?
     a. 6–8 weeks
     b. 3–4 weeks
     c. 4–6 weeks
     d. 18 days

595. What is the age of sexual maturity for rabbits?
   a. 3–4 weeks
   b. 10–12 weeks
   c. 12 months
   d. 5–8 months

596. How many canine teeth does the rabbit have?
   a. 2
   b. 4
   c. 6
   d. None, they do not contain canine teeth

597. The premolars of rabbits are also known as:
   a. Incisors
   b. Canines
   c. Cheek teeth
   d. Diastema

598. Rabbits are unable to vomit because of the arrangement of the _____ in relation to the stomach.
   a. Esophagus
   b. Pylorus
   c. Duodenum
   d. Cardia

599. The ileum in rabbits terminates at which of the following structures?
   a. Ileocecal tonsil
   b. Cecum
   c. Rectum
   d. Duodenum

600. What is the largest organ in the abdominal cavity of rabbits?
   a. Liver
   b. Spleen
   c. Cecum
   d. Colon

601. All of the following are true about rabbits, *except:*
   a. Rabbits are omnivores
   b. Rabbits are hindgut fermenters
   c. Rabbits are monogastric
   d. Rabbits are herbivores

602. Hard fibrous pellets from the digestive system of rabbits are produced within _____ hours of eating.
   a. 3
   b. 4
   c. 6
   d. 8

603. Food material of rabbits passes through the digestive system twice within ____ hours.
   a. 6
   b. 8
   c. 12
   d. 24

604. What does it mean when rabbits breathe through their mouths?
   a. Normal breathing
   b. Good prognosis
   c. Poor prognosis
   d. Rabbits never breathe through their mouths

605. How often does the nose of a rabbit twitch during general anesthesia?
   a. 10–20 times
   b. 25–50 times
   c. 50–100 times
   d. 20–120 times

606. Rabbits have _____ renal medullary pyramid(s).
   a. 1
   b. 2
   c. 6
   d. 9

607. At what age do the testes descend in the rabbit?
   a. Less than 10 days
   b. 8 weeks
   c. 12 weeks
   d. Rabbits' testes do not descend

608. The female rabbit has which type of uterus?
   a. Bicornuate
   b. Didelphic
   c. Unicornuate
   d. Septate

609. The term altricial refers to:
   a. Born hairless
   b. Born deaf
   c. Born blind
   d. All of the above

610. A male guinea pig is known as a:
   a. Doe
   b. Buck
   c. Boar
   d. Sow

611. How long is the gestational period of guinea pigs?
   a. 28–32 days
   b. 63 days
   c. 111 days
   d. 19–21 days

612. Ferrets have which type of vision?
    a. Monocular
    b. Binocular
    c. 3D
    d. Both a and b

613. What is the main source of a ferret's body odor?
    a. Fur
    b. Sebaceous glands
    c. Anal glands
    d. Mouth

614. Ferrets have _____ thoracic vertebrae.
    a. 7
    b. 15
    c. 5–6
    d. 3

615. The coccygeal vertebra of the ferret is located in which part of the body?
    a. Neck
    b. Thorax
    c. Pelvis
    d. Tail

616. The spine of a ferret is flexible and allows for the ferret to bend at an angle of at least:
    a. 15 degrees
    b. 45 degrees
    c. 90 degrees
    d. 180 degrees

617. The lumbar vertebra of the ferret is located distal to the:
    a. Thoracic vertebrae
    b. Sacrum
    c. Coccygeal vertebrae
    d. Pelvis

618. What is the average litter size of ferrets?
    a. 3–4
    b. 5–6
    c. 8–10
    d. More than 20

619. After mating occurs in ferrets, ovulation occurs within:
    a. 30 minutes
    b. 1–2 hours
    c. 30–40 hours
    d. 3 days

620. What is the average gestational period of a ferret?
    a. 28–32 days
    b. 42 days
    c. 63 days
    d. 111 days

621. A castrated male ferret is referred to as a:
    a. Jill
    b. Hobble
    c. Hob
    d. Gelding

622. Where are the lungs located in a tortoise?
    a. The ventral surface above the carapace
    b. The dorsal side below the carapace
    c. Caudal to the stomach
    d. Caudal to the heart

623. In the male tortoise, the testes are located adjacent to what other organ?
    a. Stomach
    b. Urinary bladder
    c. Kidneys
    d. Liver

624. All of the following are face bones in small animals, *except:*
    a. Zygomatic bones
    b. Pterygoid bones
    c. Vomer bone
    d. Sphenoid bone

625. The incus, malleus, and stapes are all bones that create the _____ in small animals.
    a. Ear
    b. Face
    c. Foot
    d. Cranium

626. Which bone is the most caudal bone of the skull in small animals?
    a. Parietal bone
    b. Occipital bone
    c. Interparietal bone
    d. Temporal bone

627. The spinal cord exits the skull through which structure?
    a. Temporal bone
    b. Atlas
    c. Foramen magnum
    d. Occipital condyles

628. The calcaneus of dogs is also referred to as the:
    a. Manubrium
    b. Point of hock
    c. Point of elbow
    d. Olecranon

629. The caudal end of the sternum of dogs is also referred to as the:
    a. Carpal
    b. Coxae
    c. Nuchae
    d. Xiphoid

630. The tibia and fibula of the dog are located immediately proximal to what bones?
    a. Metatarsal bones
    b. Metacarpal bones
    c. Tarsal bones
    d. Olecranon

631. The sacrum of dogs is cranial to what structure?
    a. Ligamentum nuchae
    b. Coccygeal
    c. Lumbar vertebrae
    d. Atlas

632. The mental foramen of the cat is located on which bone?
    a. Occipital bone
    b. Mandible
    c. Tympanic bulla
    d. Nasal bone

633. Which skull bone is the most rostral bone?
    a. Occipital
    b. Interparietal
    c. Incisive
    d. Lacrimal

634. A space within the lacrimal bones houses which of the following structures?
    a. Lacrimal sac
    b. Maxillary sinuses
    c. Hard palate
    d. Nasal cavity

635. The zygomatic bones of dogs are also referred to as:
    a. Premaxillary bones
    b. Hard palate
    c. Malar bones
    d. Cochlea

636. The _____ of the mandible is the horizontal portion that houses all the teeth.
    a. Ramus
    b. Shaft
    c. Palate
    d. Malar

637. Which of the following are the inner bones of the face of small animals?
    a. Vomer bone
    b. Palatine bone
    c. Pterygoid bone
    d. All of the above

638. The two small pterygoid bones support the lateral walls of what structure?
    a. Pharynx
    b. Mandibular symphysis
    c. Nasal septum
    d. Nasal conchae

639. Which animal contains the highest number of sacral vertebrae?
    a. Horse
    b. Dog
    c. Cat
    d. Pig

640. How many cervical vertebrae does the cat have?
    a. 3
    b. 7
    c. 13
    d. 18

641. The bodies of adjacent vertebrae are separated by what structure?
    a. Spinal canal
    b. Articular process
    c. Intervertebral disks
    d. Ligamentum nuchae

642. The junction between the bone and the cartilage of the ribs is referred to as the:
    a. Costochondral junction
    b. Xiphoid process
    c. Asternal ribs
    d. Manubrium

643. Which of the following is the most proximal bone of the thoracic limb?
    a. Ulna
    b. Humerus
    c. Scapula
    d. Brachium

644. Which of the following are considered to be organic molecules?
    a. Lipids
    b. Proteins
    c. Nucleic acids
    d. Carbohydrates
    e. All of the above

645. All of the following are lipids, *except:*
    a. Steroids
    b. Glycogen
    c. Triglycerides
    d. Prostaglandins

646. A sugar that contains 5 carbons is referred to as a:
    a. Monosaccharide
    b. Hexose sugar
    c. Pentose sugar
    d. Disaccharide

647. Which part of the cell contains and processes genetic information and controls cell metabolism?
    a. Nucleus
    b. Cell membrane
    c. Cilia
    d. Chromatin

648. The digestion of absorbed material is performed by which organelle?
    a. Peroxisomes
    b. Ribosomes
    c. Lysosomes
    d. Mitochondria

649. _____ move cells through fluid.
    a. Flagella
    b. Cilia
    c. Basal bodies
    d. Centrioles

650. What is the fluid of a cell called?
    a. Cytoplasm
    b. Cytosol
    c. Cytoskeleton
    d. Tubulins

651. Glucose that is not immediately used by cells is converted to glycogen and is stored in which organ?
    a. Gallbladder
    b. Pancreas
    c. Spleen
    d. Liver

652. Amphibians and reptiles are commonly referred to as ectothermic, which is correctly described by which of the following?
    a. Warm-blooded
    b. Cold-blooded
    c. Endothermic
    d. Behavioral thermoregulation

653. The term ecdysis refers to:
    a. Cold-blooded
    b. Shedding of skin
    c. Hibernation
    d. Active at night

654. When tension is generated in the muscle, muscle tone increases but the muscle does not shorten. Which of the following correctly names this action?
    a. Isotonic contraction
    b. Isometric contraction
    c. Muscle tone
    d. None of the above

655. Which of the following muscles opens the jaw and is located on the caudoventral surface of the mandible?
    a. Temporalis
    b. Dorsal rectus
    c. Digastricus
    d. Masseter

656. Which of the following muscles are responsible for side-to-side movements of the mouth?
    a. Masseter
    b. Temporalis
    c. Medial and lateral pterygoids
    d. Digastric

657. The _____ in the muscles of the jaw is responsible for closure and helps keep the mouth closed when it is not in use.
    a. Shape
    b. Length
    c. Tone
    d. Atrophy

658. Which of the following muscles originate at the zygomatic arch and inserts on the masseteric fossa on the lateral surface of the mandible?
    a. Temporalis
    b. Masseter
    c. Digastricus
    d. Medial and lateral pterygoids

659. How many extrinsic muscles of the eye are responsible for moving the eye up, down, and side to side within its socket?
    a. 1
    b. 2
    c. 3
    d. 4

660. Which muscle of the eye is responsible for rotating the eye about its visual axis?
    a. Dorsal oblique
    b. Dorsal rectus
    c. Ventral oblique
    d. Both a and c

661. What is the function of the retractor bulbi muscle?
    a. To move the eye upward
    b. To move the eye downward
    c. To move the eye outward
    d. To pull the eye deeper in the socket

662. Where do the epaxial muscles lie?
    a. Dorsal to the transverse process of the vertebrae
    b. Ventral to the transverse process of the vertebrae
    c. Between the thoracic and abdominal cavity
    d. Along each side of the linea alba

663. Which muscle originates from the caudal border of one rib and inserts on the cranial border of the rib behind it?
    a. Internal intercostals
    b. External intercostals
    c. External abdominal oblique
    d. Internal abdominal oblique

664. All of the following structures pass through the aortic hiatus, *except:*
    a. Aorta
    b. Thoracic duct
    c. Azygous vein
    d. Vagal nerve

665. Which opening lies within the central tendon and transmits the caudal vena cava?
    a. Aortic hiatus
    b. Caval foramen
    c. Esophageal hiatus
    d. Foramen magnum

666. Which canine muscle originates from the dorsal midline from C2 to C7 and inserts on the spine of the scapula?
    a. Pectoralis
    b. Trapezius
    c. Latissimus dorsi
    d. Brachiocephalicus

667. Which muscle is responsible for retracting the forelimb of dogs?
    a. Pectoralis
    b. Trapezius
    c. Latissimus dorsi
    d. Supraspinatus

668. Which muscle is responsible for stabilizing and flexing the shoulder joint?
    a. Supraspinatus
    b. Infraspinatus
    c. Triceps brachii
    d. Biceps brachii

669. Which muscle group extends the hip joint and abducts the thigh?
    a. Sartorius
    b. Gluteals
    c. Quadriceps femoris
    d. Gastrocnemius

670. Which muscle is the most medial muscle of the hamstring?
    a. Semitendinosus
    b. Gastrocnemius
    c. Semimembranosus
    d. Quadriceps femoris

671. Which muscle flexes the hock and rotates the paw medially?
    a. Gastrocnemius
    b. Anterior tibialis
    c. Pectineus
    d. Gracilis

672. All of the following are muscles of the hind limb in dogs, *except:*
    a. Biceps femoris
    b. Quadriceps femoris
    c. Semitendinosus
    d. Biceps brachii

673. The _____ is a projection of bone on the lateral edge above its condyle.
    a. Foramen
    b. Epicondyle
    c. Head
    d. Periosteum

674. The protuberances on bones, which are used for the attachment of muscles, are referred to as which of the following?
    a. Fossa
    b. Tendon
    c. Tuberosity
    d. Shaft

675. Grooves on bones that allow tendons to act as pulleys are known as:
    a. Fossa
    b. Ligament
    c. Trochlea
    d. Epicondyle

676. Which of the following dogs has a mesaticephalic head?
    a. Boxer
    b. Greyhound
    c. Beagle
    d. Bulldog

677. The _____ artery carries deoxygenated blood to the lungs.
    a. Pulmonary
    b. Carotid
    c. Subclavian
    d. Renal

678. The azygous vein drains venous blood from what structure?
    a. Head
    b. Thoracic body wall
    c. Hind limbs
    d. Liver

679. The veins that drain the stomach, intestine, and pancreas drain into which of the following?
    a. Hepatic veins
    b. Hepatic arteries
    c. Portal veins
    d. Iliac veins

680. Which artery supplies the stomach, spleen, and liver with blood?
    a. Renal artery
    b. Portal vein
    c. Hepatic vein
    d. Celiac artery

681. Which artery supplies the small intestines with blood?
    a. Celiac artery
    b. Cranial mesenteric artery
    c. Caudal mesenteric artery
    d. Femoral artery

682. Which vein returns deoxygenated blood from the pelvic region, hind limbs, and abdominal viscera?
    a. Caudal vena cava
    b. Aorta
    c. Iliac veins
    d. Pulmonary vein

683. The smallest veins are called _____.
    a. Capillaries
    b. Venules
    c. Iliacs
    d. Vessels

684. Which of the following are present in all organs/tissues and are the sites of exchange between blood and tissue fluid?
    a. Venules
    b. Capillaries
    c. Valves
    d. Lymph

685. A venous shunt within the liver that connects the umbilical vein to the caudal vena cava is known as what?
    a. Ductus venosus
    b. Ligamentum arteriosus
    c. Foramen ovale
    d. Ductus arteriosus

686. Blood leaves the right ventricle to enter what structure?
    a. Pulmonary artery
    b. Aorta
    c. Cranial vena cava
    d. Left atrium

687. Blood leaving the lungs travels to enter which section of the heart?
    a. Right atrium
    b. Left atrium
    c. Right ventricle
    d. Left ventricle

688. Which is the largest lymphoid organ?
    a. Liver
    b. Cisterna chyli
    c. Lymph node
    d. Spleen

689. When an animal becomes severely dehydrated, it loses both tissue fluid and plasma fluid. What effect would this have on the hematocrit and the PCV?
    a. Increase both values
    b. Decrease both values
    c. Increase the hematocrit but no effect on the PCV
    d. No change in either value

690. Which of the following is a short irregular tube of cartilage and muscle that connects the pharynx with the trachea?
    a. Larynx
    b. Epiglottis
    c. Bronchi
    d. Esophagus

691. Which organelle is the site of protein synthesis?
a. Golgi apparatus
b. Ribosomes
c. Endoplasmic reticulum
d. Mitochondria

692. What structure extends along the ventral midline from the xiphoid process of the sternum to the pubic symphysis?
a. Spinal cord
b. Linea alba
c. Diaphragm
d. Transversus abdominus

693. Which muscle forms the caudal half of the medial surface of the thigh?
a. Sartorius
b. Semitendinosus
c. Biceps femoris
d. Gracilis

694. Which type of cells make up bone?
a. Osteoblasts
b. Osteocytes
c. Osteoclasts
d. All of these

695. The bones of the head and trunk are referred to as the:
a. Axial skeleton
b. Appendicular skeleton
c. Visceral skeleton
d. Metacarpal bones

696. Which bone is located where the spinal cord exits the skull?
a. Interparietal
b. Occipital
c. Parietal
d. Temporal

697. The two small bones that form part of the orbit of the eye are which of the following:
a. Ossicles
b. Malleus
c. Incus
d. Lacrimal

698. The two zygomatic bones are also known as the:
a. Malar bones
b. Maxillary bones
c. Lacrimal bones
d. Nasal bones

699. Which of the following are four, thin, scroll-like bones that fill most of the space in the nasal cavity and are also called the nasal conchae?
a. Palatine bones
b. Pterygoid bones
c. Turbinates
d. Vomer bone

700. The non-floating ribs that make up the caudal part of the thorax are called:
a. The sternal ribs
b. The asternal ribs
c. The floating ribs
d. The costochondral junction

ⓔ *Answers and rationales available on Evolve*
http://evolve.elsevier.com/Prendergast/QAvettech/

Hospital Management

Brooke Lockridge, RDMS

QUESTIONS

1. Credentialed veterinary technicians are allowed to perform certain duties under the direct supervision of whom?
   a. Office manager
   b. Lead veterinary technician
   c. Veterinarian
   d. Practice owner

2. Which of the following health care team members is allowed to diagnose, prescribe medication, and perform surgery?
   a. Veterinarian
   b. Office manager
   c. Credentialed veterinary technician
   d. Veterinary technologist

3. Which of the following tasks is the responsibility of a veterinary assistant?
   a. Perform dental prophylaxis
   b. Calculate drug dosages
   c. Perform surgical procedures
   d. Maintain legible and accurate medical records

4. The term "petty cash" refers to which of the following?
   a. Change owed back to an owner on a bill
   b. Cash set aside in the practice to purchase items needed for business when a check is not available
   c. The cash balance in the drawer at the start and end of every day
   d. Payment received from a third party

5. How many components does the human voice contain?
   a. 2
   b. 4
   c. 8
   d. 10

6. Which of the following is the correct definition of a *mission statement* in a hospital?
   a. The desired future of the practice
   b. The purpose of the hospital; the fundamental reason the hospital exists
   c. Guiding principles that are not to be compromised during change
   d. None of the above

7. Which of the following are characteristics of effective leaders?
   a. Team player
   b. Effective communicator
   c. Self-confident
   d. All of the above

8. Which of the following are methods that can be used to decrease loss of revenue in the hospital?
   a. Use travel sheets to decrease missed charges
   b. Implement internal controls to prevent employee theft
   c. Manage inventory appropriately
   d. All of the above
   e. Both a and b

9. Which of the following statements is the correct definition of *rapport*?
   a. Denotes a duty or obligation that a team member is expected to uphold
   b. Mutual trust or emotional relationship that exists among team members
   c. Consideration or esteem that is given to another person
   d. All of the above

10. How many branches of veterinary ethics exist?
    a. 2
    b. 4
    c. 6
    d. 8

11. Descriptive ethics refers to which of the following?
    a. The study of the ethical views of veterinarians and veterinary professionals regarding their behavior and attitudes
    b. The creation of the official ethical standards adopted by organizations of professionals and imposed on their members
    c. The search for correct principles of good and bad, right and wrong, justice or injustice
    d. Actions by administrative government bodies that regulate veterinary practice and activities in which veterinarians engage

12. Law is divided into how many categories?
    a. 1
    b. 2
    c. 4
    d. 5

13. A noncompete agreement falls under which division of the law?
    a. Civil
    b. Criminal
    c. Both criminal and civil
    d. Neither criminal nor civil

14. Animal abuse falls under which division of the law?
    a. Civil
    b. Criminal
    c. Both criminal and civil
    d. Neither criminal nor civil

15. Which of the following correctly defines negligence?
    a. A civil offense to an opposing party in which harm has occurred
    b. An intentional action that has taken place in which harm has occurred to another member of society
    c. The performance of an act that a reasonable person under the same circumstances would not perform
    d. The unlawful activity against a member of the public that is prosecuted by a public official

16. On what are lawsuits against veterinarians almost always based?
    a. Defamation
    b. Breach of warranty
    c. Neglect
    d. Breach of contract

17. Which of the following is considered an act of malpractice?
    a. Abandonment
    b. Incorrect drug administration
    c. Disease transmission
    d. Failure to communicate
    e. All of the above

18. When a mistake is written in the medical record, what is the proper method to correct it?
    a. Erase the mistake and start over
    b. Use white-out to cover the written mistake, initial it, and rewrite it
    c. Draw a single line through the mistake, initial it, and write the correction
    d. Scratch out the mistake with ink and rewrite with initials

19. Which of the following acts was created to establish minimum wage and overtime pay standards as well as to regulate the employment of minors?
    a. Family and Medical Leave Act
    b. Fair Labor and Standards Act
    c. Equal Employment Opportunity
    d. Occupational Safety and Health Administration

20. Which of the following Laws/Acts does NOT apply to veterinary facilities?
    a. Uniformed Services Employment and Reemployment Rights Act
    b. Immigration Reform and Control Act
    c. Employee Polygraph Protection Act
    d. None of the above

21. Which of the following are considered to be employee benefits?
    a. Sick leave
    b. Veterinary care
    c. Continuing education
    d. All of the above

22. Employee discounts on services greater than what percent MUST be reported to the IRS as pay?
    a. 10%
    b. 15%
    c. 20%
    d. 50%

23. Which of the following is an example of incorporeal property?
    a. Buildings
    b. Equipment
    c. Vehicles
    d. Practice goodwill

24. What is the correct protocol for handling a pregnant veterinary technician employee?
    a. Have the employee placed on a temporary resignation status for the duration of the pregnancy
    b. Have the employee transferred to a receptionist position for the duration of the pregnancy
    c. Limit the employee on all safety issues such as lifting, anesthesia exposure, and radiation exposure
    d. Address the safety issues within the facility but allow the employee to decide their own safety level

25. Which of the following questions should NOT be asked during an interview?
    a. What is your salary requirement?
    b. Are you currently employed?
    c. Do you have any children?
    d. What are some areas you feel you need improvement on?

26. Which of the following are considered to be environmental stressors to veterinary health care team members?
    a. Noise level
    b. Inventory
    c. Equipment
    d. All of the above

27. Overproduction of neurotransmitters can cause all of the following conditions to occur, *except:*
    a. Anxiety
    b. Depression
    c. Anger
    d. Excitement

28. Excess levels of positive stress may lead to:
    a. Satisfaction
    b. Exhaustion
    c. Energy
    d. Relief

29. Which of the following descriptions are considered cognitive signs of compassion fatigue?
    a. Decreased concentration and/or ability to concentrate
    b. Questioning life's meaning
    c. Failure to develop non–work-related aspects of life
    d. Dread of working with certain co-workers

30. Which of the following correctly describes the term ergonomics?
    a. The organization of materials in a logical sequence
    b. The science that studies the relationship between people and their work environments
    c. The positioning of objects as close to the point of use as possible
    d. The amount of time and degree of motion required to perform a given task

31. All of the following are considered physiological factors of the work environment, *except:*
    a. Space
    b. Patients
    c. Acoustics
    d. Color

32. Which area of the hospital typically requires the most efficiency?
    a. Kennels
    b. Doctor's office
    c. Retail area
    d. Middle area

33. The ADA is a federal law that protects which of the following?
    a. Employees and their exposure to radiation
    b. Employees and clients with disabilities
    c. Employees and their ergonomic environment
    d. The sale and distribution of pharmaceuticals

34. A program or software that installs itself onto the computer without the user's knowledge is known as which of the following?
    a. Cookies
    b. Spam
    c. Spyware
    d. Adware

35. A program that replicates itself over a computer network and performs malicious actions that can shut down the computer system is referred to as which of the following?
    a. Host
    b. Worm
    c. Firewall
    d. Trojan horse

36. A measure of computer data storage at approximately 1 million bytes refers to which of the following?
    a. Zip drive
    b. Megabyte
    c. Gigabyte
    d. Hard drive

37. What is ethylenediaminetetraacetic acid?
    a. An anticoagulant added to blood collection tubes
    b. A serum separator agent added to blood collection tubes
    c. Rubbing alcohol added to the skin for aseptic purposes
    d. None of the above

38. When submitting a tissue sample for pathology what should the ratio of formalin to tissue volume be?
    a. 1:1
    b. 5:1
    c. 10:1
    d. 20:1

39. Serum separator tubes should NOT be used for which of the following therapeutic monitoring?
    a. Phenobarbital levels
    b. Theophylline levels
    c. Digoxin levels
    d. All of the above

40. All of the following are anticoagulants used in blood collection tubes, *except:*
    a. Potassium citrate
    b. Lithium heparin
    c. Sodium heparin
    d. ETDA

41. An anaerobic culture should be kept at room temperature and processed within how many hours of collection?
    a. 8 hours
    b. 12 hours
    c. 24 hours
    d. 48 hours

42. What does a SWOT analysis evaluate within a marketing plan?
    a. Weaknesses
    b. Opportunities
    c. Strengths
    d. All of the above

43. Which of the following is an example of internal marketing?
    a. Web page/social media
    b. Yellow pages
    c. Client education
    d. Newspaper advertisement

44. Recalls should be performed for which of the following patient scenarios?
    a. Yearly exams
    b. Vaccines
    c. Wound care/infection
    d. Surgery
    e. All of the above

45. Which of the following is NOT an example of external marketing?
    a. Outdoor building sign
    b. Lectures
    c. Media advertising
    d. Client education

46. Which message component contributes the most during communication?
    a. Verbal
    b. Nonverbal
    c. Paraverbal
    d. All components of a message are equal in contribution

47. Which of the following is an example of a nonverbal skill?
    a. Folded arms
    b. High-pitched tone
    c. Slang word choice
    d. Using "yeah" instead of "yes"

48. Which team members should present treatment plans to clients?
    a. Receptionist
    b. Office manager
    c. Veterinary technician
    d. Veterinarian

49. The percentage of clients who accept a recommendation is defined as:
    a. Quantity
    b. Turnover
    c. Retention
    d. Compliance

50. When should client grievances be addressed?
    a. After a meeting with the office manager
    b. Immediately, at the time of the grievance
    c. A week later after the pet, client, and employee have recovered
    d. Depends on the severity of the grievance

51. When a client is not present to sign a euthanasia form, to verify the euthanasia how many team members must the owner talk to?
    a. 1
    b. 2
    c. 3
    d. 4

52. Euthanasia comes from the Greek terms *eu* and *Thanatos*. What does the term *eu* stand for?
    a. Right
    b. Death
    c. Good
    d. Both a and c

53. Which of the following characteristics would be examples of a barrier to communication?
    a. Cultures
    b. Exam room tables
    c. Reception desk
    d. Constant eye contact

54. Which of the following correctly defines mass cremation?
    a. A cremation service held within a church
    b. A cremation of multiple animals without private ashes returned
    c. A cremation of a single animal with private ashes returned
    d. A cremation of a single animal without ashes returned

55. How should a pet be presented to an owner after it is has been euthanized?
    a. In a box
    b. In a trash bag
    c. In a waterproof body bag
    d. Without any covering

56. What drug is commonly used for euthanasia?
    a. Barbiturate
    b. Morphine
    c. Acepromazine
    d. Telazol

57. When scheduling appointments, which of the following factors should be considered?
    a. Number of veterinarians seeing appointments
    b. Veterinary technician appointments
    c. Length of time for client education
    d. All of the above

58. Which of the following is an example of a nonsterile procedure?
    a. Spay procedures
    b. Orthopedic surgeries
    c. Abscess debridement
    d. Exploratory surgery

59. To help reduce client overload at the front desk, appointments should be:
    a. Set every 15 minutes
    b. Set every $\frac{1}{2}$ hour
    c. Staggered every 5 minutes
    d. None of the above

60. Appointment lengths may vary for all of the following *except:*
    a. Specific client
    b. Appointment type
    c. Veterinarian
    d. Patient

61. Which of the following people must be able to read medical records?
    a. Veterinarians
    b. Team members
    c. Legal personnel
    d. All of the above

62. What are computerized medical records filed under?
    a. Pet name
    b. Clients last name
    c. Client number
    d. Both b and c

63. Which of the following is considered a disadvantage of computerized medical records?
    a. Legibility
    b. Client perceives progressive, higher-quality medicine
    c. Computer-generated records can lack medical details
    d. Can target specific clients quickly and efficiently when promoting specific services

64. Medical record entry should follow the standard SOAP format, which includes all of the following, *except:*
    a. Plan
    b. Obsession
    c. Subjective
    d. Assessment

65. Which of the following correctly defines the term prognosis?
   a. The surgical procedure
   b. The medication prescribed
   c. The prediction of the outcome of a disease
   d. The treatment plan

66. Which of the following correctly defines the objective portion of the exam?
   a. The reason for the visit, history, and observations made by the client
   b. Information gathered directly from the patient, physical exam, diagnostic workup
   c. Conclusion reached along with a definitive diagnosis
   d. Treatment, surgery, medication, and diagnostics recommended

67. Surgical patients must be examined within what time frame before anesthesia is administered?
   a. 2 hours
   b. 12 hours
   c. 24 hours
   d. 48 hours

68. Which of the following is considered the correct entry for medication?
   a. Cefazolin 0.2 mL IV
   b. 0.5 mL Cefazolin
   c. 0.4 mL Cefazolin (100 mg/mL) IV
   d. Cefazolin .3 100 mg/mL

69. When a medication is being dispensed, all of the following must be included in the medical record *except:*
   a. Drug lot number
   b. Drug strength
   c. Drug administration route
   d. Drug duration of treatment

70. An inactive medical record is defined as a client who has not been seen by the practice in how long?
   a. 6 months
   b. 12 months
   c. 3 years
   d. 7 years

71. All of the following are rules for medical records, *except:*
   a. Records can be written in any color ink desired
   b. The author of the entry must date and initial each time an entry is made
   c. Correction fluid may never be used
   d. Use standard and approved abbreviations only

72. Which of the following are considered losses associated with poor inventory management?
   a. Backorders
   b. Shrinkage
   c. Frequent ordering
   d. All of the above

73. Which of the following correctly defines "turnover rate" in reference to inventory?
   a. The most popular product used in the facility
   b. The number of times a specific product turns over in a practice
   c. How quickly the product will expire
   d. The time it takes to receive product after it has been purchased

74. Which of the following is the proper way to handle expired drugs?
   a. Prescribe them to owners to get them out the facility
   b. Flush them down the drain
   c. Combine them with cat litter for absorption and then throw away
   d. Throw them in the trash

75. What does a dispensing fee cover?
   a. The label on the bottle
   b. The vial used to package the medication
   c. The wear and tear on the label machine
   d. All of the above

76. Missed charges account for approximately how much of gross revenue?
   a. 5%
   b. 10%
   c. 25%
   d. 45%

77. Any pharmaceutical that is a controlled substance will have what letter on the bottle?
   a. A
   b. C
   c. D
   d. S

78. Controlled substance prescriptions administered to clients for classes III, IV, and V can have 5 refills available for how long?
   a. 1 month
   b. 6 months
   c. 12 months
   d. None, they cannot have refills

79. Which class level of controlled drugs has the highest potential for abuse?
    a. I
    b. IV
    c. V
    d. VII

80. Class II controlled substances can be filled for 30 days with how many refills?
    a. 1
    b. 3
    c. 5
    d. None, this class is not allowed refills on the original script

81. Which controlled substance class level does not have DEA dispensing limits?
    a. Class I
    b. Class II
    c. Class IV
    d. Class V

82. Which controlled substance class must have separate logs and invoices from other classes?
    a. I
    b. II
    c. IV
    d. V

83. All of the following information is included in drug logs, *except:*
    a. Amount of drug administered
    b. Balance of drug after use
    c. Client name
    d. Drug lot number

84. Which of the following will not be found on an inventory log?
    a. Date of purchase
    b. Date and time of inventory
    c. Client name, patient name
    d. Product name, strength, and count in a full bottle

85. When a drug loss or theft has been identified, who must be notified?
    a. DEA
    b. Police
    c. Both a and b
    d. No one. It just needs to be recorded

86. What is the correct way to dispose of controlled substances of any class?
    a. Poured down the drain
    b. Added to cat litter and then thrown away
    c. Sent through a certified "reverse distribution" company
    d. None of the above

87. A loss equal to or greater than what amount must be reported to the DEA?
    a. 1%
    b. 2%
    c. 3%
    d. 5%

88. The law requires which of the following logs?
    a. Compliance logs
    b. Controlled substance logs
    c. Laboratory logs
    d. All of the above

89. Controlled substance logs should be kept for _____ year(s) beyond the last recorded entry.
    a. 1
    b. 2
    c. 3
    d. 4

90. Accounts receivable should not be greater than what percentage of gross revenue?
    a. 1.5%
    b. 5%
    c. 10%
    d. 12.5%

91. Which of the following best describes the Fair Debt Collection Practices Act of 1996?
    a. Any facility or collecting agency is allowed to call anytime in an effort to collect its debt.
    b. Any collecting agency is allowed to state that it is a government agency attempting to collect its debt
    c. Protects the public from unethical collection procedures
    d. Protects the businesses on past-due accounts made by the patron

92. Which of the following is NOT allowed to be given to a collection agency?
    a. Client's full name, address, and telephone number
    b. Client's occupation
    c. Client's driver's license number
    d. None of the above

93. What does indemnity insurance provide?
    a. A contract for veterinarians to provide medical service at a set price
    b. A reimbursement the veterinarian collects directly from the insurance company for services rendered
    c. Compensation for treatment of injured or sick pets paid directly to the client, following the company policy
    d. None of the above

94. Which of the following correctly defines a per-incident limit?
    a. The maximum dollar amount a company will pay out on one policy for the lifetime of the pet
    b. The maximum dollar amount an insurance company will pay out per incident filed
    c. Injury or illness contracted, manifested, or incurred before the policy effective date
    d. An extension of coverage that can be purchased and added to a base medical policy

95. A team member must be able to walk to an eyewash station within what amount of time after being exposed to a chemical?
    a. 10 seconds
    b. 30 seconds
    c. 60 seconds
    d. 2 minutes

96. What is the minimum PPE that must be worn when performing x-rays?
    a. Lead gown only
    b. Lead gown and thyroid collar
    c. Lead gown, thyroid collar, and lead gloves
    d. Lead gown, thyroid collar, lead gloves, and goggles

97. Where should dosimeter badges be worn?
    a. Under the lead gown
    b. In the pocket of the team member
    c. On the outside of the PPE
    d. Dosimeter badges are not worn and should be kept outside of the x-ray room at all times

98. How long should dosimetry reports be kept in accordance with OSHA standards?
    a. 2 years
    b. 10 years
    c. 15 years
    d. 30 years

99. Noise protection should be provided for employees when noise levels reach which decibel level?
    a. 75 dB
    b. 85 dB
    c. 95 dB
    d. Ear protection is not required in the veterinary practice

100. All of the following are provided in SDS sheets, *except:*
    a. Health hazards
    b. The nearest emergency facility
    c. Permissible exposure limits
    d. Emergency first aid procedures

101. Colors on NFPA labels are used to identify:
    a. The hazards of chemicals
    b. The level of safety
    c. PPE that is required
    d. Permissible exposure limits

102. What does a NFPA label with the number 4 within a blue diamond indicate?
    a. No hazard
    b. Can cause significant irritation
    c. Can cause temporary incapacitation
    d. Can be lethal

103. A urine sediment evaluation checks for which of the following?
    a. White blood cells
    b. Crystals
    c. Epithelial cells
    d. All of the above

104. A urine dipstick analysis tests for all of the following, *except:*
    a. Glucose
    b. pH
    c. Bacteria
    d. Leukocytes

105. Which of the following diagnostic imaging procedures uses sound waves?
    a. MRI
    b. x-ray
    c. Fluoroscopy
    d. Sonography

106. Which of the following abbreviations indicates "every other day"?
    a. QID
    b. QOD
    c. BID
    d. OD

107. Drugs that reduce inflammation are termed:
    a. Anthelmintics
    b. Antimicrobials
    c. Anti-inflammatories
    d. Antifungal

108. Insulin is an example of what type of drug?
    a. Anthelmintic
    b. Gastric
    c. Endocrine
    d. Nervous

109. A positive practice culture has all of the following characteristics, *except:*
    a. Warm, welcoming environment
    b. Teamwork
    c. Gossip
    d. Team etiquette

110. When placing a caller on hold in the veterinary practice, how long is an acceptable wait time?
    a. 1 minute
    b. 2 minutes
    c. 5 minutes
    d. 10 minutes

111. What percentage of phone shoppers should become a client in each veterinary hospital?
    a. 20%
    b. 50%
    c. 70%
    d. 100%

112. Clients are expected to complete which forms?
    a. Rabies certificates
    b. Spay or neuter certificates
    c. Medical records
    d. Patient information sheet

113. When clients ask for their medical records to be released to anyone other than themselves, which ACT regulates how those records can be released?
    a. Privacy Act of 1974
    b. Family and Medical Leave Act
    c. Fair Credit and Reporting Act
    d. There is no ACT that regulates how to release medical records

114. The Red Flags Rule establishes that practices must:
    a. Give clients the option to purchase medication wherever they choose
    b. Verify identification when the client has presented credit cards to pay for services
    c. Give team members time off for jury duty
    d. Verify team member citizenship in advance of hiring

115. Which of the following are acceptable methods of payment in most veterinary practices?
    a. Credit cards
    b. Check
    c. Care Credit
    d. All of the above

116. Which of the following methods would the receptionist use to ensure the safety of both clients and patients in the reception area?
    a. Place every client and pet in an exam room when they arrive.
    b. Make sure every dog is on a leash and every cat is in a carrier.
    c. Provide signage advising of animal restraint policies
    d. Provide separate reception areas for well and ill pets.

117. Clients and visitors observe a heated argument between two staff members regarding whose responsibility it is to clean up urine from a "doggie mishap" in the reception area. This type of staff interaction will have an effect on which of the following:
    a. Etiquette
    b. Job descriptions
    c. Cleaning product selection
    d. Team culture

ⓔ *Answers and rationales available on Evolve*
http://evolve.elsevier.com/Prendergast/QAvettech/

Medical Calculations

Heather Prendergast, RVT, CVPM

QUESTIONS

1. The doctor asks you to administer 5 g of 25% mannitol to a patient. How many mL do you give?
   a. 5 mL
   b. 20 mL
   c. 40 mL
   d. 25 mL

2. Many drugs do not have X mg/mL listed on their labels but instead have their concentrations listed as a percent (e.g., X% solution). Which of the following most accurately reflects the conversion of a percentage of a solution to a weight per volume format?
   a. X% = X g/mL
   b. X% = X g/10 mL
   c. X% = X g/100 mL
   d. X% = X mg/10 mL

3. A 75-lb dog must be dewormed. If the daily dose of the dewormer is 1 tsp/25 lb of body weight for 3 days, approximately how much should be administered each day?
   a. 3 tbs
   b. 1 tbs
   c. 5 tsp
   d. 1 tsp

4. A cat on intravenous fluids must receive 30 mL/hr of normal saline. If this cat has a drip set that provides 60 drops/mL, what should the drip rate be?
   a. 1 drop/2 sec
   b. 1 drop/6 sec
   c. 3 drops/sec
   d. 16 drops/sec

5. The concentration of furosemide is 5%. How many mg are in 0.5 mL?
   a. 150 mg
   b. 2.5 mg
   c. 25 mg
   d. 50 mg

6. How many mL of a drug with a concentration of 100 mg/mL should be administered to a 75-lb dog at a dose of 1 mg/lb?
   a. 75 mL
   b. 100 mL
   c. 0.75 mL
   d. 0.34 mL

7. How many mL are in a teaspoon?
   a. 1 mL
   b. 3 mL
   c. 5 mL
   d. 10 mL

8. A prescription in which 3 mL of lactulose is administered orally twice daily will require how many ounces to last at least 30 days?
   a. 3 oz
   b. 6 oz
   c. 90 oz
   d. 180 oz

9. A commercial dog food is 420 kcal/cup. A dog weighing 60 lb fed at a rate of 70 kcal/lb/day should be fed how many cups at each meal if he is fed twice daily?
   a. 5 cups
   b. 10 cups
   c. 2 cups
   d. 1 cup

10. A cockatiel needs 100 mg/kg piperacillin via intramuscular injection. If the bird weighs 80 g, and the concentration of piperacillin is 100 mg/mL, how many mL should be administered?
    a. 0.08 mL
    b. 0.8 mL
    c. 80 mL
    d. 1.6 mL

11. A rabbit needs 300 μg/kg of a 1% ivermectin solution. If the rabbit weighs 8 lb, how many mL of ivermectin should be administered?
    a. 8 mL
    b. 10 mL
    c. 0.1 mL
    d. 0.8 mL

12. How many mL of a 50% dextrose solution are needed to make 1000 mL of a 5% dextrose solution?
    a. 1 mL
    b. 10 mL
    c. 50 mL
    d. 100 mL

13. Six 12-oz puppies need deworming medication. If the dose is 1 mL/lb, how many mL do you dispense?
    a. 12 mL
    b. 4.5 mL
    c. 6 mL
    d. 3 mL

14. The doctor asks you to start a fentanyl constant rate infusion (CRI) at 3 mcg/kg/hr in a 50-kg dog. The fentanyl you have available in the hospital is 50 mcg/mL. What will the rate per hour be?
    a. 1 mL/hr
    b. 3 mL/hr
    c. 5 mL/hr
    d. 50 mL/hr

15. To make a solution with a concentration of 15 mg/mL, how many mL of sterile water should be added to 30 g of powdered drug?
    a. 5 mL
    b. 200 mL
    c. 150 mL
    d. 2000 mL

16. A prescription reads "2 tab q4h po prn until gone." The translation of these instructions is:
    a. Two tablets are to be taken four times per day for pain until all tablets are gone
    b. Two tablets are to be taken four times per day under supervision by the veterinarian until all tablets are gone
    c. Two tablets are to be taken every 4 hours with food and water until all tablets are gone
    d. Two tablets are to be taken every 4 hours by mouth as needed until all tablets are gone

17. How many tablets would you dispense for a 30-day supply of a drug with a dose of one and one-half tablets three times daily?
    a. 500 tablets
    b. 45 tablets
    c. 135 tablets
    d. 90 tablets

18. One gram of powdered drug diluted with how many mL of sterile water will make a concentration of 20 mg/mL?
    a. 0.05 mL
    b. 0.2 mL
    c. 100 mL
    d. 50 mL

19. You regularly order six 10 mL vials per month of a drug that has a concentration of 50 mg/mL. This month that same drug is available only in 20 mL vials of 10 mg/mL. How many vials should you order this month to obtain the same total amount of drug?
    a. 150
    b. 60
    c. 10
    d. 15

20. If a dog that receives fluids at a rate of 120 mL/hr has a rate reduction of 20%, what is the new rate in mL/hr?
    a. 1.6 mL/hr
    b. 0.4 mL/hr
    c. 24 mL/hr
    d. 96 mL/hr

21. Generally 1 fluid ounce is equal to approximately how many mL of liquid?
    a. 1 mL
    b. 15 mL
    c. 30 mL
    d. 60 mL

22. A cat that weighs 5 kg is given 0.1 mL of a drug with a concentration of 10 mg/mL. What dose did this cat receive?
    a. 0.05 mg/kg
    b. 0.2 mg/kg
    c. 2 mg/kg
    d. 25 mg/kg

23. You give 5 mg of a drug to a 10-kg animal. What is the dose of the drug in mg/kg?
    a. 2 mg/kg
    b. 10 mg/kg
    c. 0.5 mg/kg
    d. 50 mg/kg

24. A bird that weighs 50 g requires a particular drug at 4 mg/kg divided twice daily. What is the morning dose?
    a. 1 mg
    b. 4 mg
    c. 0.1 mg
    d. 100 mg

25. A 1-mg/kg dose of diazepam is to be administered to a 50-lb dog. How many mg will he be given?
    a. 50 mg
    b. 22.7 mg
    c. 500 mg
    d. 2.27 mg

26. How long will it take to give a whole blood transfusion of 60 mL at a rate of 2 mL/min?
    a. 30 hr
    b. 3 hr
    c. ½ hour
    d. 1.8 hr

27. If a prescription calls for one tablet to be administered for 3 days bid, then one tablet for 5 days sid, then ½ tablet administered every other day for 2 weeks, how many tablets should be dispensed?
    a. 15 tablets
    b. 18 tablets
    c. 20 tablets
    d. 11 tablets

28. Fifty mL of a solution of 50% dextrose is added to a liter of 0.45% NaCl with 2.5% dextrose to yield a solution with a final dextrose concentration of what percent?
    a. 3%
    b. 4.8%
    c. 5%
    d. 10%

29. A dog consumes five bowls of water in a 24-hr period. Each bowl contained exactly 100 mL. If you collect 475 mL of urine over the same 24-hr period, approximately how many mL constitute insensible loss?
    a. 475 mL
    b. 500 mL
    c. 25 mL
    d. 5 mL

30. If you measure an animal and set the x-ray machine at 70 kVp and $\frac{1}{60}$ second, and the resulting radiograph is 20% too light, to what setting should the new kVp be increased?
    a. 84
    b. 87
    c. 90
    d. 114

31. Tidal volume for a dog is 15 mL/kg. If a 10-kg male dog is taking 10 breaths/min, what is his minute volume?
    a. 150 mL/min
    b. 1500 mL/min
    c. 15 mL/min
    d. 10 mL/min

32. A 10-kg dog has a diaphragmatic hernia, and his tidal volume is only 10 mL/kg. If this dog were on a ventilator, what should his breathing rate be, when a normal tidal volume is 15 mL/kg and 10 breaths/min?
    a. 15 breaths/min
    b. 5 breaths/min
    c. 8 breaths/min
    d. 100 breaths/min

33. You are asked to administer a drug that is supplied as an enteric-coated tablet at 100 mg, 50 mg, and 25 mg; you require 25 mg but have available 50-mg tablets only. You should:
    a. Use a pill splitter to divide the 100-mg tablet into quarters to obtain the smallest piece
    b. Use a pill splitter to divide the 50-mg tablet into halves to obtain the most accurate dose
    c. Administer the 50-mg tablet but then skip the next scheduled dosing
    d. Order or purchase 25-mg tablets for the dosing schedule

34. An anesthesia machine is set to deliver 1 L/min oxygen and 3% isoflurane. Approximately how many mL of isoflurane gas will be used for a 1-hr procedure?
    a. 30 mL
    b. 180 mL
    c. 2400 mL
    d. 1800 mL

35. A 300-g bird must be tube fed 2 mL liquid formula/100 g body weight three times daily. One gram of powdered formula will yield 15 mL of liquid formula after reconstitution, which is good for 24 hours only. How many mL of reconstituted formula should you measure out for a 24-hr period, assuming no waste?
    a. 0.8
    b. 0.4
    c. 2.5
    d. 1.2

36. A cat with a gastrostomy tube must receive 300 kcal daily. A 15-oz can of the prescribed diet has 1500 kcal. The prescribed diet must be diluted 50:50 with water to flow through the tube, and a maximum of 45 mL can be administered at one feeding. Approximately how many feedings does this cat need daily?
    a. 10
    b. 8
    c. 4
    d. 2

37. If the cat in the previous question requires an additional 160 mL of water daily, how many additional 45-mL boluses of water must be given?
    a. 3.5 mL boluses
    b. 2.5 mL boluses
    c. 1.5 mL boluses
    d. 5.5 mL boluses

38. Five tonometer readings in millimeters of mercury are 14, 15, 19, 14, and 18. What is the average (mean) reading?
    a. 17
    b. 18
    c. 16
    d. 15

39. A patient requires 3 units of insulin every 12 hr. If the concentration of insulin is 100 units/mL, how many mL should be given at each administration?
    a. 0.3 mL
    b. 30 mL
    c. 0.03 mL
    d. 0.15 mL

40. If the concentration of the insulin in the previous question were 30 units/mL, what would the volume of insulin given at each administration be?
    a. 0.1 mL
    b. 10 mL
    c. 0.05 mL
    d. 0.01 mL

41. A diagnostic laboratory requires 1 mL of serum to run a chemistry panel. A bird with a PCV of 50% would need how many full HCT tubes collected to have enough serum for the panel? (Each HCT tube holds 0.1 mL of whole blood.)
    a. 100
    b. 20
    c. 10
    d. 5

42. A 20-kg dog with a PCV of 40% has 300 mL of blood collected. The red blood cells are separated from the serum. What volume of saline would you add to the red cells to make a PCV of 50%?
    a. 360 mL
    b. 240 mL
    c. 180 mL
    d. 120 mL

43. You are taking the heart rate of a cat. If you count 10 beats in 5 seconds, what is the rate in beats/min?
    a. 50
    b. 120
    c. 300
    d. 220

44. Six blood pressure readings are 115, 120, 123, 121, 121, and 112 mm Hg. What is the average (mean) value?
    a. 123
    b. 120
    c. 121
    d. 119

45. A growth in the skin is 2 inches in diameter. What is the diameter of the growth in centimeters?
    a. 2.5 cm
    b. 30 cm
    c. 20 cm
    d. 5 cm

46. The veterinary dermatologist is asking you to prepare a dog for a patch test. Forty antigens need to be tested, and each antigen must be 1 cm from the next. What size patch should you shave on the dog?
    a. 4 cm × 4 cm
    b. 20 cm × 20 cm
    c. 8 cm × 5 cm
    d. 16 cm × 10 cm

47. A 16-oz bottle contains how many mL?
    a. 480 mL
    b. 240 mL
    c. 40 mL
    d. 1.6 mL

48. Four hundred pounds is how many kilograms?
    a. 880 kg
    b. 182 kg
    c. 600 kg
    d. 18 kg

49. A commercial poultry diet contains 18 g of calcium per pound of feed on an as-fed basis. If calcium carbonate, the sole calcium source, is 60% elemental calcium, how much calcium carbonate is in 1 ton of feed?
    a. 21.6 kg
    b. 30 g
    c. 6000 g
    d. 18 kg

50. How many mg are in each mL of a 24% solution?
    a. 24 mg
    b. 2.4 mg
    c. 240 mg
    d. 0.24 mg

51. In a feed that includes 20 lb of corn, 5 lb of beet pulp, 1 lb of bone meal, and 2 lb of whey, approximately what percent is corn?
    a. 98%
    b. 28%
    c. 40%
    d. 71%

52. Approximately how many ounces of bleach diluted with water make 1 gal of a 30% bleach solution (1 qt = 32 oz)?
    a. 19 oz
    b. 38 oz
    c. 3 oz
    d. 76 oz

53. A dose of 30 mEq KCl has been added to 1 L of normal saline. What drip rate would provide a patient with 2 mEq KCl/hr?
    a. 15 mL/hr
    b. 67 mL/hr
    c. 6.7 mL/hr
    d. 60 mL/hr

54. Which of the following is a concentration of a drug solution?
    a. 15 mg/kg
    b. 1000 U/mL
    c. 20 gr/mg
    d. 250 g/lb

55. You have an injectable calcium solution that is 30 mg/mL. How much do you add to 1 L of lactated Ringer solution to deliver 4 mg/hr of calcium at a fluid rate of 30 mL/hr?
    a. 133 mL
    b. 13.3 mL
    c. 4.4 mL
    d. 0.67 mL

56. A 5% dextrose solution is diluted with 100 mL of sterile water. The volume of the sterile water added is 40% of the volume of the 5% dextrose solution. What approximately is the new dextrose concentration?
    a. 1.4%
    b. 2.3%
    c. 3.6%
    d. 6.5%

57. Most pharmaceutical agents that are measured in grains have how many mg/gr?
    a. 32.4
    b. 64.8
    c. 100
    d. 120

58. The volume of an injection for a small iguana is 0.005 mL. This amount is too small to measure accurately. What dilution would allow you to give a volume of 0.05 mL?
    a. 1:10
    b. 1:100
    c. 1:1000
    d. 1:50

59. Ten cockatiels consume a total of approximately 60 mL/day of water. How many mg of tetracycline powder should you add to the daily measured drinking water so that each 100-g bird receives 10 mg/kg/day?
    a. 100 mg
    b. 10 mg
    c. 60 mg
    d. 36 mg

60. The veterinarian asks you to fill 250 mg po bid of metronidazole for 6 days. You have 500-mg tablets in stock. How many tablets will you fill?
    a. 3 tablets
    b. 6 tablets
    c. 12 tablets
    d. 24 tablets

61. You need to deworm 100 head of cattle with a pour-on product that is applied at a rate of 1 mL/100 lb and is sold in 250-mL bottles. The cattle weigh 825 to 1050 lb each. Approximately how many bottles of dewormer should you purchase?
    a. 4 bottles
    b. 8 bottles
    c. 10 bottles
    d. 16 bottles

62. The level of fluid in the 1-L IV bag reads halfway between the 4 and 5 marks. How much fluid remains in the bag?
    a. 1000 mL
    b. 550 mL
    c. 450 mL
    d. 0.5 L

63. The level of fluid in the 1-L IV bag reads at the 700 mark. How much fluid has been administered?
    a. 700 mL
    b. 300 mL
    c. 0.3 L
    d. 300 cc

64. How many pounds does a 10-kg animal weigh?
    a. 2 #
    b. 15 #
    c. 18 #
    d. 22 #

65. How many mg of dextrose does 1 mL of 50% dextrose solution contain?
    a. 5 mg/mL
    b. 50 mg/mL
    c. 500 mg/mL
    d. 5000 mg/mL

66. The doctor orders a patient to receive a CRI of fentanyl. How often will this drug be administered?
    a. Every 2 hr
    b. Every 4 hr
    c. Every 6 hr
    d. At a constant rate

67. The "French" unit is commonly used to express the diameter of a urinary catheter. Each French unit is equivalent to $\frac{1}{3}$ mm. What is the diameter of a 12-French catheter in millimeters?
    a. 3 mm
    b. 4 mm
    c. 18 mm
    d. 36 mm

68. What is the correct volume of epinephrine, in mL, to administer to a 28-lb dog, if the dose is 0.1 mg/kg and the concentration in the bottle is 1:1000 (1 mg/mL)?
    a. 2.8 mL
    b. 1.4 mL
    c. 1.3 mL
    d. 0.28 mL

69. How many mg of epinephrine are administered in the previous calculation?
    a. 0.13 mg
    b. 2.8 mg
    c. 0.41 mg
    d. 1.3 mg

70. How many mg of doxapram (Dopram) should be administered to a 7-lb cat, if the dose range is 1 to 5 mg/kg IV and the concentration in the bottle is 20 mg/mL?
    a. 9.5 mg
    b. 0.59 mg
    c. 21 mg
    d. 0.21 mg

71. How many mL will be administered in the previous calculation?
    a. 1.3 mL
    b. 2.1 mL
    c. 0.95 mL
    d. 0.48 mL

72. How many mL of a 50:50 mixture of diazepam and ketamine at a dose of 1 mL/20 lb should be administered to an 8-lb cat?
    a. 0.4 mL diazepam; 0.4 mL ketamine
    b. 0.2 mL diazepam; 0.2 mL ketamine
    c. 2 mL diazepam; 2 mL ketamine
    d. 1 mL diazepam; 1 mL ketamine

73. The suggested oxygen flow rate for a circle rebreathing system is 25 to 50 mL/kg/min and 130 to 300 mL/kg/min for a nonrebreathing system. What is the most appropriate flow setting for a 10-lb cat?
    a. 0.3 L/min
    b. 900 mL/min
    c. 3 L/min
    d. 0.9 mL/min

74. Using the same suggested oxygen flow rates as in the previous question, what is the most appropriate oxygen flow rate for a 32-lb spaniel?
    a. 8 L
    b. 1.6 L
    c. 435 mL
    d. 0.435 mL

75. You have just administered an injection of 0.02 mL of acepromazine (10 mg/mL). How many mg did you give?
    a. 2 mg
    b. 0.2 mg
    c. 20 mg
    d. 200 mg

76. You have just administered one tablet of 64.8 mg of phenobarbital. How many grains of drug did you deliver?
    a. 0.25 gr
    b. 0.5 gr
    c. 0.6 gr
    d. 1 gr

77. A 0.25 gr (grain) of phenobarbital is how many mg?
    a. 15.2 mg
    b. 14 mg
    c. 16.2 mg
    d. 32.4 mg

78. The doctor asks you to fill oral metronidazole, 10 mg/kg po bid for 7 days. The dog weighs 37.5 kg and you have 250 mg tablets available in the hospital. How many tablets do you fill?
    a. 7 tablets
    b. 14 tablets
    c. 21 tablets
    d. 42 tablets

79. 2% lidocaine is prescribed for a 13-lb beagle at a dose of 2 mg/kg IV. How many mL will you deliver?
    a. 1.6 mL
    b. 0.16 mL
    c. 0.6 mL
    d. 6 mL

80. You just administered 1.2 mL of penicillin (300,000 U/mL). How many units did you administer?
    a. 260,000 u
    b. 360,000 u
    c. 360 u
    d. 0.26 u

81. What unit of measure is most commonly used for serum potassium?
    a. French
    b. mEq
    c. International units
    d. German

82. Your patient is a 42-lb shepherd mix with a history of vomiting. The order reads: metoclopramide HCl (5 mg/mL); give 0.3 mg/kg IM q6h prn. How many mL will you deliver?
    a. 8 mL
    b. 1 mL
    c. 5 mL
    d. 2 mL

83. In the situation described in the previous question, how many mg will you deliver?
    a. 8 mg
    b. 1 mg
    c. 5.7 mg
    d. 2 mg

84. NPH insulin is labeled 100 units/mL. The order is for a 12-lb poodle and reads: NPH insulin 1 unit/kg qd. How many units do you deliver?
    a. 4 u
    b. 3 u
    c. 5.5 u
    d. 6 u

85. How many mL will you draw up to deliver the number of units in the previous question?
    a. 4 mL
    b. 3 mL
    c. 6 mL
    d. 0.05 mL

86. You are preparing an insulin drip. If you add 1 unit of insulin/100 mL of IV fluid, how many units will you add to the 1-L bag of fluids?
    a. 100 u
    b. 1 u
    c. 10 u
    d. 1000 u

87. The insulin drip prepared in the previous question is to be administered at 1 unit/hr. How many mL will this be per hour?
    a. 1 mL
    b. 10 mL
    c. 0.01 mL
    d. 100 mL

88. What would the drip rate be (per second) for 6 units of insulin using the drip prepared in Question 86 (1 unit/100 ml) administered during a 2-hour period using a 60 gtt (drops/ml) administration set?
    a. 1 gtt/sec
    b. 0.5 gtt/sec
    c. 1.5 gtt/sec
    d. 5 gtt/sec

89. A cat in end-stage renal disease is receiving epoetin (2000 units/mL). The dose is 100 units/kg. Your patient weighs 5.5 lb. How many units will you deliver?
    a. 250 u
    b. 25 u
    c. 0.25 u
    d. 100 u

90. How many mL will you draw up to administer 25 units of epoetin (2000 units/mL)?
    a. 2.5 mL
    b. 0.25 mL
    c. 0.01 mL
    d. 0.1 mL

91. Potassium gluconate is administered ¼ tsp/4.5 kg po bid. How many mL will you deliver in 1 day to a 10-lb cat?
    a. 4.5 mL
    b. 2 mL
    c. 0.15 mL
    d. 2.5 mL

92. If the potassium is labeled 5 mEq/5 mL, how many milliequivalents of potassium are delivered in 2 mL?
    a. 2.0 mEq
    b. 0.2 mEq
    c. 20 mEq
    d. 5.5 mEq

93. Chemotherapy medications are dosed by:
    a. mL/kg
    b. cc/lb
    c. Body surface area
    d. mg/mL

94. What is the fluid deficit in mL for a 33-lb dog with 9% dehydration?
    a. 297 mL
    b. 1350 mL
    c. 135 mL
    d. 330 mL

95. To prepare 128 oz of a 1:7 dilution of iodine and alcohol, you would use:
    a. 480 oz iodine, 3360 oz alcohol
    b. 12.8 oz of iodine, 115.2 oz of alcohol
    c. 128 mL of iodine, 896 mL alcohol
    d. 480 mL iodine, 3360 mL alcohol

96. What is the fluid deficit for a 10-lb cat with 12% dehydration?
    a. 120 mL
    b. 60 mL
    c. 545 mL
    d. 1200 mL

97. To prepare 1 cup of instrument milk using the suggested 1:6 dilution ratio, you would use:
    a. 1 oz milk, 6 oz water
    b. 34.3 mL milk, 205.7 mL water
    c. 30 mL milk, 210 mL water
    d. 1 mL milk, 6 mL water

98. You need to deliver 450 mL of 5% glucose. You have on hand a liter of sterile water and a 500-mL bottle of 50% glucose. Which of the following is the correct preparation?
    a. 45 mL of 50% glucose in 405 mL sterile water
    b. 0.45 mL of 50% glucose in 40.5 mL sterile water
    c. 90 mL of 50% glucose in 360 mL of sterile water
    d. 4.5 mL of 50% glucose in 445.5 mL sterile water

99. A 25% solution of sulfamethazine contains how many mg of sulfamethazine per mL?
    a. 2500 mg/mL
    b. 250 mg/mL
    c. 25 mg/mL
    d. 2.5 mg/mL

100. How much sodium chloride is required to produce 5 L of 0.85% saline solution?
    a. 42.5 mg
    b. 4.25 kg
    c. 425 mg
    d. 42.5 g

101. What volume of a 1.2% sodium hydroxide (NaOH) solution can be made from 600 mg of NaOH?
    a. 50 mL
    b. 5 mL
    c. 250 mL
    d. 500 mL

102. What volume of distilled water must be added to a 5-g vial of thiopental sodium to create a 2.5% solution?
    a. 40 mL
    b. 200 mL
    c. 250 mL
    d. 500 mL

103. A stock solution was diluted 1:5, then 1:3, then 1:2, and finally 1:6 to produce a final concentration of 0.4 mg/mL. The original concentration of the stock solution was:
    a. 0.025%
    b. 6.4 mg/mL
    c. 7.2%
    d. 7.2 mg/mL

104. What volume of water must be added to 12.5 mL of a 6% stock solution to produce a 0.5% solution?
    a. 150 mL
    b. 137.5 mL
    c. 37.5 mL
    d. 6.25 mL

105. A 30% stock solution of potassium permanganate (KMnO4) was diluted four times as follows: 0.1 mL of stock was added to 0.4 mL of distilled water; 4.5 mL of distilled water was added; the resulting solution was diluted 1:3; the resulting solution was again diluted to 0.06 L. The final concentration of the solution was:
    a. 1.36%
    b. 50 mg/mL
    c. 5 mg/mL
    d. 0.05%

106. What volume of 4.5% potassium chloride (KCl) solution is needed to prepare 0.75 L of a 9-mg/mL KCl solution?
    a. 15 mL
    b. 375 mL
    c. 1.5 mL
    d. 150 mL

107. The concentration of a culture medium produced by dissolving 2.5 g in 0.4 L of distilled water is:
    a. 0.15%
    b. 0.625%
    c. 0.16%
    d. 6.25%

108. The amount of glucose to be weighed to produce 500 mL of a 4.5% solution is:
    a. 22.5 g
    b. 2.25 g
    c. 0.225 kg
    d. 22.5 mg

109. How many mg of a drug should be administered to a patient who weighs 22 lb if the dose is 0.2 mg/kg?
    a. 2 mg
    b. 4.4 mg
    c. 20 mg
    d. 44 mg

110. A stock solution was diluted four times as follows: 18 mL of distilled water was added to 2 mL of stock; the resulting solution was diluted 1:3; 240 mL of distilled water was added; the resulting solution was diluted to 0.9 L. If the final concentration of the diluted solution was determined to be 100 µg/mL, the original concentration of the stock solution was:
    a. 4.5 mg/mL
    b. 4.5%
    c. 60 mg/mL
    d. 0.21%

111. What volume of sulfuric acid (H2SO4) is in 275 mL of a 12% v/v solution?
    a. 33 mL
    b. 22.9 mL
    c. 3.3 mL
    d. 4.36 mL

112. The concentration of a glucose solution produced when 4500 mg of glucose is dissolved in 3.6 L of water is:
    a. 0.8%
    b. 0.008%
    c. 0.125%
    d. 1.25%

113. How many cubic centimeters are in a tablespoon?
    a. 5 cc
    b. 15 cc
    c. 25 cc
    d. 30 cc

114. The basic unit of mass in the metric system is the:
    a. Kilogram
    b. Gram
    c. Milligram
    d. Microgram

115. The doctor ordered a patient to receive Unasyn, 1200 mg IV. Once reconstituted, the Unasyn has a concentration of 375 mg/mL. How many mL will you administer?
    a. 0.31 mL
    b. 1.2 mL
    c. 3.2 mL
    d. 6.4 mL

116. 50 g is equal to:
    a. 0.005 kg
    b. 0.05 kg
    c. 500,000 mg
    d. 5,000,000 µg

117. The mean cellular hemoglobin (MCH) for a particular blood sample is calculated to be 24.3 pg. This is equal to:
    a. 24,300 mg
    b. 2430 µg
    c. 24.3×10^{12} g
    d. 24.3×10^{-12} g

118. The mean corpuscular volume (MCV) for a particular blood sample is calculated to be 66.5 femtoliter (fl). This is equal to:
    a. 66.5×10^{-15} L
    b. 66.5×10^{15} mL
    c. 66.5×10^{-3} µl
    d. 66.5×10^{-9} L

119. The basic unit of length in the metric system is the:
    a. Millimeter
    b. Centimeter
    c. Meter
    d. Kilometer

120. 485 km is equal to:
    a. 4.85×10^3 m
    b. 485×10^4 mm
    c. 4.85×10^8 mm
    d. 48,500 cm

121. 250 cc is equal to:
    a. 25 mL
    b. 0.25 L
    c. 25,000 µl
    d. 2.5 L

122. One metric ton of livestock feed is equal to:
    a. 1000 lb
    b. 10,000 g
    c. 2200 lb
    d. 1,000,000 mg

123. One centimeter is:
    a. Greater than 1 mm but shorter than 1 µ (1 micron)
    b. Shorter than both 1 m and 1 mm
    c. Greater than both 1 mm and 1 µ
    d. Shorter than 1 km but greater than 1 m

124. A dog weighs 55 lb. Its weight can also be stated as:
    a. 121 kg
    b. 25 g
    c. 121 mg
    d. 25 kg

125. 8 oz is equal to approximately:
    a. 227,200 mg
    b. 454 g
    c. 227 mg
    d. 2.27 kg

126. 10 inches is equal to approximately:
    a. 25 mm
    b. 4 cm
    c. 25 cm
    d. 0.04 m

127. The volume of a stock solution required to prepare 3.5 L of a 1:40 dilution is:
    a. 0.14 L
    b. 87.5 mL
    c. 630 mL
    d. 0.875 L

128. A stock solution of atropine sulfate has a concentration of 2.2 mg/mL. It may also be used clinically as a 0.05% solution. The volume of the more concentrated atropine solution required to prepare 40 mL of the dilute solution is
    a. 17.6 mL
    b. 9.1 mL
    c. 4.4 mL
    d. 0.91 mL

129. The doctor would like to place a patient on a metoclopramide CRI at 2 mg/kg/day. He would like this added to a 1-L bag of fluids that will last 24 hr. The patient weighs 20 kg. How many mL of 5 mg/mL metoclopramide should be added to the bag?
    a. 2 mL
    b. 8 mL
    c. 20 mL
    d. 40 mL

130. The volume of a 1:25 dilution that can be prepared from 150 mL of stock solution is:
    a. 3750 mL
    b. 6 L
    c. 6000 mL
    d. 75 mL

131. If a 0.75% solution results from the addition of 380 mL of water to 20 mL of stock solution, the concentration of the stock solution is:
    a. 15%
    b. 0.375 mg/mL
    c. 14.25%
    d. 300 mg/mL

132. If you are asked to administer 0.1 mg of epinephrine to an animal with threatened cardiac collapse, how much of a 1:10,000 solution should you inject?
    a. 10 mL
    b. 0.01 mL
    c. 0.1 mL
    d. 1 mL

133. When the doctor orders an intravenous infusion, you need three pieces of information to calculate the flow rate in drops per minute. Which of the following is not relevant to this calculation?
    a. Total volume to be infused
    b. Type of fluid to be delivered
    c. Calibration of the administration set being used (in drops/mL)
    d. Duration of the infusion

134. The doctor orders an intravenous infusion to run at 20 mL/hr. Calculate the flow rate using an administration set that delivers 60 drops/mL.
    a. 30 drops/min
    b. 33 drops/min
    c. 20 drops/min
    d. More information is needed

135. Calculate the flow rate for an intravenous infusion of 1 L of fluid to run over 8 hr with a set calibrated at 20 drops/mL.
    a. 20 drops/min
    b. 42 drops/min
    c. 50 drops/min
    d. 125 drops/min

136. Calculating drug dosages involves routine conversion between units of measure within the metric system. Which of the following conversions is not correct?
    a. 3 cc = 3 mL
    b. 1 μg = 1000 mg
    c. 1 kg = 1000 g
    d. 1 L = 1000 mL

137. Which metric conversion is not correct?
    a. 3500 mL = 3.5 L
    b. 520 mg = 0.52 g
    c. 950 μg = 9.5 mg
    d. 750 cc = 0.75 L

138. Which common equivalent is not correct?
    a. 1 tbs = 3 tsp = 15 mL
    b. 1 oz = 30 mL = 2 tbs
    c. ½ gr = 64 mg
    d. 1 L of H2O = 1000 g of H2O

139. Which equivalent is not correct?
    a. 1 tbs = 1 tablespoonful = 15 mL
    b. 1 tsp = 1 teaspoonful = 5 mL
    c. 1 gtt = 1 drop
    d. 1 gr = 1 gram = 30 mL

140. A doctor's order calls for prednisone at a dosage of 2 mg/kg to be delivered orally to a 7.5-kg cat. How many 5-mg tablets of prednisone would you administer to the cat?
    a. ¼ tablet
    b. 1 tablet
    c. 2 tablets
    d. 3 tablets

141. You are asked to give a patient phenobarbital po at 2.2 mg/kg. The medication is available in ½-gr tablets. How many tablets should you give a 35-lb dog?
    a. ¼ tablet
    b. ½ tablet
    c. 1 tablet
    d. 2 tablets

142. A prescription reads "amoxicillin, 750 mg, po bid, 10 days." The drug is available in 500-mg tablets. How many tablets must you count out to fill this prescription?
    a. 30 tablets
    b. 60 tablets
    c. 90 tablets
    d. 120 tablets

143. Diphenhydramine elixir, 25 mg po, is ordered for a 12-year-old, 12.5-kg beagle. The solution contains 12.5 mg/5 mL. What volume should you give to this patient?
    a. 0.5 mL
    b. 2 mL
    c. 10 mL
    d. 20 mL

144. You are asked to give a dog with head trauma 20% mannitol at 0.5 g/kg by slow intravenous injection. You check the record and see that the dog weighs 44 lb. What volume should you give?
    a. 10 mL
    b. 25 mL
    c. 50 mL
    d. 250 mL

145. How much drug does 100 mL of a 10% solution contain?
    a. 0.1 g
    b. 1 g
    c. 10 g
    d. More information is needed

146. You are asked to draw up 2 mL of 50% dextrose in water to give to a hypoglycemic kitten. What volume should you draw into the syringe?
    a. 1 mL
    b. 2 mL
    c. 10 mL
    d. More information is needed

147. To mix a 4% solution in a bottle that contains 5 g of drug powder, how much water should you add?
    a. 12.5 mL
    b. 50 mL
    c. 125 mL
    d. 500 mL

148. To prepare a dose of 0.2 mg of atropine using a solution that contains 400 μg/mL, how much do you draw into the syringe?
    a. 0.05 mL
    b. 0.2 mL
    c. 0.5 mL
    d. 2 mL

149. You are asked to administer intravenously 20 mg of furosemide. The solution contains 25 mg/mL. What volume should you draw into the syringe?
    a. 0.8 mL
    b. 1.25 mL
    c. 2.5 mL
    d. The weight of the patient must be known

150. You are asked to prepare 20 mEq of KCl for addition to a 1-L bag of lactated Ringer solution. The solution contains 30 mEq/15 mL. How much should you draw into a syringe to add to the fluid bag?
    a. 10 mL
    b. 20 mL
    c. 30 mL
    d. 40 mL

151. You are asked to infuse fluids intravenously at 50 mL/hr. The administration set is calibrated at 60 drops/mL. How fast should you set the drip rate?
    a. 1 drop/min
    b. 10 drops/min
    c. 50 drops/min
    d. 60 drops/min

152. You are asked to infuse intravenously 3 L of 0.9% saline during 24 hr. The administration set is calibrated at 15 drops/mL. How fast should you set the drip rate?
    a. 200 drops/min
    b. 125 drops/min
    c. 31 drops/min
    d. 15 drops/min

153. You are asked to infuse fluids intravenously at 60 drops/min. The drip rate is currently at 7 drops/15 sec. What adjustment in the drip rate is necessary?
    a. No adjustment is necessary
    b. Double the flow rate
    c. Reduce the flow rate by 50%
    d. Increase the flow rate by 25%

154. You are asked to infuse intravenously 1 L of fluids at 25 drops/min throughout 10 hr. After 5 hr you observe that 650 mL have been administered. What adjustment in the drip rate is necessary?
    a. No action is necessary; the IV infusion will be completed on schedule
    b. Rate must be slowed from 25 drops/min to 18 drops/min to complete the infusion as ordered
    c. Rate must be increased from 25 drops/min to 32 drops/min to complete the infusion as ordered
    d. Rate must be slowed from 100 mL/hr to 60 mL/hr to complete the infusion as ordered

155. You are asked to infuse intravenously 750 mL of fluids throughout 6 hr. The administration set is calibrated at 20 drops/mL. After 2 hr you observe that 300 mL have been infused. What should the adjusted drip rate be?
    a. 8 drops/min
    b. 19 drops/min
    c. 27 drops/min
    d. 38 drops/min

156. You are asked to infuse intravenously 500 mL of fluids throughout 6 hr. The administration set is calibrated at 20 drops/mL. After 4 hr you observe that only 150 mL have been given. What should the adjusted drip rate be?
    a. 19 drops/min
    b. 25 drops/min
    c. 39 drops/min
    d. 58 drops/min

157. How much 50% dextrose must be added to 1 L of lactated Ringer solution to make a solution that contains 5% dextrose?
    a. 5 mL
    b. 50 mL
    c. 55 mL
    d. 110 mL

158. Diphenhydramine elixir is prescribed at 12.5 mg po q8h. The drug is available in 30-mL bottles that contain 25 mg/5 mL. How long will one bottle last?
    a. 2 days
    b. 4 days
    c. 6 days
    d. 1 week

159. You are asked to prepare a bottle of heparinized saline with a concentration of 4 IU heparin/mL to flush indwelling catheters. The stock sodium heparin solution contains 1000 IU/mL. How much heparin must be added to each 250-mL bottle of sterile physiologic saline (0.9% NaCl) to make the flushing solution?
    a. 1 mL
    b. 2 mL
    c. 3 mL
    d. 4 mL

160. A 1-L sample contains:
    a. 1 mL
    b. 10 mL
    c. 100 mL
    d. 1000 mL

161. A 10-cc syringe can hold:
    a. 1 mL
    b. 10 mL
    c. 100 mL
    d. 1000 mL

162. A 5-kg dog weighs approximately:
    a. 2.5 lb
    b. 5 lb
    c. 7.5 lb
    d. 11 lb

163. A 354-g rat weighs:
    a. 0.0354 kg
    b. 0.354 kg
    c. 3.54 kg
    d. 35.4 kg

164. A 450-μg sample contains:
    a. 4.5 g
    b. 0.45 g
    c. 0.045 g
    d. 0.00045 g

165. A 3700-cc sample contains:
    a. 370 mL
    b. 37 L
    c. 0.37 L
    d. 3.7 L

166. An 11-lb cat weighs approximately:
    a. 22 kg
    b. 5 kg
    c. 500 g
    d. 5000 g

167. A 6.2-g sample contains:
    a. 3 kg
    b. 3100 mg
    c. 6,200,000 μg
    d. 6200 μg

168. A 0.5 g/mL sample contains:
    a. 5 mg/mL
    b. 50 g/100 mL
    c. 5 g/100 mL
    d. 500 mg/100 mL

169. A 500-kg horse weighs approximately:
    a. 250 lb
    b. 750 lb
    c. 1100 lb
    d. 1000 lb

170. A 20-dram vial of digitalis contains approximately:
    a. 1.5 oz
    b. 2 oz
    c. 2.5 oz
    d. 4 oz

171. A 120-gr aspirin contains approximately:
    a. 7.8 mg
    b. 78 mg
    c. 780 mg
    d. 7800 mg

172. A solution of 45 gr/30 mL contains approximately:
    a. 100 mg/mL
    b. 450 mg/mL
    c. 10 g/mL
    d. 1 g/100 mL

173. A 12-fl dram bottle contains approximately:
    a. 36 mL
    b. 45 mL
    c. 68 mL
    d. 120 mL

174. A $\frac{1}{120}$-gr tablet contains approximately:
    a. 0.005 mg
    b. 0.05 mg
    c. 0.5 mg
    d. 5 mg

175. A 2-qt container holds:
    a. 12 oz
    b. 18 oz
    c. 32 oz
    d. 64 oz

176. A 14-oz bottle contains approximately:
 a. 420 mL
 b. 210 mL
 c. 105 mL
 d. 56 mL

177. A 6-tbs dose administered bid requires:
 a. 2 oz/day
 b. 240 mL/day
 c. 1.8 L for a 10-day supply
 d. 2.6 L for a 2-week supply

178. A dosage of 1 tbs daily requires:
 a. 2 oz for a 14-day supply
 b. 5 oz for a 14-day supply
 c. 7 oz for a 14-day supply
 d. 10 oz for a 14-day supply

179. A dosage of 2 tbs bid requires approximately:
 a. 16 oz for a 16-day supply
 b. 1 qt for a 16-day supply
 c. 36 oz for a 16-day supply
 d. 2.5 pt for a 16-day supply

180. A dosage of 1.5 tsp bid requires:
 a. 8 tbs for a 2-week supply
 b. 1 oz for a 2-week supply
 c. 10 tbs for a 2-week supply
 d. 14 tbs for a 2-week supply

181. A dosage of 5 mL tid equals approximately:
 a. 1 tsp/day
 b. 2 tsp/day
 c. 3 tsp/day
 d. 5 tsp/day

182. A dosage of 1 tbs every other day requires approximately:
 a. 45 mL for a 2-week supply
 b. 90 mL for a 2-week supply
 c. 105 mL for a 2-week supply
 d. 210 mL for a 2-week supply

183. A 554-kg mare needs sulfadimethoxine at 10 mg/lb daily. It is available as a 40% solution. How much sulfadimethoxine should be administered daily?
 a. 13.85 mL
 b. 138.5 mL
 c. 45.32 mL
 d. 30.5 mL

184. Fenbendazole liquid is available as a 22.2% concentration, and a 45-lb German shorthaired pointer needs 50 mg/lb. How many teaspoons does it require?
 a. 1 tsp
 b. 1.5 tsp
 c. 2 tsp
 d. 3 tsp

185. Procaine penicillin is available in a concentration of 300,000 IU/mL and is administered at 20,000 IU/kg. How much do you give a 900-lb Arabian gelding?
 a. 2.7 mL
 b. 27 mL
 c. 60 mL
 d. 132 mL

186. Altrenogest for horses is available as a 0.22% solution. The daily dosage is 0.044 mg/kg. If you treated a 990-lb Morgan mare for 15 days, how much would you dispense for the client?
 a. 9 mL
 b. 135 mL
 c. 165 mL
 d. 254 mL

187. A 9-month-old female Great Dane is admitted for a routine ovariohysterectomy. The animal weighs 65 lb, and the veterinarian wants to use the following preanesthetic regimen: butorphanol (10 mg/mL) IM at 0.2 mg/kg; acepromazine (10 mg/mL) IM at 0.05 mg/kg; and atropine (0.02% solution) SC at 0.02 mg/kg. How much butorphanol should be administered?
 a. 0.6 mL
 b. 1.3 mL
 c. 2.9 mL
 d. 6 mL

188. A 9-month-old female Great Dane is admitted for a routine ovariohysterectomy. The animal weighs 65 lb, and the veterinarian wants to use the following preanesthetic regimen: butorphanol (10 mg/mL) IM at 0.2 mg/kg; acepromazine (10 mg/mL) IM at 0.05 mg/kg; and atropine (0.02% solution) SC at 0.02 mg/kg. How much acepromazine should be administered?
 a. 0.15 mL
 b. 0.3 mL
 c. 0.7 mL
 d. 1.5 mL

189. A 9-month-old female Great Dane is admitted for a routine ovariohysterectomy. The animal weighs 65 lb, and the veterinarian wants to use the following preanesthetic regimen: butorphanol (10 mg/mL) IM at 0.2 mg/kg; acepromazine (10 mg/mL) IM at 0.05 mg/kg; and atropine (0.02% solution) SC at 0.02 mg/kg. How much atropine should be administered?
    a. 1.43 mL
    b. 3.0 mL
    c. 6.5 mL
    d. 14.3 mL

190. A yearling paint colt is admitted for castration. The animal weighs 700 lb, and the veterinarian wants to use the following regimen: butorphanol (10 mg/mL) IV at 0.02 mg/kg; xylazine (10 mg/mL) IV at 0.2 mg/kg; and ketamine (100 mg/mL) IV at 2.2 mg/kg. How much butorphanol should be administered?
    a. 0.6 mL
    b. 1.4 mL
    c. 3.1 mL
    d. 6 mL

191. A yearling paint colt is admitted for castration. The animal weighs 700 lb, and the veterinarian wants to use the following regimen: butorphanol (10 mg/mL) IV at 0.02 mg/kg; xylazine (10 mg/mL) IV at 0.2 mg/kg; and ketamine (100 mg/mL) IV at 2.2 mg/kg. How much xylazine should be administered?
    a. 3.2 mL
    b. 6.4 mL
    c. 14 mL
    d. 31 mL

192. A yearling paint colt is admitted for castration. The animal weighs 700 lb, and the veterinarian wants to use the following regimen: butorphanol (10 mg/mL) IV at 0.02 mg/kg; xylazine (10 mg/mL) IV at 0.2 mg/kg; and ketamine (100 mg/mL) IV at 2.2 mg/kg. How much ketamine should be administered?
    a. 2.8 mL
    b. 7.0 mL
    c. 15.4 mL
    d. 34 mL

193. A pet needs 100 mg of a tablet, and the medication is available as a 50-mg tablet. How many tablets will be needed?
    a. 0.5 tablet
    b. 1 tablets
    c. 2 tablets
    d. 4 tablets

194. A pet needs 35 mg of a solution, and the medication is available as a 100-mg/mL solution. How many mL will be needed?
    a. 0.03 mL
    b. 0.35 mL
    c. 3.5 mL
    d. 35 mL

195. A pet needs medication at a dose of 5 mg/kg, and the medication is available in 25-mg tablets. The pet weighs 10 lb. How many tablets will be administered?
    a. 1 tablet
    b. 2 tablets
    c. 5 tablets
    d. 10 tablets

196. A pet needs a medication at a dose of 100 mg/kg, and the medication is available in a 100-mg/mL solution. The pet weighs 25 lb. How many mL will be administered?
    a. 1 mL
    b. 11 mL
    c. 12 mL
    d. 114 mL

197. A pet needs 25 mg of a 2% solution. How many mL will be administered? 2% solution = 20 mg/mL
    a. 25 mL
    b. 20 mL
    c. 1.25 mL
    d. 0.1 mL

198. A pet needs butorphanol for pain at a dose of 0.04 mg/kg and the medication is available in a 10-mg/mL solution. The pet weighs 4 lb. How many mLs will be administered?
    a. 1.8 mL
    b. 0.07 mL
    c. 0.1 mL
    d. 0.01 mL

199. A veterinarian writes a script for 25 mg of acepromazine to be administered every 8 hr for 5 days, and the medication is available in 25-mg tablets. How many tablets will be dispensed?
    a. 3 tablets
    b. 5 tablets
    c. 10 tablets
    d. 15 tablets

200. A pet needs 5 mg/kg of Albon po sid on day 1, then 2.5 mg/kg po sid for 5 more days. The medication is available in 125-mg tablets and the pet weighs 25 lb. How many tablets will be dispensed for the owner?
    a. 0.5 tablets
    b. 1 tablet
    c. 2 tablets
    d. 5 tablets

201. A 22-lb dog needs IV fluids at a maintenance rate of 66 mL/kg/24 hr. How many mL/hr will the patient receive?
    a. 660 mL/hr
    b. 60 mL/hr
    c. 27.5 mL/hr
    d. 2.7 mL/hr

202. A 7-lb cat will have a dental procedure and needs IV fluids at the surgical rate of 11 mL/kg/hr. How many mL/hr will the patient receive?
    a. 1.5 mL/hr
    b. 3 mL/hr
    c. 11 mL/hr
    d. 35 mL/hr

203. A 120-lb dog is experiencing vomiting and diarrhea and must have IV fluids at two times maintenance (132 mL/kg/24 hr). How many mL will he receive per hour?
    a. 132 mL/hr
    b. 54 mL/hr
    c. 300 mL/hr
    d. 400 mL/hr

204. A 32-lb dog needs IV fluids at a surgical rate (11 mL/kg/hr). How many mL/hr will the patient receive?
    a. 32 mL/hr
    b. 15 mL/hr
    c. 100 mL/hr
    d. 160 mL/hr

205. A 50-lb dog needs IV fluids at two times maintenance (132 mL/kg/24 hr). How many fluids will the patient receive in a 24-hour period?
    a. 125 mL
    b. 132 mL
    c. 2200 mL
    d. 3000 mL

206. A 4.5-lb cat requires maintenance fluids (66 mL/kg/24 hr). How many mL/hr will be administered in a 24-hour period?
    a. 5 mL
    b. 28 mL
    c. 132 mL
    d. 300 mL

207. Lidocaine at 2% is prescribed for a 33-lb beagle at a dose of 2 mg/kg IV. How many mL will you deliver?
    a. 1.5 mL
    b. 0.15 mL
    c. 0.5 mL
    d. 5 mL

208. You just administered 3.2 mL of penicillin (300,000 U/mL). How many units did you administer?
    a. 960,000 units
    b. 96,000 units
    c. 960 units
    d. 0.96 units

209. Your patient is a 66-lb shepherd mix with a history of vomiting. The order reads: metoclopramide HCl (5 mg/mL); give 0.6 mg/kg IM q8h prn. How many mL will you deliver?
    a. 5 mL
    b. 1 mL
    c. 0.36 mL
    d. 3.6 mL

210. In the situation in the previous question, how many mg will you deliver?
    a. 18 mg
    b. 8 mg
    c. 1 mg
    d. 3.6 mg

211. Vetsulin insulin is labeled 40 units/mL. The order is for a 12-lb poodle and reads: Vetsulin 2 units/kg qd. How many units do you deliver?
    a. 1 u
    b. 2 u
    c. 8 u
    d. 11 u

212. How many mL will you draw up to deliver the number of units in the previous question?
    a. 0.27 mL
    b. 0.5 mL
    c. 1 mL
    d. 11 mL

213. A cat on intravenous fluids must receive 20 mL/hr normal saline. If this cat has a drip set that provides 60 drops/mL, what should the drip rate be?
    a. 1 drop/2 sec
    b. 1 drop/3 sec
    c. 3 drops/sec
    d. 16 drops/sec

214. The concentration of furosemide is 10%. How many mg's are in 1.2 mL?
    a. 120 mg
    b. 100 mg
    c. 25 mg
    d. 8.3 mg

215. How many mL of a drug with a concentration of 200 mg/mL should be administered to a 60-lb dog at a dose of 3 mg/lb?
    a. 90 mL
    b. 9 mL
    c. 3 mL
    d. 0.9 mL

216. A prescription in which 3 mL of cisapride is administered orally three times daily will require how many ounces to last at least 30 days?
    a. 3 oz
    b. 9 oz
    c. 90 oz
    d. 270 oz

217. A commercial cat food is 120 kcal/cup. A cat weighing 6 lb that is fed at a rate of 40 kcal/lb/day should be fed how many cups at each meal if he is fed twice a day?
    a. 5 cups
    b. 10 cups
    c. 2 cups
    d. 1 cup

218. A cockatiel needs 80 mg/kg piperacillin via intramuscular injection. If the bird weighs 30 g, and the concentration of piperacillin is 100 mg/mL, how many mL should be administered?
    a. 0.03 mL
    b. 0.3 mL
    c. 3 mL
    d. 30 mL

219. A dose of 40 mEq KCl has been added to 1 L of normal saline. What drip rate would provide a patient with 1 mEq KCl/hr?
    a. 2.5 mL/hr
    b. 20 mL/hr
    c. 25 mL/hr
    d. 40 mL/hr

220. You have an injectable calcium solution that is 50 mg/mL. How much do you add to 1 L of lactated Ringer solution to deliver 5 mg/hr of calcium at a fluid rate of 50 mL/hr?
    a. 200 mL
    b. 20 mL
    c. 2 mL
    d. 0.2 mL

221. A 45-kg animal weighs how many pounds?
    a. 2.2
    b. 20
    c. 45
    d. 99

222. How many mg of dextrose does 6 mL of 50% dextrose solution contain?
    a. 3 mg/mL
    b. 30 mg/mL
    c. 300 mg/mL
    d. 3000 mg/mL

ⓔ *Answers and rationales available on Evolve*
http://evolve.elsevier.com/Prendergast/QAvettech/

QUESTIONS

1. What is the correct term for an intact male cat?
   a. Sire
   b. Tom
   c. Dam
   d. Stud

2. Which of the following correctly defines the prefix *poly-*?
   a. Joint
   b. Many
   c. Disease
   d. Cartilage

3. A group of turkeys is referred to as which of the following?
   a. Poult
   b. Rafter
   c. Paddling
   d. Gaggle

4. The study of the cause of disease correctly corresponds to which term?
   a. Etiopathology
   b. Neogenic
   c. Pathology
   d. Idiopathic

5. Which of the following prefixes refers to bone?
   a. *Myelo-*
   b. *Corpo-*
   c. *Osteo-*
   d. *Cerebro-*

6. Which of the following correctly defines kaliopenia?
   a. Presence of an excess amount of sodium in the blood
   b. Presence of an excess amount of potassium
   c. Excretion of an abnormal amount of sodium in the urine
   d. Presence of a less than normal amount of potassium

7. A group of cats is also referred to as:
   a. Clowder
   b. Cluster
   c. Pounce
   d. All of the above

8. An atypical heart sound associated with a functional or structural valve abnormality is known as:
   a. Arrhythmia
   b. Fibrillation
   c. Murmur
   d. Infarct

9. A whelp is referred to as which of the following?
   a. An intact female dog
   b. A young feline
   c. A young canine
   d. The male parent of his offspring

10. The prefix *myring-* refers to which of the following?
    a. Ear
    b. Eardrum
    c. Embryo
    d. Empty

11. What is the correct term for an intact male horse older than 4 years?
    a. Gelding
    b. Mare
    c. Colt
    d. Stallion

12. An equine that is about to turn one year old is referred to as a:
    a. Yearling
    b. Foaling
    c. Weanling
    d. Filly

13. A male donkey that has not been castrated and is capable of breeding is referred to as a:
    a. Jenny
    b. Dam
    c. Jack
    d. Sire

14. A female calf (usually sterile) born twin to a bull calf is referred to as a:
    a. Freshening
    b. Freemartin
    c. Heifer
    d. Cow

15. Which of the following definitions correctly defines the term *wether*?
    a. An intact male sheep
    b. A young ovine
    c. The process of giving birth to lambs
    d. A castrated/neutered male ovine

16. The process of giving birth to pigs is referred to as:
    a. Stag
    b. Freshening
    c. Farrowing
    d. Kidding

17. A young female pig that has not yet given birth is referred to as:
    a. Dam
    b. Gilt
    c. Sow
    d. Stag

18. A young male chicken between 10 and 32 weeks of age is referred to as:
    a. Rooster
    b. Cockerel
    c. Capon
    d. Pullet

19. An egg-type chicken more than 32 weeks of age is referred to as a:
    a. Roaster
    b. Layer
    c. Hen
    d. Chick

20. Which of the following correctly defines the term *drake*?
    a. An intact male duck
    b. An intact female duck
    c. An immature duck of either sex
    d. A young turkey

21. An intact male ferret is known as a:
    a. Gib
    b. Jill
    c. Sprite
    d. Hob

22. The prefix *blephar-* refers to which of the following?
    a. Eye
    b. Eyelid
    c. False
    d. Fat

23. A disease that is transmitted from animals to humans is defined as:
    a. Zoology
    b. Zoonotic
    c. Enzootic
    d. Epizootic

24. The number of animals within a population that become sick can be defined as:
    a. Morbidity
    b. Mortality
    c. Chronic
    d. Acute

25. The suffix *-itis* refers to:
    a. Disease
    b. Inflammation
    c. False
    d. Bone

26. *Chondro-* refers to what structure?
    a. Bone
    b. Many
    c. Cartilage
    d. Inflammation

27. The prefix *hyster-* refers to which of the following?
    a. Oviduct
    b. Uterus
    c. Ovary
    d. Surgical removal

28. The suffix *-ac* refers to which of the following?
    a. Pertaining to
    b. Condition
    c. Structure
    d. To act on

29. Which of the following terms means *within a living body*?
    a. Benign
    b. In vivo
    c. Infection
    d. In vitro

30. Becoming progressively worse, recurring, and/or leading to death refers to:
    a. Remission
    b. Malignant
    c. Exacerbation
    d. Idiopathic

31. Chondrology correctly corresponds with which definition?
    a. The study of cartilage
    b. The study of malignancy
    c. The study of the cardiovascular system
    d. The study of bones

32. Neoplasm refers to which of the following?
    a. The process of abnormal or difficult growth
    b. A malignant growth of tissue
    c. Any new and abnormal growth
    d. Death of tissue

33. What is the correct term for the resting phase of a heartbeat that occurs between filling of the lower chamber of the heart and the start of contraction?
    a. Diastole
    b. Systole
    c. Arrhythmia
    d. Tachycardia

34. Which of the following terms correctly corresponds with the phrase *toward the median plane*?
    a. Medial
    b. Lateral
    c. Anterior
    d. Posterior

35. The term *rostral* refers to which of the following definitions?
    a. Toward the head end of the body
    b. Toward the nose when referring to the head
    c. Toward the tail end of the body
    d. Posterior surface of the body

36. The transverse plane correctly divides the body into which parts?
    a. Anterior/posterior
    b. Cranial/caudal
    c. Left/right
    d. Transverse refers to a position on a limb closer to the point of attachment

37. A collection of blood in the cranial portion of the ventral cavity is known as:
    a. Pneumothorax
    b. Pneumonia
    c. Hematothorax
    d. Hemostasis

38. An abnormal presence of tissue cells in the blood is known as:
    a. Histology
    b. Histiocytosis
    c. Karyogenic
    d. Homeostasis

39. The term *myodysplasia* refers to which of the following?
    a. A specialized cell for the storage of fat
    b. An abnormal growth of tissue
    c. An abnormal development of muscles
    d. Slower than normal heartbeat

40. The term *abrasion* refers to which of the following descriptions?
    a. A localized collection of pus
    b. A group of furuncles in adjacent hairs
    c. Loss of hair, wool, or feathers
    d. A skin scrape

41. Blood leaking from a ruptured vessel into subcutaneous tissue is known as:
    a. Cicatrix
    b. Ecchymosis
    c. Eschar
    d. Fissure

42. The term *excoriate* refers to:
    a. Scratching the skin
    b. A boil or skin abscess
    c. Dried serum, blood, or pus
    d. A scar

43. An overgrowth of scar tissue at the site of injury is known as:
    a. Papule
    b. Petechia
    c. Laceration
    d. Keloid

44. A circumscribed craterlike lesion of the skin or mucous membrane is known as:
    a. Wheal
    b. Suppurate
    c. Ulcer
    d. Papule

45. Which of the following suffixes refers to a blood condition that is usually abnormal?
    a. *-staxis*
    b. *-emia*
    c. *-clast*
    d. *-pnea*

46. A bridge that forms as part of the healing process across the two halves of a bone fracture is known as a:
    a. Condyle
    b. Callus
    c. Crest
    d. Cull

47. What term is defined as a joint dislocation when the joint is displaced or goes out of alignment?
    a. Fracture
    b. Luxation
    c. Olecranon
    d. Subluxation

48. A rough projection on a bone is known as a:
    a. Suture
    b. Wing
    c. Tuberosity
    d. Trochanter

49. Osteomalacia is known as the:
    a. Hardening of bones
    b. Softening of bones
    c. Collection of abnormal cells that accumulate within the bones
    d. Thickened skin

50. Which term is defined as the incomplete development or underdevelopment of an organ or tissue?
    a. Osteoporosis
    b. Hypoplasia
    c. Hyperplasia
    d. Ankylosis

51. A small opening or perforation is referred to as which of the following?
    a. Fossa
    b. Foramen
    c. Exacerbation
    d. Process

52. What structure connects muscles to bones?
    a. Ligaments
    b. Tendons
    c. Foramen
    d. Process

53. Which of the following provides a smooth joint surface, allowing the bones to move freely over one another?
    a. Cartilage
    b. Ligaments
    c. Callus
    d. Fossa

54. The prefix *chondro-* refers to which of the following?
    a. Bone
    b. Muscle
    c. Cartilage
    d. Cheek

55. A rare benign tumor derived from striated muscle is known as:
    a. Cervicomuscular
    b. Rhabdomyoma
    c. Myopathology
    d. Rhabdomyosarcoma

56. Myofibrosis is correctly defined as which of the following?
    a. Spasm of the muscle
    b. Abnormal condition of muscle fibers
    c. A disorder in which muscles are slow to relax
    d. A technique used for evaluating and recording the electrical activity produced by skeletal muscles

57. A connective tissue membrane that surrounds each muscle fiber is referred to as:
    a. Epimysium
    b. Endomysium
    c. Myopathy
    d. Sarcoma

58. The prefix *cephal-* refers to which of the following?
    a. Hard
    b. Head
    c. Hearing
    d. Heart

59. Skeletal muscle is also known as:
    a. Striated muscle
    b. Smooth muscle
    c. Cardiac muscle
    d. None of these

60. The term *ipsilateral* refers to which of the following?
    a. Opposite side affected
    b. Located on or affecting the same side of the body
    c. Near or connected to the maxilla or jawbone
    d. Movement away from the point of origin

61. Pain affecting half of the body is known as which of the following?
    a. Semiconscious
    b. Hemialgia
    c. Analgesia
    d. Bicaudal

62. The presence of four digits on one foot is known as:
    a. Tetradactyly
    b. Polydactyl
    c. Multiarticular
    d. Quadrilateral

63. Inflammation of all bones or inflammation of every part of one bone is known as:
    a. Panosteitis
    b. Polypathia
    c. Pandemic
    d. Osteoporosis

64. The word root *digitorum* refers to which of the following?
    a. Rib
    b. Wrist
    c. Digit
    d. Thigh

65. The word root *brachii* refers to which of the following?
    a. Shin bone
    b. Thigh
    c. Upper foreleg
    d. Shoulder blade

66. Which type of muscle attaches the limb to the body?
    a. Intrinsic muscles
    b. Extrinsic muscles
    c. Adductor muscles
    d. Abductor muscles

67. The term *amyoplasia* refers to the:
    a. Lack of muscle formation or development
    b. Paralysis of muscles
    c. Muscular weakness or partial paralysis restricted to one side of the body
    d. Any disease of a muscle

68. _____ is known as the destruction of the rod-shaped muscle cells?
    a. Hypertrophy
    b. Rhabdomyolysis
    c. Hypoplasia
    d. Necrosis

69. The term *aponeurosis* refers to which of the following definitions?
    a. An acute tendon injury in which the tendon is forcibly torn away from its attachment side on the bone
    b. Temporary muscular stiffening that follows death
    c. Rapid involuntary muscle contractions that release waste heat
    d. Sheetlike dense fibrous collagenous connective tissue that binds muscles together or connects muscle to bone

70. The prefix *onych-* refers to which of the following?
    a. Claw, nail
    b. Cell
    c. Clotting process
    d. Cornea

71. Clonic spasm refers to:
    a. An acute involuntary muscle contraction
    b. A continuous spasm
    c. Alternating spasm and muscle relaxation
    d. Painful, sustained muscle contractions caused by toxins

72. The term *atrophy* refers to:
    a. All four limbs
    b. Wasting away
    c. Muscle stretch
    d. Inflammation of muscles

73. The term *tetraparesis* refers to the:
    a. Muscular weakness in all four limbs
    b. Inflammation of nerves
    c. Inflammation of many muscles
    d. A continuous spasm

74. The suffix *-rrhage* refers to which of the following?
    a. Expansion, dilation
    b. Excessive flow
    c. Sensation
    d. Flow, flowing

75. The term *acardia* refers to which of the following?
    a. Disease affecting the muscles of the heart
    b. Excessive growth of the auricles
    c. Absence of the heart
    d. Pertaining to the heart and to the blood vessels

76. Which of the following terms pertains to the upper and lower chambers of the heart?
    a. Atriotomy
    b. Atrioventricular
    c. Valvulosis
    d. Avascular necrosis

77. Hydremia refers to which of the following?
    a. Inadequate supply of blood to a part of the body
    b. Disorder in which there is an excess of fluid in the blood
    c. Low red blood cell count
    d. The narrow pointed bottom of the heart

78. The prefix *eu-* refers to which of the following?
    a. Glucose
    b. Gland
    c. Good
    d. Hair

79. The demarcation line that separates the left and right ventricles of the heart is termed as an:
    a. Interventricular septum
    b. Atrium
    c. Interventricular groove
    d. Auricle

80. Which vessel carries blood to the lungs?
    a. Aorta
    b. Inferior vena cava
    c. Pulmonary artery
    d. Carotid artery

81. The inside surface of the chamber of the heart is lined by a thin membrane known as the:
    a. Pericardium
    b. Endocardium
    c. Atrium
    d. Epicardium

82. The bicuspid valve is also known as the _____ valve.
    a. Tricuspid
    b. Semilunar
    c. Mitral
    d. Atrioventricular

83. Which of the following suffixes refers to crushing or grinding?
    a. *-tripsy*
    b. *-lytic*
    c. *-osis*
    d. *-pathy*

84. A benign tumor that is composed of newly formed blood vessels is known as:
    a. Hemangioma
    b. Hamartoma
    c. Hepatoma
    d. Hepatocellular carcinoma

85. The rupture of an artery is known as:
    a. Hemorrhage
    b. Arteriorrhexis
    c. Arteriostasis
    d. Venostasis

86. Which of the following is the largest artery in an animal's body?
    a. Carotid artery
    b. Pulmonary artery
    c. Aorta
    d. Inferior vena cava

87. The prefix *ultra-* refers to which of the following definitions?
    a. Beyond, excess
    b. Below, decrease
    c. Black
    d. Back surface of rear limb

88. The term *bradycardia* refers to:
    a. A slower than normal heart rate
    b. An abnormally rapid heart rate
    c. An irregular heart rate
    d. Narrowing of the arteries

89. Enlargement of the heart is termed:
    a. Agnathia
    b. Cardiomegaly
    c. Dactyledema
    d. Pericarditis

90. The accumulation of fluid in the abdominal cavity is defined as:
    a. Auscultate
    b. Infarct
    c. Ascites
    d. Edema

91. What is the term for the inflammation of a vein?
    a. Arteritis
    b. Stenosis
    c. Phlebitis
    d. Venostasis

92. An increase in arterial blood pressure is defined as:
    a. Hypertension
    b. Hypotension
    c. Edema
    d. Pleural effusion

93. Pericardiocentesis refers to which of the following definitions?
    a. Abnormal buildup of fluid within a space
    b. Buildup of fluid between the layer of the pericardial sac and the epicardium
    c. When the pericardial sac is full of fluid that the heart can no longer beat
    d. The removal of fluid via a needle inserted into the pericardial sac

94. The suffix -ptosis refers to which of the following?
    a. To act on
    b. Downward placement
    c. Enzyme
    d. Engage in a specific activity

95. _____ is defined as the extensive loss of blood resulting from bleeding.
    a. Hematology
    b. Exsanguination
    c. Electrohemostasis
    d. Anemia

96. An abnormal new growth of plasma cells is known as:
    a. Plasmacytoma
    b. Plasmocyte
    c. Serosanguineous
    d. Polycythemia

97. Karyoclastic refers to which of the following definitions?
    a. The rupture of a nucleus
    b. A cell that breaks down cartilage
    c. The breaking up of a cell nucleus
    d. The condition of many cells in the blood

98. _____ refers to redness of the skin.
    a. Erythrocyte
    b. Erythematous
    c. Leukocyte
    d. Leukocytosis

99. Which of the following prefixes refers to the chest?
    a. Baso-
    b. Chyl-
    c. Col-
    d. Steth-

100. A blood cell that has both pale red and blue granules visible in the cytoplasm is known as a/an:
    a. Basophil
    b. Neutrophil
    c. Eosinophil
    d. Agranulocyte

101. Inflammation of the lymph vessels is known as:
    a. Leukocytosis
    b. Lymphangitis
    c. Lymphoma
    d. Immunocyte

102. Difficulty in eating or swallowing is termed:
    a. Dysphagia
    b. Dystocia
    c. Dysraphism
    d. Aphagia

103. _____ is a primitive blood cell.
    a. Hematopoiesis
    b. Hematoblast
    c. Hemoglobin
    d. Hemolysis

104. An abnormally low white blood cell count is referred to as:
    a. Normocytic
    b. Leukocytosis
    c. Leukopenia
    d. Anemia

105. The term idiopathic refers to:
    a. A general term for an abnormality
    b. A disease that has an unknown cause
    c. An uncoordinated and dehydrated patient
    d. A blood clot that forms and adheres to the wall of a blood vessel

106. The prefix cox- refers to which of the following?
    a. Heat
    b. Hip
    c. Hernia
    d. Humerus

107. The increased destruction of RBCs within the vascular system is known as:
    a. Macrocytic anemia
    b. Hemolytic anemia
    c. Polychromasia
    d. Hypochromic anemia

108. An abnormally low number of neutrophils refers to:
    a. Pancytopenia
    b. Neutropenia
    c. Monocytosis
    d. Eosinophilia

109. The measure of the percent of red blood cells in a volume of blood is known as:
    a. Hematocrit
    b. Packed cell volume
    c. Total protein
    d. Both a and b

110. Hematopoiesis is defined as:
    a. The formation of blood cells in the body
    b. An abnormally low number of neutrophils in the blood
    c. A high number of white blood cells
    d. Resembling a white blood cell

111. The destruction of a blood clot is known as:
    a. Exsanguination
    b. Monocyte
    c. Thrombolysis
    d. Leukemia

112. Which of the following defines neutropenia?
    a. An abnormal condition of too many white blood cells
    b. The formation of blood cells in the body
    c. An abnormally low number of neutrophils in the blood
    d. An abnormal increase in the number of platelets

113. An increased amount of carbon dioxide in the blood refers to:
    a. Olfaction
    b. Hypercapnia
    c. Hyperemia
    d. Hypoxia

114. The term *apnea* refers to which of the following?
    a. Absence of breathing
    b. A collection of air in the chest from a wound or tear in the lung
    c. Surgical puncture of the lung
    d. The abnormal development of the air sacs of the lung

115. The last breath taken near or at death is referred to as:
    a. Emphysema
    b. Agonal breathing
    c. Asthma
    d. Furcation

116. _____ is defined as a nosebleed.
    a. Cardiectasis
    b. Epistaxis
    c. Atelectasis
    d. Tussiculation

117. A lack of digestion is referred to as which of the following?
    a. Bradypeptic
    b. Apepsia
    c. Monogastric
    d. Anastomosis

118. A pathological softening of any of the structures of the mouth is known as:
    a. Hyperphagia
    b. Polydipsia
    c. Cheilophagia
    d. Stomatomalacia

119. The term *buccal* refers to which of the following?
    a. Pertaining to toward the side of the mouth or cheek
    b. Oriented toward the tongue
    c. Toward the nose
    d. Away from midline

120. The act of spitting up blood is known as:
    a. Esophagoplegia
    b. Hemoptysis
    c. Xerostomia
    d. Hypoptyalism

121. A surgical fixation of the stomach of a ruminant to the body wall is referred to as which of the following?
    a. Gastropexy
    b. Abomasopexy
    c. Omasal stenosis
    d. Laparosplenotomy

122. An infection of the common bile duct is known as:
    a. Hepatitis
    b. Pancreatitis
    c. Cholangitis
    d. Cholecystitis

123. A generalized wasting of the body as a result of disease is known as:
    a. Eructation
    b. Anemia
    c. Necrosis
    d. Cachexia

124. The term *melena* refers to which of the following?
    a. Passing of dark, tarry feces containing blood that has been acted on by bacteria in the intestines
    b. A semifluid mass of partially digested food that enters the small intestine from the stomach
    c. A protein produced by living cells that initiates a chemical reaction but is not affected by the reaction
    d. To fall back into a disease state after an apparent recovery

125. A progressive wave of contraction and relaxation of the smooth muscles in the wall of the digestive tract that moves food through the digestive tract is known as:
    a. Ingesta
    b. Rumination
    c. Retrograde
    d. Peristalsis

126. Which of the following definitions correctly describes incisor teeth?
    a. Teeth that are used for tearing food
    b. The most rostral teeth that are used for grasping food
    c. The most caudal teeth in the mouth that are used for grinding food
    d. Baby teeth or temporary teeth

127. A large amount of fat in the feces is known as which of the following?
    a. Lipase
    b. Steatorrhea
    c. Lipolysis
    d. Malodorous

128. The pathological condition that results from a stone is referred to as:
    a. Enteroptosis
    b. Lithiasis
    c. Lipolysis
    d. Lithogenesis

129. Tube feeding through a stomach tube is known as which of the following terms?
    a. Emesis
    b. Gavage
    c. Emetic
    d. Enema

130. Slipping or telescoping of one part of a tubular organ into a lower portion, causing the type of obstruction typically seen in the intestines, is known as what?
    a. Impaction
    b. Nosocomial
    c. Intussusception
    d. Ileus

131. Which of the following refers to an overdistention of the reticulorumen as a result of rumen gas being trapped in the rumen when the ruminant is unable to eructate?
    a. Ruminal tympany
    b. Retch
    c. Volvulus
    d. Torsion

132. Total parenteral nutrition is correctly defined as which of the following?
    a. No food or water given
    b. Nutrition must be administered by means other than the mouth
    c. Specialized diet for a certain disease process
    d. Giving as much food as you have to for the desired result

133. Hair loss is referred to as which of the following?
    a. Abrasion
    b. Alopecia
    c. Proud flesh
    d. Aphagia

134. The destruction of skeletal muscle is referred to as which of the following?
    a. Papule
    b. Osteochondritis
    c. Rhabdomyolysis
    d. Pneumothorax

135. A disease of the nerves is known as:
    a. Neuropathy
    b. Enchondroma
    c. Neuromyelitis
    d. Poliomyelitis

136. The prefix *sarc-* refers to which of the following?
    a. Flesh
    b. Femur
    c. Flank
    d. First

137. The wasting away of the brain tissue is referred to as which of the following?
    a. Meningocele
    b. Cerebroatrophy
    c. Necrosis
    d. Neuromyelitis

138. A head that is abnormally small or thin is referred to as which of the following?
    a. Ataxia
    b. Arachnoid
    c. Leptocephaly
    d. Hydrocephalus

139. The term *aberrant* refers to which of the following?
    a. To carry to or bring toward a place
    b. Abnormal, deviating from the usual or ordinary
    c. To carry out or take away from a place
    d. An abnormal convex curvature of the spine

140. The _____ is the second largest portion of the brain.
    a. Corpus callosum
    b. Cortex
    c. Cerebrum
    d. Cerebellum

141. A *syrinx* refers to which of the following?
    a. The part of the brain that relays sensory impulses to the cerebral cortex
    b. A pathological tube-shaped lesion in the brain or spinal cord
    c. The junction across which a nerve impulse passes from an axon to another neuron, to a muscle cell, or to a gland cell
    d. The space or cavity that can exist between two adjacent body parts that are not tightly adjoined

142. _____ are short, fine-branching fibers that extend from the cell body.
    a. Dendrites
    b. Perikarya
    c. Axons
    d. Microglial cells

143. A protein manufactured by the liver that maintains the osmotic fluid balance between capillaries and tissues is referred to as which of the following?
    a. Aldosterone
    b. Albumin
    c. Alkaline
    d. Acetylcholine

144. The recognition by the nervous system of an injury or painful stimulus is known as:
    a. Nociperception
    b. Proprioception
    c. Anesthesia
    d. Visceral sensation

145. A painful response to a normally nonpainful stimulus is defined as:
    a. Allodynia
    b. Proprioception
    c. Nociperception
    d. Tactile agnosis

146. Normal digestion is described by the term:
    a. Rhinitis
    b. Eupepsia
    c. Malodorous
    d. Anosmia

147. The surgical removal of the eardrum is:
    a. Splenectomy
    b. Cholecystectomy
    c. Nephrectomy
    d. Myringectomy

148. Pertaining to the eyes and the skin is referred to as which of the following?
    a. Ophthalmology
    b. Oculocutaneous
    c. Audiology
    d. Blepharospasm

149. Palpebration is defined as:
    a. An abnormal contraction of the eyelid
    b. The method of feeling with fingers or hands during the physical examination
    c. Inflammation of the cornea
    d. Flow of tears mixed with pus

150. An abnormal dilation of the pupil of the eye is defined as:
    a. Iridocele
    b. Keratitis
    c. Corneitis
    d. Corectasis

151. An inflammation affecting both the optic nerve and the retina is known as:
    a. Neuroretinitis
    b. Conjunctivitis
    c. Cholecystitis
    d. Hepatitis

152. Prolonged constriction of the pupil of the eye is referred to as which of the following?
    a. Mydriasis
    b. Iridocele
    c. Miosis
    d. Canthus

153. Which of the following statements correctly describes a pheromone?
    a. A nerve ending that responds to a stimulus, found in the internal or external environment of an animal
    b. An animal that is active at night
    c. A surrounding substance in which something else is contained
    d. A liquid substance released in small quantities by an animal, which causes a specific response if it is detected by another animal of the same species

154. An ear flap is also known as a:
    a. Pinna
    b. Papilla
    c. Callus
    d. Canthus

155. _____ is defined as pertaining to the study of cells.
    a. Cytology
    b. Morphology
    c. Zoology
    d. Oncology

156. Difficult or labored breathing is also known as:
    a. Epistaxis
    b. Lysis
    c. Leukopenic
    d. Dyspnea

157. The blood cells that carry oxygen to body cells are known as:
    a. White blood cells
    b. Red blood cells
    c. Neutrophils
    d. Eosinophils

158. A stone found in the stomach is a:
    a. Hepatolith
    b. Cholelith
    c. Coprolith
    d. Gastrolith

159. A stone found within the artery is referred to as which of the following?
    a. Arteriolith
    b. Cardiolith
    c. Hysterolith
    d. Broncholith

160. A surgical puncture of the vagina is referred to as which of the following?
    a. Vaginodynia
    b. Colpocentesis
    c. Paracentesis
    d. Cystocentesis

161. Crushing of a stone into fragments that may pass through natural channels is known as:
    a. Lithogenesis
    b. Lithologist
    c. Lithiasis
    d. Lithoclasty

162. Which of the following terms describes a substance produced by one tissue or by one group of cells that is carried by the bloodstream to another tissue or organ to affect its physiological functions such as metabolism or growth?
    a. Hormone
    b. Endorphin
    c. Protein
    d. Enzyme

163. The disease of a gland is referred to as:
    a. Amyotrophy
    b. Adenopathy
    c. Adrenomegaly
    d. Cardiomyopathy

164. The surgical removal of the thyroid gland is a(n):
    a. Splenectomy
    b. Oophorectomy
    c. Thyroidectomy
    d. Cholecystectomy

165. Which of the following hormones is responsible for testosterone production in males and estrogen production and ovulation in females?
    a. Prolactin
    b. Thyroid-stimulating hormone
    c. Follicle-stimulating hormone
    d. Luteinizing hormone

166. A nephroblastoma refers to which of the following?
    a. A record made of the kidney, such as an x-ray
    b. A rapidly developing tumor the of the kidney that is most often malignant
    c. A tumor of the soft tissue usually found in the muscle
    d. A tumor found within the liver

167. The term *uremia* is defined as:
    a. Painful urination
    b. Surgical repair of the kidney pelvis
    c. Urine constituents that are found in the blood
    d. Blood found in the urine

168. Pain felt in the ureter is termed:
    a. Cystitis
    b. Ureteralgia
    c. Dysuria
    d. Menorrhagia

169. Crushing of a stone is referred to as which of the following terms?
    a. Lithogenesis
    b. Lithotripsy
    c. Lithiasis
    d. Lithology

170. The downward displacement of the kidney is referred to as which of the following terms?
     a. Nephrectomy
     b. Nephroptosis
     c. Nephrostomy
     d. Nephrology

171. A concretion is correctly described as:
     a. A solid or calcified mass formed by disease found in a body cavity or tissue
     b. A stone
     c. A chemical element that carries an electrical charge when dissolved in water
     d. The functional tissue of an organ

172. The act or urination is referred to as:
     a. Micturition
     b. Concretion
     c. Voiding
     d. Both a and c

173. The term *denude* refers to which of the following?
     a. The process in the kidney whereby blood pressure forces material through a filter
     b. A tube for injecting or removing fluids
     c. The loss of epidermis, caused by exposure to urine, feces, body fluids, drainage, or friction
     d. The end product of muscle metabolism; waste product excreted in urine

174. Painful urination as a result of muscle spasms in the urinary bladder and urethra is referred to as:
     a. Dysuria
     b. Stranguria
     c. Urea
     d. Slough

175. The lack of voluntary urination or defecation is referred to as:
     a. Urolithiasis
     b. Uremia
     c. Incontinence
     d. Anuria

176. The term *azotemia* refers to:
     a. The presence of urinary calculi
     b. The lack of voluntary urination
     c. The increased production of urine
     d. The buildup of nitrogenous waste material in the blood

177. The excess dilution of urine is defined as:
     a. Oliguresis
     b. Albuminuria
     c. Hydruria
     d. Hydrocephalus

178. A higher than normal blood level of nitrogen-containing compounds in the blood is described as:
     a. Bilirubinuria
     b. Azotemia
     c. Hydruria
     d. Natriuresis

179. When the amount of glycogen in the liver is depleted, it is known as:
     a. Hypoglycemia
     b. Hyperglycemia
     c. Ketosis
     d. Sepsis

180. A diseased condition of pus within the ureter is defined as:
     a. Ureteropyosis
     b. Bacterium
     c. Ketonuria
     d. Pyometra

181. Nephrolithotomy refers to the:
     a. Surgical removal of the gallbladder
     b. Surgical incision into the kidney to remove a stone
     c. Surgical removal of a kidney
     d. Surgical removal of spleen

182. A cystocentesis refers to the:
     a. Microscopic examination of a urine sample
     b. Collection of urine directly from the bladder through a surgical puncture
     c. Surgical incision into the bladder
     d. Removal of free fluid from the abdominal cavity

183. Hypokalemia is defined as:
     a. High sodium level
     b. Low sodium level
     c. High potassium level
     d. Low potassium level

184. _____ is the surgical removal of testicles.
     a. Orchectomy
     b. Oophorectomy
     c. Cryptorchidism
     d. Hysterectomy

185. *Spermaturia* refers to which of the following?
     a. Pertaining to sperm
     b. The presence of sperm in the urine
     c. Presence of blood in the urine
     d. Painful urination

186. The surgical removal of the penis is:
     a. Castration
     b. Penectomy
     c. Hysterectomy
     d. Oophorectomy

187. Inflammation of the penis is referred to as a:
  a. Priapitis
  b. Megalopenis
  c. Micropenis
  d. Hypospadias

188. Phimosis is defined as a/an:
  a. Persistent erection of the penis
  b. Idiopathic protrusion of the nonerect penis with the inability to retract it
  c. Inability to extend the penis
  d. Hypertrophy of the penis

189. _____ is defined as the release of an egg from the ovary.
  a. Ovum
  b. Ovulation
  c. Oocyte
  d. Paraphimosis

190. Which of the following terms correlates with bleeding from the ovary?
  a. Ovariectomy
  b. Oophorrhagia
  c. Menorrhagia
  d. Vaginodynia

191. Inflammation of the vulva is referred to as which of the following?
  a. Vulvitis
  b. Cystitis
  c. Vaginitis
  d. Pyometra

192. The term *corpus* refers to the:
  a. Horn
  b. Flared end of a funnel-shaped duct
  c. Body
  d. A sensitive female external organ homologous to the penis

193. The _____ is described as a fringelike structure found in the infundibulum.
  a. Caruncle
  b. Fimbria
  c. Oviduct
  d. Follicle

194. The prefix *hetero-* refers to which of the following?
  a. Digestion
  b. Digit
  c. Different
  d. Disease

195. The surgical removal of an animal in the early stages of development in the womb is known as:
  a. Hysterectomy
  b. Oophorectomy
  c. Embryectomy
  d. Penectomy

196. A false pregnancy is known as:
  a. Primigravida
  b. Pseudocyesis
  c. Pseudoaneurysm
  d. Uniparous

197. The term *bipara* refers to what?
  a. The period of time just after the birth of offspring
  b. A false pregnancy
  c. A female that has given birth twice in two separate pregnancies
  d. A female that has never given birth

198. Which term refers to the capability of producing offspring?
  a. Fetus
  b. Natal
  c. Perineum
  d. Fecund

199. A vascular membranous organ in the womb between a mother and her offspring is known as the:
  a. Fecund
  b. Perineum
  c. Placenta
  d. Umbilical cord

200. The injection of semen into the vagina or uterus by the use of syringe is termed:
  a. Copulation
  b. In vitro fertilization
  c. In vivo fertilization
  d. Artificial insemination

201. Which of the following refers to a species that has two estrous cycles per year?
  a. Monestrous
  b. Polyestrous
  c. Diestrous
  d. Anestrous

202. An abnormally slow or difficult birth is referred to as which of the following?
  a. Dysuria
  b. Dystocia
  c. Ectopic
  d. Pyometra

203. When an animal is not able to produce offspring it is referred to as:
    a. Stillborn
    b. Sterile
    c. Pseudocyesis
    d. Hermaphroditism

204. The term _____ pertains to the skin of animals.
    a. Zoogenous
    b. Zoogamous
    c. Endozoic
    d. Zoodermic

205. Which of the following terms refers to feeding on animals?
    a. Zoophile
    b. Zooplasty
    c. Zooid
    d. Zoophagy

206. Any human disease that may be transmitted from an animal is referred to as which of the following?
    a. Zooscopy
    b. Zootomy
    c. Zoonosis
    d. Zootrophic

207. An _____ is a substance that prevents blood from clotting when it is added to the blood.
    a. Anticodon
    b. Anticoagulant
    c. Antigen
    d. Anticonvulsant

208. The bare area of the skin of birds where feathers do not originate is referred to as what?
    a. Apteria
    b. Aponeurosis
    c. Anuria
    d. Ataxia

209. The lack of normal muscle tone is known as:
    a. Atrophy
    b. Auricle
    c. Atony
    d. Ataxia

210. The term *avascular* refers to which of the following terms?
    a. Blood clot
    b. Increased amount of blood supply
    c. Decreased amount of blood supply
    d. Without a blood supply

211. A lower respiratory tract infection affecting the lining of the larger air passageways in the lungs is known:
    a. Pneumonia
    b. Bronchitis
    c. Pleural effusion
    d. Conjunctivitis

212. The dorsal shell of turtles and tortoises is the:
    a. Canthus
    b. Capsular space
    c. Carapace
    d. Cardia

213. The movement of white blood cells into an area of inflammation in response to chemical mediators released by injured tissue or other white blood cells at the site is referred to as:
    a. Leukocytosis
    b. Chemotaxis
    c. Anemia
    d. Leukopenia

214. The term *circumduction* refers to which of the following?
    a. The removal of the male testicles
    b. A joint motion whereby the distal end of an extremity moves in a circle
    c. A reservoir that stores fluid
    d. The movement of a joint where the distal end of the extremity moves away from the body.

215. The initial secretion of the mammary gland before milk is produced is known as:
    a. Colloidal
    b. Columella
    c. Colostrum
    d. Cisterna

216. The process of shaping or trimming a bird's beak is referred to as:
    a. Corium
    b. Coping
    c. Culling
    d. Crop

217. The process by which white blood cells leave the blood vessel and enter tissue by squeezing through the tiny spaces between the cells' lining is defined as:
    a. Leukopenia
    b. Diapedesis
    c. Leukocytosis
    d. Chemotaxis

218. A freely moveable synovial joint is known as a:
    a. Diastole
    b. Diestrous
    c. Diarthrosis
    d. Diaphysis

219. The prefix *dys-* refers to which of the following definitions?
    a. Before, anterior
    b. Painful, defective
    c. Below
    d. Between

220. An immature goose of either sex is referred to as which of the following?
    a. Poult
    b. Rafter
    c. Gosling
    d. Gander

221. *Ovariohysterectomy* is correctly defined as which of the following?
    a. Surgical removal of the ovaries
    b. Surgical removal of the uterus
    c. Surgical removal of the testicles
    d. Surgical removal of the uterus and oviducts/ovaries

222. Pruritus refers to:
    a. Swelling of tissue
    b. Itching
    c. Containing or consisting of pus
    d. An overgrowth of scar tissue

223. Red blood cells that remain pale after staining indicates which of the following?
    a. Hypochromic
    b. Hemoglobin
    c. Agranulocytes
    d. Anucleate

224. The auditory canal is also referred to as the:
    a. Humerus
    b. Cochlea
    c. Eustachian tube
    d. Pinna

225. A surgical incision into the windpipe is defined as:
    a. Glottis
    b. Epistaxis
    c. Tracheotomy
    d. Endoscope

226. _____ describes an increase in urine production.
    a. Dysuria
    b. Diuresis
    c. Polyuria
    d. Anuria

227. The excretion of an abnormal amount of sodium in the urine is referred to as:
    a. Hypernatremia
    b. Natriuresis
    c. Hydruria
    d. Albuminuria

228. Pain within the testicle is termed:
    a. Orchectomy
    b. Orchialgia
    c. Menorrhagia
    d. Myalgia

229. _____ is known to be the thickest layer of the uterine wall.
    a. Perimetrium
    b. Endometrium
    c. Myometrium
    d. Caruncle

230. The prefix *atel-* refers to which of the following?
    a. Injury
    b. Intestines
    c. Incomplete
    d. Inward

(e) *Answers and rationales available on Evolve*
http://evolve.elsevier.com/Prendergast/QAvettech/

PART TWO
VTNE Review

Pharmacology

Brandy Tabor, BS, CVT, VTS (ECC)

QUESTIONS

1. Neonatal animals are less tolerant of some drugs than older animals, because in neonates the drugs are:
   a. Biotransformed more rapidly
   b. Absorbed more slowly from the gastrointestinal tract
   c. Not biotransformed
   d. Biotransformed more slowly

2. Decreased function of what organ would have the greatest effect on the biotransformation of most drugs?
   a. Kidney
   b. Liver
   c. Pancreas
   d. Spleen

3. The generic name for a drug is also called the:
   a. Trade name
   b. Chemical name
   c. Proprietary name
   d. Nonproprietary name

4. You are asked to administer a drug that is supplied as an enteric-coated tablet at 100 mg, 50 mg, and 25 mg; you require 25 mg but have available 50-mg tablets only. You should:
   a. Use a pill splitter to divide the 100-mg tablet into quarters to have the smallest piece.
   b. Use a pill splitter to divide the 50-mg tablet into halves to have the most accurate dose.
   c. Administer the 50-mg tablet but then skip the next scheduled dosing.
   d. Order or purchase 25-mg tablets for the dosing schedule.

5. A prescription reads "2 tab q4h po prn until gone." The translation of these instructions is:
   a. Two tablets are to be taken four times per day for pain until all tablets are gone.
   b. Two tablets are to be taken four times per day under supervision by the veterinarian until all tablets are gone.
   c. Two tablets are to be taken every 4 hr with food and water until all tablets are gone.
   d. Two tablets are to be taken every 4 hr by mouth as needed until all tablets are gone.

6. Ten mL of a 2.5% solution of thiopentone contains:
   a. 2.5 mg of thiopentone
   b. 25 mg of thiopentone
   c. 250 mg of thiopentone
   d. 2500 mg of thiopentone

7. The percentage of the total dose that ultimately reaches the bloodstream is called:
   a. Absorption
   b. Bioavailability
   c. Clearance
   d. Distribution

8. Cholinergic agents do all of the following *except:*
   a. Cause bradycardia
   b. Control vomiting
   c. Increase intraocular pressure
   d. Increase gastrointestinal motility

9. The nonsteroidal anti-inflammatory drug (NSAID) that is extremely toxic to cats is:
   a. Aspirin
   b. Acetaminophen
   c. Carprofen
   d. Flunixin

10. The most common adverse side effect(s) of aminoglycoside antimicrobials are:
    a. Nephrotoxicity
    b. Nephrotoxicity and ototoxicity
    c. Ototoxicity and neurotoxicity
    d. Nephrotoxicity, ototoxicity, and neurotoxicity

11. Which statement regarding tetracyclines is true?
    a. They are bactericidal
    b. They alter the permeability of the cell wall and cause lysis
    c. Currently many bacteria are resistant to tetracyclines
    d. They are unable to penetrate the bacterial cell wall

12. Cephalosporins are closely related to what other drug class?
    a. Tetracyclines
    b. Sulfas
    c. Penicillins
    d. Fluoroquinolones

13. Because of the manner in which they are excreted, sulfonamides are often effective against infections of:
    a. Nervous tissue
    b. Urinary tract
    c. Skin
    d. Joint capsules

14. The Food and Drug Administration does not approve the use of fluoroquinolones in:
    a. Dogs
    b. Cats
    c. Poultry
    d. Birds

15. The antibiotic that should be avoided in all food-producing animals is:
    a. Lincosamides
    b. Cephalexin
    c. Enrofloxacin
    d. Chloramphenicol

16. Penicillins are primarily excreted by the:
    a. Small intestine
    b. Liver
    c. Kidney
    d. Stomach

17. Acepromazine must be used with caution or not at all in:
    a. Bitches
    b. Tomcats
    c. Heifers
    d. Stallions

18. The benzodiazepine derivative diazepam is often administered in combination with:
    a. Droperidol
    b. Morphine
    c. Ketamine
    d. Xylazine

19. If using a regular disposable-type syringe, which of the following drugs should not be preloaded and left for a time before use?
    a. Acepromazine
    b. Atropine
    c. Diazepam
    d. Ketamine

20. A 10-kg dog has inadvertently been administered a dose of xylazine hydrochloride intended for a 30-kg dog. The correct reversal agent for this overdose is:
    a. Atropine
    b. Flumazenil
    c. Naloxone
    d. Yohimbine

21. Griseofulvin acts on:
    a. Gram-positive bacteria
    b. Gram-negative bacteria
    c. Gram-negative and gram-positive bacteria
    d. Dermatophytes

22. Which of the following is not a side effect of sulfonamides?
    a. Crystalluria
    b. Keratoconjunctivitis sicca
    c. Seizures
    d. Thrombocytopenia

23. Which class of antibiotics, when administered to juvenile animals, can impair cartilage development?
    a. Cephalosporins
    b. Fluoroquinolones
    c. Macrolides
    d. Penicillins

24. Potentiated penicillins:
    a. Have a narrow spectrum of action relative to regular penicillins
    b. Include cephalosporins
    c. Are active against beta-lactamase–producing bacteria
    d. Are not used in treating mastitis

25. If you are instructed to give a medication IP, you will inject the medication into:
    a. The jugular vein
    b. The popliteal artery
    c. The abdominal cavity
    d. A major muscle mass

26. Which of the following statements is true when considering the use of xylazine?
    a. It is safe in all dogs
    b. It can be reversed with naloxone
    c. It provides some analgesia
    d. It can cause priapism in stallions

27. Which of the following statements is true when considering the use of propofol?
    a. It is a potent analgesic
    b. It can be given via the IM and IV routes
    c. It is best administered as a single bolus
    d. It can be given in incremental doses

28. Which of the following statements is true when considering the use of butorphanol?
    a. It is an antibiotic
    b. It is an antitussive
    c. It can be reversed using yohimbine
    d. It is contraindicated in the cat

29. Which of the following statements is true regarding an iodophor?
    a. It has a longer action than basic iodine compounds
    b. Organic materials do not inactivate it
    c. It is not an irritant at concentrations generally used
    d. It provides adequate disinfection with a single application

30. Heartgard contains ivermectin, which:
    a. Prevents dogs from developing congestive heart failure
    b. Is also effective in treating tapeworms
    c. Is used to prevent heartworm infection
    d. Can be administered orally only

31. The active drug in ProHeart is moxidectin, and it is a member of which drug class?
    a. Arsenical
    b. Organophosphate
    c. Milbemycin
    d. Pyrantel

32. A risk to veterinary technicians who administer prostaglandins is:
    a. Acne
    b. Liver failure
    c. Kidney damage
    d. Inducing an asthma attack

33. Loop diuretics such as furosemide:
    a. Cause dehydration in normal animals
    b. Cannot be used simultaneously with ACE inhibitors
    c. Are unsafe for use in animals with pulmonary edema
    d. May cause hypokalemia with chronic use

34. Pain receptors are known as:
    a. Nociceptors
    b. C fibers
    c. Proprioceptors
    d. Prostaglandins

35. If it is accidentally administered as an IV bolus, lidocaine may cause:
    a. Full body numbness
    b. Seizures
    c. Sinus arrest
    d. Polyuria

36. Which of these opioids is an agonist/antagonist?
    a. Oxymorphone
    b. Meperidine
    c. Butorphanol
    d. Fentanyl

37. Acepromazine maleate causes:
    a. Respiratory depression
    b. Tachycardia
    c. Hypotension
    d. Reduced salivation

38. What is the ratio between the toxic dose and therapeutic dose of a drug used as a measure of the relative safety of the drug for a particular treatment?
    a. Toxic index
    b. LD50
    c. ED50
    d. Therapeutic index

39. Aspirin may be safely used in cats as an NSAID, but it should be noted that its half-life in this species is approximately:
    a. 10 hr
    b. 20 hr
    c. 30 hr
    d. 40 hr

40. Which statement is most accurate pertaining to insect growth regulators?
    a. They prevent the female from laying eggs
    b. They effectively kill all adult stages
    c. They interfere with development
    d. They are neurotoxic to mammals

41. What drug is approved for the treatment of old dog dementia?
    a. Clomipramine
    b. Meloxicam
    c. Diazepam
    d. Anipryl

42. What is not a short-term effect of corticosteroid therapy?
    a. Polyuria
    b. Polyphagia
    c. Delayed healing
    d. Osteoporosis

43. A common side effect of antihistamine drugs such as diphenhydramine is:
    a. Polyuria
    b. Sedation
    c. Pruritus
    d. Panting

44. The H2 receptors are found in the:
    a. Gastric mucosa
    b. Saliva
    c. Carotid arteries
    d. Aortic arch

45. Thiobarbiturates should be administered with great care, or not at all, to:
    a. Collies
    b. Greyhounds
    c. Rottweilers
    d. Spaniels

46. What drug is not used in the treatment of glaucoma?
    a. Chloramphenicol
    b. Carbachol
    c. Latanoprost
    d. Pilocarpine

47. A chronotropic agent affects the:
    a. Force of a contraction
    b. Rate of a contraction
    c. Rhythm of a contraction
    d. Rate of relaxation

48. Puppies born via cesarean section that are not breathing well may benefit from _____ drops administered sublingually.
    a. Diazepam
    b. Digitalis
    c. Dobutamine
    d. Doxapram

49. Parenteral administration of phenylbutazone should be only via:
    a. Subcutaneous injection
    b. Intramuscular injection
    c. Intradermal injection
    d. Intravenous injection

50. Intradermal injections are used primarily for:
    a. Allergy testing
    b. Antibiotics
    c. Insulin
    d. Vaccinations

51. Most biotransformation of drugs occurs in the:
    a. Liver
    b. Kidney
    c. Lungs
    d. Skin

52. The main reason that generic forms of drugs are less expensive than trademark name drugs is because generic brands:
    a. Use less expensive ingredients
    b. Are not advertised heavily
    c. Do not incur the expense of developing a new drug
    d. Do not work as well as trademark name drugs

53. Repository forms of parenteral drugs:
    a. Contain a special coating that protects the drug from the harsh, acidic environment of the stomach
    b. Are formulated to prolong absorption of the drug from the site of administration
    c. Are composed of specially prepared plant or animal parts rather than being manufactured from chemicals
    d. Are extremely irritating to the tissues

54. All of the following organs may facilitate the elimination of drugs *except* the:
    a. Kidneys
    b. Liver
    c. Lungs
    d. Spleen

55. What liquid form of drug is administered intravenously?
    a. Emulsion
    b. Solution
    c. Suspension
    d. Elixir

56. When a drug is said to have a narrow therapeutic range, it means that:
    a. The dose range that is effective is small
    b. It may be used for treatment of a few disorders only
    c. It must be dosed frequently
    d. It must be given in greater concentrations to be effective

57. The regulatory agency that oversees the development and approval of animal topical pesticides is the:
    a. FDA
    b. EPA
    c. USDA
    d. DEA

58. A drug that has extreme potential for abuse and no approved medicinal purpose in the United States is classified as:
    a. C-I
    b. C-II
    c. C-IV
    d. C-V

59. A drug given by which of the following routes reaches its peak plasma concentration the fastest?
    a. Orally
    b. Intramuscularly
    c. Subcutaneously
    d. Intravenously

60. Which of these drugs is not an antifungal drug?
    a. Fluconazole
    b. Clotrimazole
    c. Ketoconazole
    d. Sulfadimethoxine

61. An example of an antibiotic that is considered to be a βeta-lactamase inhibitor is:
    a. Amoxicillin
    b. Clavamox
    c. Tetracycline
    d. Penicillin

62. In what class of antibiotic drugs are nephrotoxicity and ototoxicity potential side effects?
    a. Aminoglycosides
    b. Barbiturates
    c. Dissociative anesthetics
    d. Phenothiazine tranquilizers

63. The best means of assuring that a particular antibiotic treatment will be successful is to:
    a. Treat for no less than a full 2-week course
    b. Collect a sample from the infected area for culture and sensitivity
    c. Use the highest dose that is considered nontoxic
    d. Use a broad-spectrum antibiotic

64. Dr. Blackman prescribed a particular antibiotic for a rabbit with a Pasteurella infection and asked you to educate the client regarding special instructions for administration of the drug. You told the client that she should wear gloves when handling this medication, because it has been associated with a rare adverse reaction in humans: aplastic anemia. Based on this information, the drug that you dispensed was most likely:
    a. Gentamicin
    b. Tetracycline
    c. Erythromycin
    d. Chloramphenicol

65. A useful group of broad-spectrum drugs, whose popularity has recently declined because of numerous potential side effects, including keratoconjunctivitis sicca, polyarthritis (especially in Doberman pinschers), hematuria, allergic reactions, thrombocytopenia, and leukopenia, is the:
    a. Sulfonamides
    b. Macrolides
    c. Tetracyclines
    d. Fluoroquinolones

66. Which of the following statements about tetracyclines is true?
    a. Tetracyclines are bacteriocidal.
    b. Oral absorption of tetracyclines is increased in the presence of food.
    c. Tetracyclines are potentially nephrotoxic and ototoxic.
    d. Tetracyclines may lead to bone or teeth problems if given to young animals.

67. A 50-lb dog is to be given 1 mg/kg dose of diazepam. How many milligrams should he receive?
    a. 50 mg
    b. 22.7 mg
    c. 500 mg
    d. 2.27 mg

68. Amoxicillin (Amoxi-Drop) was prescribed for Tallulah, a 4-year-old female Chihuahua, who was being discharged after hospitalization. Dr. Segal asks you to provide her owner with discharge instructions. You advise the client of all of the following, *except:*
    a. She should call if she notices any adverse side effects as a result of the medication.
    b. She should complete all the medication dispensed, even if Tallulah is feeling well and her symptoms have resolved.
    c. She must administer the medication on an empty stomach, even if Tallulah vomits.
    d. The medication should be refrigerated.

69. Antimicrobial drugs such as enrofloxacin, marbofloxacin, and orbifloxacin all belong to which group of antibiotics?
    a. Fluoroquinolones
    b. Cephalosporins
    c. Penicillins
    d. Aminoglycosides

70. Which of the following drugs is least likely to kill the normal flora in the gut of a rabbit, thus avoiding severe diarrhea?
    a. Clavamox
    b. Clindamycin
    c. Cefotaxime
    d. Enrofloxacin

71. Guaifenesin is an example of a(n):
    a. Expectorant
    b. Antitussive
    c. Bronchodilator
    d. Decongestant

72. Which of the following drugs is available over the counter as an antitussive?
    a. Codeine
    b. Dextromethorphan
    c. Hydrocodone
    d. Butorphanol

73. Dr. Charles is performing a C-section on Sadie, a 3-year-old Dalmatian. The smallest pup was not breathing spontaneously, so the doctor asks you administer which of the following drugs as a respiratory stimulant?
    a. Theophylline
    b. Albuterol
    c. Doxapram HCl
    d. Terbutaline

74. Butorphanol tartrate is an example of a drug that functions on more than one body system. It is both an analgesic and a(n) _____.
    a. Antitussive
    b. Expectorant
    c. Tranquilizer
    d. Emetic

75. The type of drug that would be most helpful for a patient with a productive cough is:
    a. Antitussive
    b. Antihistamine
    c. Expectorant
    d. Analgesic

76. The anticoagulant diluted in saline or sterile water for injection to form a flush solution for preventing blood clots in intravenous catheters is:
    a. Heparin
    b. EDTA
    c. Coumarin
    d. Acid citrate dextrose (ACD)

77. Sox, a 10-year-old M/C Siamese X, was brought to the emergency hospital, crying in pain and unable to walk. He was diagnosed with an aortic thromboembolism secondary to cardiomyopathy. The drug class used to treat this condition is:
    a. Anticoagulant
    b. Fibrinolytic
    c. Hematinic
    d. Hemostatic

78. The diuretic drug used most commonly in patients with congestive heart failure is:
    a. Mannitol
    b. Spironolactone
    c. Chlorothiazide
    d. Furosemide

79. The function of epinephrine is to:
    a. Increase the heart rate
    b. Decrease the heart rate
    c. Decrease the blood pressure
    d. Reverse the effects of acepromazine

80. The most common side effect of drugs that cause vasodilation is:
    a. Anorexia, vomiting, and diarrhea
    b. Cardiac arrhythmias
    c. Bradycardia
    d. Hypotension

81. Cosmo, an 11-year-old M/C pug, has been diagnosed with mitral insufficiency and was referred to a veterinary cardiologist. The specialist decided to initiate treatment with digoxin, which is a positive inotrope and negative chronotrope. This means that it:
    a. Increases the force of contraction and decreases the heart rate
    b. Increases the peripheral vascular resistance and decreases the cardiac output
    c. Increases the blood pressure and decreases the cardiac output
    d. Increases the heart rate and decreases the blood pressure

82. Scooter, a 13-year-old miniature schnauzer, has arrested under anesthesia for routine dentistry. You run to the crash cart and grab what you know to be the drug of choice for cardiac arrest, which is:
    a. Epinephrine
    b. Lidocaine
    c. Sodium bicarbonate
    d. Dobutamine

83. A 3-month-old chow chow is presented to the pet emergency clinic because it has eaten a box of warfarin-based rat poison. Which of the following would be most useful to treat this toxicity?
    a. Protamine sulfate
    b. Coumarin
    c. Streptokinase
    d. Vitamin K

84. Which statement is true about the drugs used for cancer chemotherapy?
    a. They are usually given by mouth
    b. They usually have relatively low margins of safety
    c. They are available over the counter
    d. They are all nephrotoxic

85. Which of the following side effects is commonly seen with many cancer chemotherapeutic drugs?
    a. Hyperglycemia
    b. Immunosuppression
    c. Constipation
    d. Hyperphagia

86. Which of the following would be the least common side effect expected with common cancer chemotherapeutic drugs?
    a. Myelosuppression
    b. Vomiting and diarrhea
    c. Pruritus
    d. Alopecia

87. Common drugs of plant origin, such as digoxin and atropine, are ineffective in a cow when administered orally because of:
    a. Eructation
    b. The large size of the rumen
    c. Methane gas
    d. Digestive microorganisms

88. Which of these tissues is not a normal site for drugs to accumulate to be released later, thereby prolonging the effect of the drug?
    a. Pancreas
    b. Fat
    c. Bone
    d. Liver

89. Chronic use of moderate-to-high doses of glucocorticoids may result in the development of:
    a. Hypoadrenocorticism
    b. Hyperadrenocorticism
    c. Hypothyroidism
    d. Hyperthyroidism

90. Glucocorticoids are often used in veterinary medicine for the treatment of all of the following conditions *except:*
    a. Allergies
    b. Musculoskeletal problems
    c. Infections
    d. Immune-mediated disease

91. Glucocorticoids have different durations of activity, a fact that plays an important role in their risk of side effects with long-term use. Which of the following glucocorticoids has the shortest duration of activity?
    a. Hydrocortisone
    b. Prednisone
    c. Dexamethasone
    d. Triamcinolone

92. Which of the following statements about glucocorticoids is true?
    a. If adverse effects are seen after long-term administration, treatment should be discontinued immediately
    b. They are generally considered safer to use than NSAIDs
    c. They are a type of NSAID
    d. They may cause immune-system suppression

93. What drug is not an NSAID?
    a. Prednisone
    b. Flunixin
    c. Phenylbutazone
    d. Aspirin

94. Flunixin meglumine (Banamine) is an NSAID most commonly used in:
    a. Dogs for the treatment of chronic osteoarthritis
    b. Horses for the treatment of colic
    c. Horses for reducing fever
    d. Dogs for its anticoagulant activity

95. The species that generally clears NSAIDs most slowly is:
    a. Dog
    b. Cat
    c. Horse
    d. Ruminant

96. What NSAID is administered to cats with a dosing interval of 2 days or more?
    a. Aspirin
    b. Ibuprofen
    c. Carprofen
    d. Naproxen

97. The most common side effect of NSAIDs is:
    a. Polyuria
    b. Gastrointestinal ulceration
    c. Diarrhea
    d. Constipation

98. What precautions should you take when applying DMSO to an animal's skin?
    a. Wear a facial mask to avoid inhaling the fumes
    b. Apply a bandage to cover the area of application
    c. DMSO is irritating and should not be applied to skin
    d. Wear latex gloves to avoid contact with the drug

99. The surgeon has completed Buffy's surgical procedure and asks you to discontinue the inhalant anesthesia. What is absolutely necessary to do when terminating anesthesia in a patient that has been receiving nitrous oxide?
    a. Give an injection of the reversal agent
    b. Observe carefully for signs of seizures
    c. Allow the patient to recuperate in a quiet, dark area
    d. Oxygenate for 5 to 10 minutes

100. Which of the following is not a controlled substance?
    a. Apomorphine
    b. Diazepam
    c. Ketamine
    d. Hydromorphone

101. Malignant hyperthermia is a phenomenon associated primarily with the use of what inhalant anesthetic?
    a. Nitrous oxide
    b. Sevoflurane
    c. Halothane
    d. Isoflurane

102. What drug is in the same class as thiopental?
    a. Ketamine
    b. Diazepam
    c. Phenobarbital
    d. Atropine

103. An opioid analgesic often used in transdermal patches to control postsurgical pain is:
    a. Fentanyl
    b. Pentazocine
    c. Meperidine
    d. Butorphanol

104. Mrs. Stillman's poodle Roxy has been diagnosed with idiopathic epilepsy. In the event of a seizure at home, which drug has the doctor decided to dispense, which Mrs. Stillman can administer per rectum?
    a. Pentobarbital
    b. Phenobarbital
    c. Diazepam
    d. Acepromazine

105. A recent graduate veterinary technician is concerned that a sedated patient has a heart rate of 50 beats/min when the heart rate in a dog is normally 60 to 120 beats/min. She also mentions that the blood pressure is normal. You ask her which sedative the veterinarian used and you were not surprised when she told you that the drug used was_____.
    a. Dexmedetomidine
    b. Diazepam
    c. Ketamine
    d. Acepromazine

106. All of the following drugs are antagonists and are used to reverse the effects of another drug, *except:*
    a. Yohimbine
    b. Detomidine
    c. Flumazenil
    d. Naloxone

107. For which gas does anesthesia demand the greatest degree of patient monitoring, because the anesthetic depth changes occur most rapidly?
    a. Desflurane
    b. Sevoflurane
    c. Halothane
    d. Isoflurane

108. Norepinephrine, epinephrine, and dopamine are the primary neurotransmitters for the:
    a. Parasympathetic nervous system
    b. Sympathetic nervous system
    c. Central nervous system
    d. Peripheral nervous system

109. Beuthanasia solution is back-ordered at the distributor so your employer asks you to order a different euthanasia solution. In researching the available drugs, you are reminded that the active ingredient in most euthanasia solutions is:
    a. Phenobarbital
    b. Pentobarbital
    c. Methohexital
    d. Thiopental

110. You are working with an equine veterinarian on a breeding farm. You will be sedating a young stallion for an oral examination. Which tranquilizer are you well aware that the veterinarian will probably not use for the procedure?
    a. Xylazine
    b. Diazepam
    c. Detomidine
    d. Acepromazine

111. The newly hired veterinary assistant is cleaning up after a procedure and returns an opened bottle of propofol to the refrigerator, stating that it can be used the next day on another patient. You explain to her that:
    a. Propofol should be stored at room temperature rather than in the refrigerator.
    b. The bottles are designed to contain only enough drug for one patient, and there likely will not be enough drug left to anesthetize another patient the next day.
    c. Bacteria will readily grow in propofol and will produce endotoxins, so it is unwise to use the remains of an opened bottle.
    d. The bottle has been contaminated from the first patient, and there is a possibility that contagious diseases can be transmitted in this way.

112. You are on an ambulatory call to Milkman's Dairy with Dr. Burrows. You are asked to bring the xylazine from the truck to sedate the patient. You are aware that when using this drug in the bovine, you must:
    a. Use adequate doses, because cattle tend to be resistant to its effects
    b. Always use it concurrently with a barbiturate to achieve adequate analgesia
    c. Not use xylazine because it is contraindicated in this species
    d. Use it at about $\frac{1}{10}$ of the equine dose

113. You were assigned to work the front office at the hospital today. When you walk back to the treatment area, you notice a cat under anesthesia. The cat has eyes wide-open, lack of blinking, the limbs are stiffly distended, and is salivating profusely. Your highly educated guess is that this cat was anesthetized using which of the following drugs?
    a. Xylazine
    b. Medetomidine
    c. Ketamine
    d. Propofol

114. A cow is accidentally dosed with an equine dose of xylazine. What drug should be immediately administered?
    a. None; the equine and bovine doses of xylazine are the same
    b. Epinephrine
    c. Naloxone
    d. Yohimbine

115. Acepromazine should be avoided in:
    a. Patients with a history of seizures
    b. Aggressive patients
    c. Geriatric patients
    d. Doberman pinschers

116. The behavioral drug group that may be sent home to stimulate appetite in cats is:
    a. Benzodiazepines
    b. Tricyclic antidepressants
    c. Selective serotonin reuptake inhibitors
    d. Progestins

117. A progestin was often used in the past for the treatment of inappropriate elimination in cats, and it has now fallen out of favor because of serious potential side effects, including mammary hyperplasia and adenocarcinoma. This drug is known as:
    a. Megestrol acetate
    b. Oxazepam
    c. Amitriptyline
    d. Fluoxetine

118. Which tricyclic antidepressant is now approved for use in dogs and cats to control separation anxiety?
    a. Buspirone
    b. Selegiline
    c. Paroxetine
    d. Clomipramine

119. A 12-year-old spayed female golden retriever is brought into your clinic with a history of waking up in her bed in a puddle of urine. A complete blood count (CBC), profile, and urinalysis show no sign of urinary tract disease. The doctor tells you to fill a prescription for phenylpropanolamine. The doctor is choosing this drug because it treats:
    a. Bladder atony by increasing bladder tone
    b. Urinary incontinence by decreasing urethral sphincter tone
    c. Urinary incontinence by increasing urethral sphincter tone
    d. Bladder atony by decreasing bladder tone

120. Erythropoietin is primarily used in the following feline patients:
    a. Cats with anemia because of chronic renal failure
    b. Cats with anemia resulting from rodenticide toxicity
    c. Cats with aortic thromboembolism secondary to cardiomyopathy
    d. Cats suffering from Tylenol toxicity

121. Which of the following drugs is used to decrease gastric acid production by blocking histamine receptors in the stomach?
    a. Famotidine
    b. Sucralfate
    c. Omeprazole
    d. Misoprostol

122. Amphojel and Basaljel are drugs in the general category of:
    a. Potassium supplements
    b. Antihypertensives
    c. Urinary acidifiers
    d. Phosphate binders

123. A heartworm preventative that is also approved for the treatment of ear mites and sarcoptic mange is:
    a. Diethylcarbamazine
    b. Milbemycin
    c. Ivermectin
    d. Selamectin

124. If a drug package insert states that the drug is a coccidiostat, against what group of parasites will this drug be effective?
    a. Ascarids (Toxocara, Toxascaris)
    b. Tapeworms (Taenia)
    c. Protozoa (Eimeria, Isospora)
    d. Flukes (liver fluke, lung fluke)

125. Which of the following drugs can cause severe tissue necrosis if administered perivascularly?
    a. Phenylbutazone
    b. Oxymorphone
    c. Dexmedetomidine
    d. Ketamine

126. Which statement about organophosphates is incorrect?
    a. They are neurotoxic
    b. They are used for control of endoparasites and ectoparasites
    c. They have a narrow margin of safety
    d. They have relatively few side effects

127. In cases of uncomplicated diabetes, by what route is insulin usually administered?
    a. Intramuscular
    b. Subcutaneous
    c. Intravenous
    d. Oral

128. Insulin concentration is measured in:
    a. Milligrams per milliliter
    b. Milliequivalents per milliliter
    c. Units per milliliter
    d. Grams per milliliter

129. Oral hypoglycemic drugs, such as glipizide (Glucotrol), are used to treat:
    a. Diabetic ketoacidosis
    b. Non–insulin-dependent diabetes
    c. Hypoglycemia
    d. Pancreatitis

130. The primary function of insulin is to:
    a. Regulate the metabolic processes of the body
    b. Regulate digestion through secretion of gastrointestinal hormones
    c. Facilitate the entry of glucose into cells
    d. Control reproductive function

131. Resuspension of NPH insulin is achieved by:
    a. Gently rolling the bottle
    b. Vigorously shaking the bottle
    c. Gently heating the bottle in warm water
    d. Refrigerating the bottle

132. Altrenogest, which is used for estrus synchronization in female animals, is a synthetic:
    a. Estrogen
    b. Androgen
    c. Progestin
    d. Follicle-stimulating hormone (FSH)

133. When diethylstilbestrol (DES), a synthetic estrogen, is used at higher doses, it can have the potentially dangerous side effect of:
    a. Gastric ulceration
    b. Cardiac arrhythmias
    c. Bone marrow suppression
    d. Hepatopathy

134. Kaolin, pectin, and bismuth subsalicylate are examples of:
    a. Narcotic analgesics
    b. Antispasmodics
    c. Anticholinergics
    d. Protectants

135. Psyllium and Metamucil are examples of:
    a. Saline cathartics
    b. Bulk laxatives
    c. Lubricants
    d. Irritant cathartics

136. What is not a potential side effect of the phenothiazine antiemetics?
    a. CNS depression
    b. Diarrhea
    c. Lowering of the seizure threshold
    d. Hypotension

137. A stool softener that often helps patients recovering from anal surgery is:
    a. Docusate sodium succinate (DSS)
    b. Magnesium hydroxide
    c. Mineral oil
    d. Bran

138. The most widely used type of antiemetic drug to prevent motion sickness in dogs and cats is the:
    a. Phenothiazine
    b. Antihistamine
    c. Anticholinergic
    d. Antispasmodic

139. The emetic of choice in cats is:
    a. Xylazine
    b. Syrup of ipecac
    c. Apomorphine
    d. Hydrogen peroxide

140. The emetic of choice in dogs is:
    a. Xylazine
    b. Syrup of ipecac
    c. Apomorphine
    d. Hydrogen peroxide

141. Spike the dog ingested his owner's cardiac medication about a half-hour ago. The veterinarian instructs you to give him an emetic that may be administered into the conjunctival sac, and then flush as necessary. The name of the drug is:
    a. Xylazine
    b. Syrup of ipecac
    c. Apomorphine
    d. Hydrogen peroxide

142. A coating agent that forms an ulcer-adherent complex at the ulcer site is:
    a. Kaopectate
    b. Sucralfate
    c. Cimetidine
    d. Misoprostol

143. In what species are Fleet (sodium phosphate) enemas contraindicated?
    a. Horses
    b. Ruminants
    c. Cats
    d. Pigs

144. The principal site of drug biotransformation is the:
    a. Liver
    b. Kidney
    c. Stomach
    d. Small intestine

145. What drug is most likely to be prescribed to prevent motion sickness in dogs and cats?
    a. Apomorphine
    b. Syrup of ipecac
    c. Atropine
    d. Acepromazine

146. A veterinarian prescribes erythropoietin for use in a dog in terminal renal failure. Why was this drug prescribed?
    a. For its fibrinolytic activity
    b. For its immunosuppressive activity
    c. For its ability to stimulate red blood cell production and release
    d. For its ability to reduce hypertension

147. Which of the following drugs is considered a biologic response modifier?
    a. Interferon
    b. Streptokinase
    c. Cephalosporin
    d. EDTA

148. Atropine is often given as a preanesthetic agent. It is classified as an anticholinergic drug. That means that it will likely have the following effects on an animal receiving the drug:
    a. Decreased heart rate, decreased salivation, and decreased GI motility
    b. Increased heart rate, increased salivation, and increased GI motility
    c. Increased heart rate, decreased salivation, and decreased GI motility
    d. Decreased heart rate, increased salivation, and increased GI motility

149. A drug classified as an antagonist may exert its influence by:
    a. Mimicking the activity of the neurotransmitter used in the impulse
    b. Preventing the breakdown of the neurotransmitter used in the impulse
    c. Blocking the neurotransmitter receptor on the effector organ
    d. Enhancing the release of the neurotransmitter used in the impulse

150. A client is advised to discontinue aspirin therapy in his dysplastic dog before the dog undergoes surgery to remove a mammary tumor. The client asks you why this request was made. You tell him:
    a. Aspirin decreases platelet aggregation and may increase the likelihood of hemorrhage
    b. Aspirin may result in gastrointestinal ulceration
    c. Aspirin may adversely affect hepatic biotransformation
    d. Aspirin has an anti-inflammatory effect

151. Duragesic (Fentanyl) transdermal patches are used most commonly in veterinary medicine to control:
    a. Diarrhea
    b. Vomiting
    c. Seizures
    d. Pain

152. Acetylcysteine (Mucomyst) is an antidote for what type of drug toxicity?
    a. Opioid
    b. Acetaminophen
    c. Lidocaine
    d. Digoxin

153. An expectorant is a drug that acts to:
    a. Suppress a productive cough
    b. Liquefy and dilute viscous secretions in the respiratory tract
    c. Suppress inflammatory cells in the respiratory tract
    d. Reduce the allergic component of respiratory disease

154. The therapeutic range of a drug refers to which of the following?
    a. The plasma concentration at which therapeutic benefits should be observed
    b. The relationship of a drug's ability to achieve a desired effect versus causing a toxic effect
    c. The range of curative properties that a drug may exhibit
    d. The frequency of idiosyncratic reactions

155. Which of the following drugs are contraindicated in a patient that has a history of seizures?
    a. Diazepam
    b. Thiopental
    c. Acepromazine
    d. Fentanyl

156. Nutraceuticals is a category of drugs that includes which of the following characteristics?
    a. Genetically derived materials that enhance immune function
    b. Drugs that are derived from humans for use in animals
    c. Drugs that are undergoing clinical trials before FDA approval
    d. Nontoxic food components that have proven health benefits

157. What is the reversal agent for xylazine?
    a. Fentanyl
    b. Naloxone
    c. Acepromazine
    d. Yohimbine

158. The reversal agent used for opioid toxicity is:
    a. Naloxone (Narcan)
    b. Yohimbine
    c. Acetylcysteine
    d. Diazepam

159. One of the adverse side effects of opioid administration is:
    a. Increased seizure activity in epileptic animals
    b. Induction of cardiac arrhythmias
    c. Significant respiratory depression
    d. Systemic hypertension

160. In which of the following circumstances should a thiobarbiturate drug be avoided?
    a. In a patient with respiratory alkalosis
    b. In obese patients
    c. In sight hounds and very thin patients
    d. In hyperproteinemic animals

161. What is a potential electrolyte imbalance that can occur as a result of administering a loop diuretic to a small animal?
    a. Hypokalemia
    b. Hyperkalemia
    c. Hypercalcemia
    d. Hypocalcemia

162. Which of the following drugs is used to treat feline hypertension?
    a. Amlodipine
    b. Erythromycin
    c. Amitriptyline
    d. Atropine

163. A cat is given ketamine as an anesthetic induction agent. The veterinary technician monitoring this animal may observe which of the following side effects?
    a. Bradycardia
    b. Hypotension
    c. Apneustic breathing
    d. Flaccid muscle tone

164. The category of drugs classified as ACE inhibitors has which of the following effects on the body?
    a. Increases preload and afterload on the heart
    b. Decreases preload and afterload on the heart
    c. Enhances fluid retention in the body
    d. Enhances the production of angiotensin II

165. Nitroglycerin is administered primarily to achieve which of the following effects?
    a. Vasodilation
    b. Vasoconstriction
    c. Antiarrhythmic effect
    d. ACE inhibitor effect

166. For cats diagnosed with hypertrophic cardiomyopathy, a calcium channel blocker is often prescribed to relax the heart in an attempt to improve cardiac output. Which of the following drugs falls in this category?
    a. Procainamide
    b. Diltiazem
    c. Lidocaine
    d. Digoxin

167. Lidocaine is primarily used to control which of the following abnormalities?
    a. Supraventricular bradycardia
    b. Ventricular tachycardia
    c. Hypertension
    d. Supraventricular tachycardia

168. In dogs that have been receiving long-term glucocorticoid therapy (months to years), a sudden discontinuation of the drug may result in which of the following medical problems?
    a. Immunosuppression
    b. Iatrogenic addisonian crisis
    c. Polyuria and polydipsia
    d. Iatrogenic thyroid disease

169. In dogs that have been receiving long-term glucocorticoid therapy (months to years), which of the following endocrinopathies can occur?
    a. Hypothyroidism
    b. Hyperthyroidism
    c. Iatrogenic Cushing disease/hyperadrenocorticism
    d. Estrogen-responsive incontinence

170. Which of the following is/are not a side effect of oral glucocorticoid administration in dogs?
    a. Polyuria and polydipsia
    b. Polyphagia
    c. Hyperglycemia
    d. Vomiting

171. Glucocorticoids are often used to treat all of the following conditions, *except:*
    a. Autoimmune skin disease
    b. Asthma
    c. Lymphocytic neoplasia
    d. Hyperadrenocorticism

172. An example of an anticholinergic drug is:
    a. Acetylcholine
    b. Pilocarpine
    c. Atropine
    d. Nicotine

173. The term drug compounding refers to which of the following activities?
    a. Diluting or combining drugs for ease of administration
    b. Delivering a drug via a different route than is directed on the label
    c. Delivering a drug at a different dose than is directed on the label
    d. Delivering the drug to a different species than is directed on the label

174. Which of the following drugs is most commonly used to treat urinary incontinence in dogs?
    a. Phenylpropanolamine
    b. Diethylcarbamazine
    c. Acepromazine
    d. Bethanechol

175. Which of the following drugs is classified as an osmotic diuretic and is often used to reduce intracranial pressure or treat oliguric renal failure?
    a. Furosemide
    b. Propranolol
    c. Mannitol
    d. Bethanechol

176. Which of the following drugs does not have an antiemetic action?
    a. Chlorpromazine
    b. Metoclopramide
    c. Meclizine
    d. Apomorphine

177. Which of the following antibiotics should not be given to an animal that demonstrates an allergic response to penicillin administration?
    a. Clindamycin
    b. Cephalosporins
    c. Sulfonamides
    d. Fluoroquinolones

178. Griseofulvin is used in cats, dogs, and horses to treat which of the following disorders?
    a. Dermatophytosis
    b. Staphylococcal pyoderma
    c. Rickettsial disease
    d. Nematode infection

179. Which of the following drugs provides analgesic relief to a patient who undergoes a painful procedure?
    a. Acepromazine
    b. Diazepam
    c. Thiopental
    d. Fentanyl

180. Which of the following drugs is used as an adulticide to treat a heartworm-positive dog?
    a. Melarsomine
    b. Ivermectin
    c. Milbemycin
    d. Moxidectin

181. The antidote for warfarin poisoning is:
    a. Vitamin C
    b. Naloxone
    c. Vitamin K
    d. 4-methylpyrazole

182. An example of an alpha-2 agonist is:
    a. Xylazine
    b. Propranolol
    c. Hydralazine
    d. Epinephrine

183. The number of species of bacteria that are affected by an antibiotic is known as the antibiotic's:
    a. Effectiveness
    b. Efficacy
    c. Spectrum
    d. Affinity

184. Which of the following drugs does not have an immunosuppressive effect?
    a. Cyclosporine
    b. Azathioprine
    c. Prednisone
    d. Ivermectin

185. An example of an aminoglycoside antibiotic is:
    a. Erythromycin
    b. Ampicillin
    c. Neomycin
    d. Doxycycline

186. A reported side effect of fluoroquinolone administration (Baytril) in cats given SID dosing at a higher dosing schedule is:
    a. Retinal damage
    b. Hypertension
    c. Renal failure
    d. Hepatic failure

187. Which of the following clinical signs may indicate that an animal is experiencing lidocaine toxicity?
    a. CNS signs: drowsiness, ataxia, muscle tremors
    b. Renal signs: oliguria
    c. Hepatic signs: jaundice, clotting problems
    d. Respiratory signs: labored respirations, bronchoconstriction

188. An asthmatic cat may receive which of the following drugs for its bronchodilatory effect?
    a. Histamine
    b. Digoxin
    c. Prednisone
    d. Theophylline

189. The class of antibiotics most commonly prescribed to treat rickettsial infections, such as Rocky Mountain spotted fever, is:
    a. Tetracyclines
    b. Penicillins
    c. Aminoglycosides
    d. Sulfonamides

190. What drug will not cause nephrotoxicity?
    a. Aminoglycosides
    b. Banamine
    c. Cisplatin
    d. Oxymorphone

191. Why is it an accepted practice for cats receiving aspirin therapy to be dosed on a 2-day interval schedule only (i.e., a minimal dose every 2 days)?
    a. Liver metabolism of salicylates occurs at a very slow rate in comparison to other species, thereby making cats extremely susceptible to overdose in comparison to dogs.
    b. Salicylates cause severe respiratory depression in cats.
    c. Salicylates often result in severe hypertension.
    d. Salicylates may result in hypercoagulable states in cats.

192. A cat diagnosed with hyperthyroidism may be offered a number of treatment options, including all of the following, *except:*
    a. Radioactive iodine-131 treatment
    b. Methimazole medical management
    c. Thyroidectomy surgery
    d. Levothyroxine

193. Triple sulfas were developed to the avert _____ that was/were seen with single sulfonamide toxicity.
    a. Diarrhea
    b. Crystalluria
    c. Bronchospasms
    d. Seizures

194. A dog diagnosed with a mast cell tumor is scheduled for surgery. The veterinarian chooses to pretreat the dog with an H1 blocker to prevent the negative effects of histamine release when the tumor is manipulated. Which of the following drugs may be chosen?
    a. Diphenhydramine
    b. Methimazole
    c. Vincristine
    d. Sulfasalazine

195. Which of the following drugs is used for its sedative, antiseizure, and appetite-stimulant effects?
    a. Diazepam
    b. Cyproheptadine
    c. Ketamine
    d. Potassium bromide

196. A cat is given methionine to alter the pH of his urine in an effort to dissolve his struvite stones. The drug has which of the following intended effects?
    a. Acidification of the urine
    b. Alkalinization of the urine
    c. Dilution of urine
    d. Concentration of the urine

197. Which of the following types of insulin provides the longest duration of action?
    a. NPH insulin
    b. Regular insulin
    c. Glargine insulin
    d. PZI insulin

198. It is essential for veterinary technicians to educate clients expecting to treat their pets with insulin. Which of the following statements is true?
    a. Insulin can be stored at room temperature between uses
    b. The bottle of insulin should be shaken before use
    c. The injection is given in the same site each time
    d. Insulin should be given with a meal

199. Which type of antimicrobial drug would be effective against organisms such as Giardia or Eimeria?
    a. Bactericidal
    b. Virucidal
    c. Antiprotozoal
    d. Fungistatic

200. Many antibiotic drug inserts (information included in packages of drugs) make reference to the MIC at which the antibiotic is effective. What is the MIC?
    a. Minimum inflammatory concentration
    b. Maximum infusion concentration
    c. Minimum inhibitory concentration
    d. Maximum inhalation concentration

201. Antimicrobial drugs such as neomycin, gentamicin, and amikacin each belong to what group of antibiotics?
    a. Penicillins
    b. Cephalosporins
    c. Quinolines
    d. Aminoglycosides

202. Aminoglycosides, if given at high dosages or by continuous IV infusion, cause damage to the:
    a. Lungs and liver
    b. Liver and inner ear
    c. Kidney and liver
    d. Inner ear and kidney

203. Bacterial resistance to antibiotics is a significant problem in veterinary medicine. What factor is not considered to be a significant contributor to the development of bacterial resistance?
    a. Prolonged levels of higher-than-recommended dosages of antibiotics
    b. Normal dosages of antibiotics for half the recommended duration
    c. Low dosages of antibiotics in the feed for prolonged periods
    d. Antibiotics that do not reach the infection site in concentrations that exceed MIC

204. Which of the following drug groups is most likely to provoke an allergic reaction in treated animals?
    a. Aminoglycosides
    b. Quinolines
    c. Penicillins
    d. Tetracyclines

205. Antimicrobial drugs that work against bacterial deoxyribonucleic acid (DNA) have the potential for causing birth defects or other problems in the host animal if they also alter mammalian DNA. One group of antimicrobial agents known for this tendency is:
    a. Antifungals
    b. Antibacterials
    c. Antivirals
    d. Antiprotozoals

206. Unlike many other penicillins, penicillin G is not recommended for use by mouth. Why?
    a. It upsets the stomach.
    b. It is destroyed by gastric acid.
    c. It causes severe diarrhea and intestinal cramping.
    d. It is ineffectively absorbed from the gastrointestinal tract.

207. Which type of adverse reaction is most commonly observed when penicillins are administered to rabbits?
    a. Kidney damage and subsequent change in urine production
    b. Hives and swelling of the face from allergic reaction
    c. High fever and severe depression
    d. Severe diarrhea

208. Certain bacteria, especially Staphylococcus, produce an enzyme (β-lactamase) that destroys many penicillin drugs. Which is one of the penicillins not destroyed by β-lactamase?
    a. Penicillin G
    b. Unasyn
    c. Amoxicillin
    d. Hetacillin

209. What is added to amoxicillin to make it resistant to the penicillin-destroying β-lactamase enzymes produced by some bacteria?
    a. Trimethoprim
    b. Clavulanic acid
    c. Piperonyl butoxide
    d. Ormetoprim

210. Some penicillin G injectable products contain procaine or benzathine, and some penicillin G products contain neither. What effects do procaine and benzathine have on penicillin G?
    a. They act as a local anesthetic to decrease the pain of injection.
    b. They prolong absorption of penicillin G from the injection site.
    c. They increase the rate at which penicillin G enters the bloodstream.
    d. They enhance the bacterial killing activity of the penicillin.

211. Ceftiofur is classified on the package insert as a third-generation cephalosporin antibiotic; cefadroxil is classified as a first-generation cephalosporin. How do third-generation cephalosporins differ from first-generation cephalosporins?
    a. Third-generation drugs are better absorbed when given orally.
    b. Third-generation drugs have better gram-negative activity.
    c. Third-generation drugs last longer in the body; they are given once daily only.
    d. Third-generation drugs have fewer side effects and adverse reactions.

212. Aminoglycoside antibiotics (e.g., amikacin and gentamicin) are powerful agents against bacteria. Unfortunately, they do not seem to work well in deep puncture wounds or in the lumen of the colon. Why?
    a. These are anaerobic sites, and bacteria require oxygen to take up aminoglycosides.
    b. These sites often have enzymes that inactivate aminoglycosides.
    c. Gram-positive bacteria commonly infect these sites, and aminoglycosides are ineffective against gram-positive bacteria.
    d. The DNA of bacteria at these sites is resistant to aminoglycosides.

213. How can a drug such as neomycin, which has severe risk of nephrotoxicity when administered by injection, have little risk when administered topically or orally?
    a. Some species are resistant to kidney damage that may result from the drug.
    b. Little of the drug is absorbed through the skin.
    c. Absorbed drug is excreted so quickly that it does not have time to damage the kidneys.
    d. Subcutaneous enzymes inactivate the drug.

214. What antibiotic is most likely to cause damage to the ear?
    a. Amoxicillin
    b. Gentamicin
    c. Tetracycline
    d. Enrofloxacin

215. What route of administration of amikacin or gentamicin causes the highest risk for nephrotoxicity?
    a. Per os
    b. Intramuscular
    c. Continuous intravenous infusion
    d. Intravenous bolus

216. What can a technician do to recognize early signs of nephrotoxicity in an animal that receives aminoglycosides?
    a. Monitor blood urea nitrogen (BUN) and creatinine levels
    b. Monitor the CBC and total protein level
    c. Monitor feces for change in consistency
    d. Monitor urine for casts and protein

217. Why is it important that pus-filled wounds or ear canals with purulent debris be thoroughly cleaned before applying a topical aminoglycoside (e.g., gentamicin)?
    a. Purulent material shields bacteria from the antibiotic.
    b. The alkaline nature of the purulent material reduces bacterial uptake of the drug.
    c. Nucleic acids in the cellular debris bind the aminoglycoside.
    d. Irritation from the purulent material causes the tissue to produce enzymes against the aminoglycoside.

218. What drugs are considered fluoroquinolones?
    a. Oxytetracycline, doxycycline
    b. Danofloxacin, enrofloxacin
    c. Sulfadimethoxine, sulfamethazine
    d. Chloramphenicol, lincomycin

219. What organ blocks the entrance of many drugs because of a barrier similar to the blood-brain barrier?
    a. Prostate gland
    b. Thyroid gland
    c. Pancreas
    d. Spleen

220. In what animal is the use of enrofloxacin safest?
    a. 1-year-old Dutch rabbit
    b. 3-month-old Doberman puppy
    c. 6-month-old quarter horse colt
    d. 2-year-old Siamese cat

221. What is the drug group of choice for treating Lyme disease (borreliosis)?
    a. Antifungal
    b. Antiviral
    c. Antibiotic
    d. Antiprotozoal

222. With what type of diet should oral tetracyclines not be administered?
    a. High fat
    b. Low sodium
    c. High calcium
    d. Low potassium

223. Why should tetracycline use be avoided in pregnant bitches?
    a. It may cause changes in the joint cartilage that may result in arthritis at an older age in the pup.
    b. It may be deposited in dental enamel and give the pup's teeth a mottled yellow appearance.
    c. It may impair normal central nervous system development in the pups that may show up as behavioral changes later in life.
    d. It may damage the developing pups and may result in liver impairment later in life.

224. What is the effect of prostaglandin F_2 alpha on the reproductive system?
    a. Ovulation
    b. Luteolysis
    c. Follicle stimulation
    d. Corpus luteum formation

225. What drug readily penetrates the blood-brain barrier and achieves therapeutic concentrations of antibiotic in the central nervous system?
    a. Amoxicillin
    b. Enrofloxacin
    c. Oxytetracycline
    d. Chloramphenicol

226. Which drug will have a prolonged half-life when used with chloramphenicol?
   a. Phenobarbital
   b. Penicillin
   c. Sulfadimethoxine
   d. Tetracycline

227. Why is chloramphenicol used with extreme caution in cats and neonates?
   a. It can bind with dietary calcium and become deactivated.
   b. The liver is unable to metabolize chloramphenicol effectively in these animals.
   c. It can alter developing bone, enamel, and cartilage.
   d. It may drastically alter gut bacterial flora, resulting in fatal diarrhea.

228. What fatal reaction to chloramphenicol has been reported in cats and people?
   a. Kidney failure
   b. Aplastic anemia
   c. Pulmonary edema
   d. Liver failure

229. When are drugs such as sulfadimethoxine, sulfadiazine, and other sulfa drugs most likely to cause kidney problems?
   a. When an animal is receiving intravenous fluids and it has a diuretic effect on the kidneys
   b. When an animal is dehydrated
   c. When an animal has only one functional kidney
   d. When an animal has a bladder infection

230. What are trimethoprim and ormetoprim?
   a. Agents that are growth regulators
   b. Agents that enhance bactericidal activity of sulfonamides
   c. Agents that enhance the spectrum of the activity of penicillins
   d. Agents that reduce the risk of liver damage from hepatotoxic drugs

231. Within the past few years there have been reports of dogs having adverse reactions to sulfadiazine, which is a commonly used sulfonamide. What reaction should clients and veterinary professionals watch for?
   a. Cardiac arrest
   b. Sudden liver failure
   c. Decreased tear production
   d. Increased urination

232. What antibacterial drug is also effective against protozoa such as Giardia?
   a. Clindamycin
   b. Griseofulvin
   c. Metronidazole
   d. Monensin

233. Ketoconazole, miconazole, and griseofulvin are effective against:
   a. Viruses
   b. Flukes
   c. Intestinal nematodes
   d. Fungi

234. What drug is used intravenously to treat status epilepticus?
   a. Potassium bromide
   b. Levetiracetam
   c. Diazepam
   d. Phenobarbital

235. What anticonvulsant drug is converted by the liver primarily to phenobarbital, which accounts for most of its anticonvulsant activity?
   a. Diazepam
   b. Primidone
   c. Phenytoin
   d. Clonazepam

236. What traditional anticonvulsant is now being used simultaneously with phenobarbital in dogs that are nonresponsive to phenobarbital alone?
   a. Diazepam
   b. Potassium bromide
   c. Phenytoin
   d. Strychnine

237. What drug is a respiratory stimulant?
   a. Oxytocin
   b. Dobutamine
   c. Propranolol
   d. Doxapram

238. Drugs that effectively block the cough reflex are called:
   a. Mucolytics
   b. Expectorants
   c. Antitussives
   d. Decongestants

239. Drugs that reduce the viscosity of secretions in the respiratory tract are called:
   a. Anti-inflammatories
   b. Expectorants
   c. Antitussives
   d. Antihistamines

240. Drugs used to increase airflow, through respiratory passageways narrowed by the relaxation of smooth muscle around them, are called:
   a. Bronchodilators
   b. Expectorants
   c. Antitussives
   d. Antihistamines

241. Butorphanol and hydrocodone are examples of:
    a. Mucolytics
    b. Expectorants
    c. Antitussives
    d. Antihistamines

242. What effect do beta-receptor agonists have on the respiratory tree?
    a. Increase the volume of watery secretions
    b. Increase the volume of sticky mucoid secretions
    c. Cause bronchoconstriction
    d. Cause bronchodilatation

243. Terbutaline, albuterol, and metaproterenol are used in veterinary medicine to:
    a. Treat feline asthma or other bronchoconstrictive diseases
    b. Treat low blood pressure caused by shock
    c. Suppress a productive cough, such as in bronchopneumonia
    d. Stimulate secretions within the respiratory tree to aid the mucociliary apparatus

244. Methylxanthines are often used to improve breathing in cardiac patients and patients with respiratory disease. Which of the following drugs are methylxanthines used for this purpose?
    a. Theophylline and aminophylline
    b. Codeine and dextromethorphan
    c. Hydrocodone and butorphanol
    d. Guaifenesin and propranolol

245. Most drugs that control arrhythmias of the heart are said to be "negative inotropes." What does this mean?
    a. They increase the heart rate.
    b. They decrease the heart rate.
    c. They increase the force of contractions.
    d. They decrease the force of contractions.

246. What drug reduces tachyarrhythmias by blocking sodium and decreasing automaticity of the cardiac cells?
    a. Propranolol
    b. Lidocaine
    c. Procainamide
    d. Digoxin

247. Hyperthyroid cats have heart rates of more than 200 beats per minute because of the large numbers of alpha-1 sympathetic receptors in their hearts, which make the heart more sensitive to epinephrine and norepinephrine. This high heart rate is an anesthetic risk. What drug is used to slow the heart rate and decrease arrhythmias associated with alpha-1 receptor stimulation?
    a. Lidocaine
    b. Propranolol
    c. Quinidine
    d. Digoxin

248. Digoxin has a narrow therapeutic index. What does this mean?
    a. Plasma drug concentrations that produce toxicity are very low.
    b. Plasma drug concentrations required to achieve a beneficial effect are very high.
    c. Plasma drug concentrations that produce toxicity are very close to the minimum concentration at which a beneficial effect occurs.
    d. Plasma drug concentrations are extremely variable from animal to animal.

249. Because digoxin has a narrow therapeutic index, veterinary technicians and owners of animals that receive digoxin must be able to detect early signs of digoxin toxicity, such as:
    a. Increased urination and increased water consumption
    b. Increased coughing and difficulty breathing
    c. Decreased appetite, anorexia, diarrhea, and vomiting
    d. Wobbly gait, fainting (syncope), and disorientation

250. Some drugs commonly used to treat veterinary patients with cardiovascular disease alter the electrolyte levels (Na+, K+, Cl⁻) within the body. Which electrolyte change greatly enhances the risk of digoxin toxicity?
    a. Hypernatremia
    b. Hyperkalemia
    c. Hypochloremia
    d. Hypokalemia

251. What drug would be most effective against dermatophytes?
    a. Tylosin
    b. Enrofloxacin
    c. Sulfadimethoxine
    d. Itraconazole

252. Drugs classified as ACE inhibitors have what effect on the body?
    a. Increase the strength of heart contractions
    b. Cause vasodilatation
    c. Cause bronchodilatation
    d. Increase the heart rate

253. Captopril is an example of a(n):
    a. Positive inotrope
    b. Antiarrhythmic
    c. Bronchodilator
    d. Vasodilator

254. Nitroglycerin is sometimes used as a paste applied to the pinna or to the abdominal skin in dogs with cardiovascular disease. Nitroglycerin has what therapeutic effect?
    a. Increases strength of heart contractions
    b. Causes vasodilation
    c. Causes bronchodilation
    d. Decreases the heart rate

255. Spironolactone, chlorothiazide, and furosemide are classified as:
    a. Diuretics
    b. Positive inotropes
    c. Antiarrhythmics
    d. Vasodilators

256. What controlled substance rating indicates a drug with the greatest potential for abuse?
    a. C-III
    b. C-II
    c. C-V
    d. C-IV

257. For what reason is apomorphine used in canine patients in emergency veterinary medicine?
    a. To keep blood pressure elevated for animals in shock
    b. To alleviate pain
    c. To produce emesis after ingestion of a toxin
    d. To maintain kidney function during periods of reduced blood flow to the kidneys

258. What drug is most likely to be prescribed to prevent motion sickness?
    a. Apomorphine
    b. Maropitant
    c. Xylazine
    d. Diphenhydramine

259. For what is syrup of ipecac used?
    a. To stimulate defecation to flush out poisons from the distal bowel
    b. To induce vomiting
    c. To stimulate duodenal movement to overcome constipation
    d. To increase blood supply to the gastrointestinal tract

260. Why should apomorphine and activated charcoal not be given simultaneously?
    a. The resultant vomiting is too severe and too prolonged
    b. Each cancels the beneficial effects of the other
    c. The patient will vomit and may aspirate the charcoal
    d. Severe diarrhea and intestinal cramping result

261. What effect are anticholinergic drugs expected to have on the gastrointestinal tract?
    a. Increased secretions by the bowel
    b. Increased movement of feces through the bowel
    c. Decreased ability of compounds to irritate the bowel wall
    d. Decreased bowel motility

262. Bismuth subsalicylate is the active ingredient in a common over-the-counter (OTC) preparation used for some types of gastrointestinal disease, to what effect?
    a. Mild laxative
    b. Antiemetic
    c. Antidiarrheic
    d. Emetic

263. Nonsteroidal anti-inflammatory drugs (NSAIDs) often produce side effects in the gastrointestinal tract with long-term use or high-dosage use, especially in dogs. What are the side effects?
    a. Increased bowel motility, resulting in fluid diarrhea
    b. Decreased ability to digest fat, resulting in fatty stool (steatorrhea)
    c. Ulcers or gastritis from decreased mucus production
    d. Decreased bowel motility, resulting in constipation

264. Cimetidine and ranitidine are used as:
    a. Antidiarrheals
    b. Laxatives
    c. Rumen stimulants
    d. Antacids

265. What type of medication is sucralfate (Carafate)?
    a. Antiulcer
    b. Antidiarrheal
    c. Antibloat
    d. Anticonstipation

266. The drug most commonly used in treating animals with hypothyroidism is:
    a. Thyroid-stimulating hormone (TSH)
    b. Thyroid extract
    c. Synthetic levothyroxine (T$_4$)
    d. Synthetic liothyronine (T$_3$)

267. For what disease is methimazole used?
    a. Hypothyroidism in dogs
    b. Hyperadrenocorticism in dogs
    c. Hyperthyroidism in cats
    d. Hypoadrenocorticism in dogs

268. What drug is used to return a mare to proestrus from diestrus through lysis of the corpus luteum?
    a. Progesterone
    b. Estrogen
    c. Prostaglandin
    d. Gonadotropin

269. What hormone is given to mares or cows for several days to mimic diestrus and then withdrawn to mimic natural lysis of the corpus luteum and a return to proestrus?
    a. Estradiol cypionate
    b. Prostaglandin F$_2$ alpha
    c. Human chorionic gonadotropin
    d. Progestin

270. What drug is used as a contraceptive in dogs and sometimes for the correction of behavioral problems in cats (e.g., inappropriate urination)?
    a. Altrenogest
    b. Megestrol acetate
    c. Estradiol cypionate
    d. Dinoprost tromethamine

271. Which of the following is most likely to cause gastrointestinal ulcerations?
    a. Aspirin
    b. Deracoxib
    c. Carprofen
    d. Meloxicam

272. The glucocorticoid drug commonly used orally to treat immune-mediated diseases in dogs and cats is:
    a. Hydrocortisone
    b. Prednisone
    c. Triamcinolone
    d. Dexamethasone

273. Predictable, short-term side effects of glucocorticoid therapy of which every client should be aware include:
    a. Polyuria and polydipsia
    b. Cough and nasal discharge
    c. Anorexia and diarrhea
    d. Dry skin and skin irritations

274. Commonly used glucocorticoids affect the CBC. What are the effects of glucocorticoid use on the CBC?
    a. Neutrophils decreased, eosinophils increased, lymphocytes decreased
    b. Neutrophils increased, eosinophils increased, lymphocytes increased
    c. Neutrophils increased, eosinophils decreased, lymphocytes decreased
    d. Neutrophils decreased, eosinophils decreased, lymphocytes increased

275. Chronic administration of high doses of glucocorticoids can cause iatrogenic:
    a. Renal failure
    b. Addison disease
    c. Cushing disease
    d. Johne disease

276. In what species might dexamethasone administration lead to abortion during the last few weeks of gestation?
    a. Horses and cattle
    b. Pigs and dogs
    c. Dogs and cats
    d. Horses and cats

277. NSAIDs are most likely to cause side effects in what two organ systems?
    a. Renal and pulmonary
    b. Renal and gastrointestinal
    c. Pulmonary and cardiac
    d. Cardiac and hepatic

278. Which NSAID, when administered perivascularly in horses, can cause skin necrosis and sloughing?
    a. Phenylbutazone
    b. Etodolac
    c. Carprofen
    d. Meclofenamic acid

279. One of the following anti-inflammatory drugs is sometimes applied topically. Care must be taken to clean the area where it is applied because it readily penetrates the skin and can carry bacterial toxins or other chemicals with it into the body. What drug is this?
   a. Dexamethasone
   b. Dimethyl sulfoxide
   c. Flunixin meglumine
   d. Hydrocortisone

280. Which of these drugs most recently became controlled?
   a. Butorphanol
   b. Buprenorphine
   c. Fentanyl
   d. Tramadol

281. A drug's package insert states that the drug is an anticestodal. Against what type of parasite will this drug be effective?
   a. Ascarids (Toxocara, Toxascaris)
   b. Tapeworms (Taenia)
   c. Protozoa (Eimeria, Giardia)
   d. Flukes (liver fluke, lung fluke)

282. What breed of dog has a blood-brain barrier that allows ivermectin to reach toxic concentrations within the brain more readily than in other breeds?
   a. German shepherd
   b. Collie
   c. Schnauzer
   d. Cocker spaniel

283. What drug is used most commonly as a microfilaricide in the treatment of heartworm disease?
   a. Thiacetarsamide
   b. Melarsomine
   c. Ivermectin
   d. Piperazine

284. If an animal receives an overdose of organophosphate insecticide (from dips, powders, sprays), what is the treatment of choice?
   a. Diphenhydramine
   b. Corticosteroids
   c. Intravenous fluids
   d. Atropine

285. What insecticide is effective in treating demodectic mange?
   a. Fenoxycarb
   b. Amitraz
   c. Pyrethrin
   d. Allethrin

286. Methoprene and fenoxycarb are ingredients increasingly found in flea and other insect products. What are they?
   a. Insecticides
   b. Repellents
   c. Insect growth regulators
   d. Synergists

287. The following information was provided for a prescription written by a veterinarian: "Dr. Pete Bill, Veterinary Associates, Inc., 325 Sentry Highway, West Lafayette, IN 47907. Indiana License Number #4xxx. (317) 555-8636. For: Mr. R. K. Jones, 111, Melrose Place, Loomisville, IN 47905. Canine patient Ruby, Amoxicillin 100 mg tablets, Sig: 1 tab q8h po prn 2 refills. Date: 1/5/16. Signature: Pete Bill." What vital information is missing from this prescription?
   a. Veterinarian's Drug Enforcement Administration (DEA) license number
   b. Pet's name
   c. Owner's telephone number
   d. Number of tablets

288. The following information was provided for a prescription written by a veterinarian: "Canine patient, Amoxicillin 100 mg tablets, Sig: 1 tab q8h po prn 2 refills. Date: 1/5/16." In the prescription what does po mean?
   a. Administer every other day
   b. Administer by mouth
   c. Administer as needed
   d. Administer on an empty stomach

289. The following information was provided for a prescription written by a veterinarian: "Canine patient, Amoxicillin 100 mg tablets, Sig: 1 tab q8h po prn 2 refills. Date: 1/5/16." How many times a day is this medication to be given?
   a. Once
   b. Twice
   c. Three times
   d. Four times

290. The following information was provided for a prescription written by a veterinarian: "Canine patient, Amoxicillin 100 mg tablets, Sig: 1 tab q8h po prn 2 refills. Date: 1/5/16." What does prn mean?
   a. Administer every other day
   b. Administer by mouth
   c. Administer as needed
   d. Administer on an empty stomach

291. The abbreviations od and os on a prescription refer to:
    a. Administer by mouth and by rectum
    b. Right eye and left eye
    c. Administer every other day and every 3 days
    d. Administer with food and without food

292. What do 15 gr and 10 g mean on a prescription?
    a. 15 grains and 10 grams
    b. 15 grains and 10 grains
    c. 15 grams and 10 grams
    d. 15 grams and 10 grains

293. Most pharmaceutical agents that are measured in grains have how many milligrams per grain?
    a. 32.4
    b. 64.8
    c. 100
    d. 120

294. Which of the following is a concentration of a drug solution?
    a. 15 mg/kg
    b. 1000 U/mL
    c. 20 gr/mg
    d. 250 g/lb

295. How many milliliters are in a teaspoon?
    a. 1
    b. 3
    c. 5
    d. 10

296. How many cubic centimeters are in a tablespoon?
    a. 5
    b. 15
    c. 25
    d. 30

297. Which equivalent is correct?
    a. q12h = QD
    b. q6h = QID
    c. q4h = TID
    d. q8h = BID

298. A 10-kg animal weighs how many pounds?
    a. 2
    b. 15
    c. 18
    d. 22

299. What dosage form must be shaken before administration to an animal?
    a. Solution
    b. Ointment
    c. Gel
    d. Suspension

300. When a drug is used by an alternative route in a species, or for an indication other than what is specified by the manufacturer, this use is termed:
    a. A felony offense
    b. An extra-label use
    c. Prohibited by the AVMA
    d. An implied consent from the manufacturer

301. Each drug approved for use in food-producing animals has a time period given on the label between the last dose and when the animal can be slaughtered for food or when the milk can be sold. What is this period called?
    a. Half-life period
    b. Secretion period
    c. Refractory period
    d. Withdrawal period

302. Sometimes drugs are first administered in a large dose and then given as a series of smaller doses. What is the first dose called?
    a. Initial dose
    b. Loading dose
    c. Distribution dose
    d. Bolus dose

303. Many drugs do not have X mg/mL listed on their labels but instead have their concentrations listed as a percent (e.g., X% solution). Which of the following most accurately reflects the conversion of a percentage of a solution to a weight per volume format?
    a. X% = X g/mL
    b. X% = X g/10 mL
    c. X% = X g/100 mL
    d. X% = X mg/10 mL

304. How many milligrams are in each milliliter of a 24% solution?
    a. 24
    b. 2.4
    c. 240
    d. 0.24

305. What class of drugs generally poses the greatest potential health threat to those handling the medication?
    a. Antibiotic
    b. Antineoplastic
    c. Antinematodal
    d. Antiprotozoal

306. What effect does renal failure or compromised liver function have on the pharmacokinetics of many drugs?
    a. Decreased absorption of drugs given orally
    b. Increased elimination rate of drugs from the body
    c. Decreased volume of distribution of drugs
    d. Increased half-life of drugs

307. Controlled substances are drugs that:
    a. Cannot be used in any animal intended for use as human food
    b. Have a high potential for abuse
    c. Are very hazardous to anyone handling them
    d. Are environmentally hazardous

308. Drugs that are administered intra-articularly are injected into the:
    a. Bone marrow
    b. Subdural space
    c. Heart
    d. Joint

309. Extravasation of a chemotherapeutic agent should first be treated by:
    a. Applying a tourniquet to prevent movement of the drug up the leg
    b. Infiltrating the area with sterile saline or another sterile isotonic fluid
    c. Withdrawing as much drug as possible from the intravenous catheter
    d. Stopping the injection

310. Generally, 1 fluid ounce is equal to approximately how many milliliters of liquid?
    a. 1
    b. 15
    c. 30
    d. 60

311. Which of the following interferes with the development of an insect's chitin?
    a. Griseofulvin
    b. Lufenuron
    c. Methoprene
    d. Spinosad

312. The trade name for diphenhydramine is:
    a. Benadryl
    b. Prozac
    c. Dulcolax
    d. Panacur

313. Which of the following will not be used to decrease the potassium in a cat with a urethral obstruction?
    a. Calcium gluconate
    b. Dextrose
    c. Insulin
    d. Sodium bicarbonate

314. Which of the following medications was approved for use in the United States in 2014 and is being compared to propofol?
    a. Alfaxalone
    b. Etomidate
    c. Thiopental
    d. Telazol

315. Malignant hyperthermia is a possible side effect of which of the following?
    a. Etomidate
    b. Fentanyl
    c. Halothane
    d. Propofol

316. The specific treatment for malignant hyperthermia is:
    a. Dexmedetomidine
    b. Dantrolene
    c. Diazepam
    d. Acepromazine

317. Diffusion of drug molecules across the cell membrane that does not require energy, and is a result of a difference in the concentration of that drug on the inside side of the cell versus the outside, is called:
    a. Active transport
    b. Diffusive transport
    c. Passive transport
    d. Facilitated transport

318. Maropitant is the active ingredient in:
    a. Carafate
    b. Cerenia
    c. Flagyl
    d. Reglan

319. What can be done to decrease the risk of esophageal lesions in cats secondary to oral medications?
    a. Do not give oral medications
    b. Crush the medications
    c. Advise the owner to bring in the cat for medicating
    d. Follow the medication with water

320. Lidocaine is in which cardiac drug class?
    a. IA
    b. II
    c. IV
    d. IB

321. Which fibers in the central nervous system are responsible for sharp, localized pain?
    a. A
    b. A delta
    c. C
    d. C delta

322. Cyclooxygenase-1 (COX-1) is associated with:
    a. Blood flow to the kidney
    b. Healing
    c. Inflammation
    d. Pain

323. Which of the following will decrease the efficacy of lidocaine when used to address cardiac arrhythmias?
    a. Hypocalcemia
    b. Hypochloremia
    c. Hypokalemia
    d. Hyponatremia

324. A drug's tendency to bind to a receptor is called its:
    a. Affinity
    b. Efficacy
    c. Specificity
    d. Effective dose

325. Transport of a drug molecule that occurs when the majority of the cell surrounds the molecule, engulfs it, and brings it into the cell is referred to as:
    a. Facilitated
    b. Passive
    c. Phagocytosis
    d. Pinocytosis

326. Carprofen is the active ingredient in:
    a. Deramaxx
    b. Previcox
    c. Metacam
    d. Rimadyl

327. Cyclooxygenase-2 (COX-2) is associated with:
    a. Blood flow to the kidney
    b. Maintenance of the gastric mucosa
    c. Inflammation
    d. Normal physiological function

328. Furosemide is the active ingredient in:
    a. Lasix
    b. Osmitrol
    c. Aldactone
    d. HydroDIURIL

329. Which of the following is associated with central nervous signs if it is overdosed?
    a. Carprofen
    b. Chloramphenicol
    c. Furosemide
    d. Metronidazole

330. Levetiracetam is the active ingredient in:
    a. Keppra
    b. Valium
    c. Luminal
    d. Zonegran

331. The mode of action in which Enrofloxacin works by is:
    a. Inhibiting cell wall synthesis
    b. Inhibiting DNA
    c. Inhibiting protein synthesis
    d. Inhibiting the metabolic pathway

332. Diffusion of a drug molecule that involves a carrier protein but does not require energy is known as:
    a. Facilitated
    b. Passive
    c. Active
    d. Pinocytosis

333. The veterinarian asks you to fill metronidazole 250 mgs po BID for 6 days. You have 500 mg tablets in stock. How many tablets will you fill?
    a. 3
    b. 6
    c. 12
    d. 24

334. Baytril is the trade name for:
    a. Acepromazine
    b. Cephalexin
    c. Enrofloxacin
    d. Gabapentin

335. With regard to the plasma concentration of a drug, what is the highest point in the concentration called?
    a. Peak
    b. Max
    c. Trough
    d. Min

336. What does it mean when a drug is at a steady state?
    a. The owner is giving the drug on a regular basis
    b. The patient is responding as expected
    c. The peak and trough are steady
    d. The patient has been on the drug more then 6 months

337. In a dog with a bite wound on the forelimb, which of the following will increase blood flow and thus delivery of a drug to the area of interest?
    a. Acute inflammation
    b. Shock
    c. Necrosis
    d. Hemorrhage

338. Metronidazole is the active ingredient in:
    a. Carafate
    b. Cerenia
    c. Flagyl
    d. Reglan

339. A patient is hospitalized for vomiting and diarrhea. The doctor orders metronidazole to be given BID. What is the most likely route the doctor will use?
    a. PO
    b. IV
    c. IM
    d. SQ

340. How long should a patient with pneumonia be on antibiotics?
    a. Two weeks past resolution of clinical signs
    b. Two weeks past resolution of radiographic signs
    c. Four weeks, no matter the clinical or radiographic signs
    d. Six weeks, no matter the clinical or radiographic signs

341. Why are prophylactic antibiotics given during surgery?
    a. To prevent contamination when the skin is entered
    b. To prevent contamination when a hollow viscous is entered
    c. To prevent contamination from the surgeon
    d. To prevent contamination from the instruments

342. Reglan is the trade name for:
    a. Metronidazole
    b. Dolasetron
    c. Maropitant
    d. Metoclopramide

343. After surgery has begun, how often should antibiotics be administered?
    a. Every 15–30 minutes
    b. Every 30–60 minutes
    c. Every 60–90 minutes
    d. Every 90–120 minutes

344. Of the following drugs, which must be in an anaerobic environment to be effective?
    a. Chloramphenicol
    b. Clindamycin
    c. Metronidazole
    d. Neomycin

345. Which of the following is generally used for infections not susceptible to other antibiotics?
    a. First-tier antibiotics
    b. Second-tier antibiotics
    c. Third-tier antibiotics
    d. Negative-tier antibiotics

346. An owner gives you a list of products and asks you which is most likely to prevent her dog from acquiring Rocky Mountain spotted fever. What would you advise her?
    a. Advantix
    b. Heartgard
    c. Revolution
    d. Interceptor

347. Which drug listed belongs in the drug class imidazole?
    a. Amoxicillin
    b. Cephalexin
    c. Enrofloxacin
    d. Ketoconazole

348. Which of the following is most likely to be used against *Malassezia*?
    a. Griseofulvin
    b. Itraconazole
    c. Metronidazole
    d. Tetracycline

349. Acylovir is an:
    a. Antibacterial
    b. Antifungal
    c. Antiparasitic
    d. Antiviral

350. Which of the following should be avoided or at least diluted out 1:100 when cleaning an ear?
    a. Chlorhexidine
    b. Saline solution
    c. Vinegar and water
    d. Cleaning solution

351. In response to hyperkalemia, calcium gluconate will:
    a. Cause potassium to move into the cell
    b. Increase urination to excrete potassium
    c. Protect the heart from the effects of the potassium
    d. Cause potassium to move out of the cell

352. Of the following antibiotics, which one is best suited to treat tetanus caused by *Clostridium tetani*?
    a. Enrofloxacin
    b. Metronidazole
    c. Neomycin
    d. Penicillin G

353. Cardiac drugs that belong in class IA act by:
    a. Stabilizing myocardial cells
    b. Blocking beta receptors
    c. Decreasing myocardial automaticity
    d. Blocking calcium channels

354. Propranolol is a:
    a. Beta-1 blocker
    b. Beta-2 blocker
    c. A nonselective beta blocker
    d. Not a beta blocker

355. Which drug class does diltiazem belong in?
    a. Beta-1 blocker
    b. Beta-2 blocker
    c. Calcium channel blocker
    d. Sodium channel blocker

356. Which of the following drugs can be used to increase platelet numbers?
    a. Chlorambucil
    b. Doxorubicin
    c. Vinblastine
    d. Vincristine

357. Which of the following products will provide oxygen-carrying capacity?
    a. Cryoprecipitate
    b. Fresh frozen plasma
    c. Frozen plasma
    d. Oxyglobin

358. The doctor ordered a patient to receive Unasyn, 1200 mg IV. After reconstitution, the Unasyn has a concentration of 375 mg/mL. How many mL will you administer?
    a. 0.31 mL
    b. 1.2 mL
    c. 3.2 mL
    d. 6.4 mL

359. How many half-lives does a drug go through before reaching a steady state?
    a. 2
    b. 3
    c. 4
    d. 5

360. The doctor asks you to fill oral metronidazole, 10 mg/kg po BID for 7 days. The dog weighs 37.5 kg and you have 250-mg tablets available in the hospital. How many tablets do you fill?
    a. 7
    b. 14
    c. 21
    d. 42

361. Cardiac drugs that belong in class IB act by:
    a. Stabilizing myocardial cells
    b. Blocking beta receptors
    c. Decreasing myocardial automaticity
    d. Blocking calcium channels

362. Of the fluids listed, which has the lowest sodium content?
    a. 0.9% NaCl
    b. D5W
    c. 0.45% NaCl
    d. Lactated ringers

363. The doctor orders a dose of calcium gluconate be administered to a patient. In addition to drawing up the medication, what other procedure should you prepare for?
    a. To monitor an EKG
    b. To monitor the BP
    c. To monitor the SpO2
    d. To monitor the temperature

364. The transport mechanism requiring a carrier protein that also requires energy is called:
    a. Facilitated
    b. Passive
    c. Active
    d. Pinocytosis

365. What type of fluid is Hetastarch considered?
    a. Blood product
    b. Crystalloid
    c. Natural colloid
    d. Synthetic colloid

366. Potassium-sparing diuretics, such as Spirolactone, act on what part of the kidneys?
    a. Loop of Henle
    b. Collecting duct
    c. Proximal tubule
    d. Bowman capsule

367. Esmolol is:
    a. A nonselective beta blocker
    b. A beta-1 blocker
    c. A beta-2 blocker
    d. Not a beta blocker

368. The doctor expresses concern that a patient's cardiac output is poor and he is considering something to increase the contractility of the heart. You know he will want to use a:
    a. Positive inotrope
    b. Negative inotrope
    c. Positive chronotrope
    d. Negative chronotrope

369. The doctor asks you to fill acepromazine, 50 mg po TID for seven days. You have 25-mg tablets available in the hospital. How many tablets do you fill?
    a. 14
    b. 21
    c. 28
    d. 42

370. Cardiac drugs that belong in class II act by:
    a. Stabilizing myocardial cells
    b. Blocking beta receptors
    c. Decreasing myocardial automaticity
    d. Blocking calcium channels

371. Which of the following processes will decrease the efficacy of an antibiotic in a dog with a bite wound on the forelimb?
    a. Acute inflammation
    b. Shock
    c. Necrosis
    d. Chronic inflammation

372. Cisapride is a(n):
    a. Antiemetic
    b. Prokinetic
    c. GI protectant
    d. Antidiarrheal

373. What condition does dirlotapide treat?
    a. Obesity in dogs
    b. Obesity in cats
    c. Anorexia in dogs
    d. Anorexia in cats

374. Ondansetron is an antiemetic that belongs in which drug class?
    a. Anticholinergic
    b. Barbiturate
    c. Phenothiazine
    d. Serotonin antagonist

375. Lactulose can be given to a patient with a portosystemic shunt to help:
    a. Decrease gastrointestinal transit time
    b. Convert ammonia to ammonium
    c. Prevent diarrhea
    d. Prevent water loss though the colon

376. The drug that treats autoimmune diseases and pruritus associated with atopic dermatitis is known as:
    a. Cyclosporine
    b. Interferon omega
    c. Ketoconazole
    d. Phytosphingosine

377. Atopica is the brand name for:
    a. Anzemet
    b. Cyclosporine
    c. Dolasetron
    d. Furosemide

378. Which of the following is a benzodiazepine tranquilizer?
    a. Fentanyl
    b. Ketamine
    c. Medetomidine
    d. Midazolam

379. Which type of diuretic is used to treat increased intracranial pressure?
    a. Loop
    b. Osmotic
    c. Potassium-sparing
    d. Thiazide

380. Which of the following medications is an opioid?
    a. Buprenorphine
    b. Carprofen
    c. Lidocaine
    d. Naloxone

381. The doctor orders a patient to receive a CRI of fentanyl. How often will this drug be administered?
    a. Every 2 hr
    b. Every 4 hr
    c. Every 6 hr
    d. At a constant rate

382. Which of the following drugs is a synthetic analog of codeine?
    a. Dextromethorphan
    b. Gabapentin
    c. Methocarbamol
    d. Tramadol

383. You are placing an intravenous catheter to administer chemotherapy. When placing the catheter you go through the vein, but you are able to reposition it and place it successfully. What should you do next?
    a. Use the catheter, but monitor it closely during the injection
    b. Pull the catheter and place it in a different vein
    c. Pull the catheter and place it higher up in the same vein
    d. Use it without concern

384. L-asparaginase, a chemotherapeutic, is used most commonly for:
    a. Hemangiosarcoma
    b. Mast cell tumors
    c. Lymphoma
    d. Osteosarcoma

385. A solution that contains so much solute that it cannot be dissolved is known as:
    a. Concentrated
    b. Dilute
    c. Saturated
    d. Supersaturated

386. Regarding the concentration of a solution, molality is known as:
    a. The number of moles per liter of solution
    b. The amount of solute per kilogram of solvent
    c. The grams per liter of solution
    d. The number of solute particles per liter

387. The doctor asks you to start a fentanyl CRI at 3 mcg/kg/hr in a 50-kg dog. The fentanyl you have available in the hospital is 50 mcg/mL. What will the rate per hour be?
    a. 1 mL/hr
    b. 3 mL/hr
    c. 5 mL/hr
    d. 50 mL/hr

388. Which injectable anesthetic is not recommended in patients with neurological disease?
    a. Barbiturates
    b. Etomidate
    c. Ketamine
    d. Propofol

389. Which of the following antiseizure medications should be avoided in a patient with existing liver disease?
    a. Levetiracetam
    b. Phenobarbital
    c. Potassium bromide
    d. Gabapentin

390. Which of the following anesthetics has the fewest cardiorespiratory effects?
    a. Etomidate
    b. Propofol
    c. Ketamine
    d. Thiopental

391. Methocarbamol is labeled as an adjunctive therapy for:
    a. Seizures
    b. Skeletal muscle trauma
    c. Increased intracranial pressure
    d. Joint pain

392. What medication can be used to confirm a diagnosis of acquired myasthenia gravis?
    a. Acepromazine
    b. Metoclopramide
    c. Tensilon
    d. Theophylline

393. Bloat-Pac is indicated for frothy bloat in:
    a. Cattle
    b. Dogs
    c. Pigs
    d. Horses

394. Which of the following should never be used in cats?
    a. Carboplatin
    b. Hydroxyurea
    c. 5-Fluorouracil
    d. Procarbazine

395. Robaxin-V is the brand name for:
    a. Gabapentin
    b. Methocarbamol
    c. Methimazole
    d. Methionine (S-Adenosyl)

396. Cardiac drugs that belong in class IV act by:
    a. Stabilizing myocardial cells
    b. Blocking beta receptors
    c. Decreasing myocardial automaticity
    d. Blocking calcium channels

397. Antibiotics should be administered when abdominal surgery is longer than:
    a. 30 minutes
    b. 60 minutes
    c. 90 minutes
    d. 120 minutes

398. The doctor asks you to administer 5 g of 25% mannitol to a patient. How many mL do you give?
    a. 5 mL
    b. 20 mL
    c. 40 mL
    d. 25 mL

399. Which of the following drugs is most likely to require therapeutic drug monitoring?
    a. Enrofloxacin
    b. Metoclopramide
    c. Metronidazole
    d. Phenobarbital

400. An aerotolerant organism is one that:
    a. Is not affected by the presence or absence of oxygen
    b. Can tolerate elevated temperatures
    c. Prefers an environment that is dehydrated
    d. Is tolerant of environments lacking moisture

401. Some bacteria have an outer layer defined as a biopolymer matrix. This layer is called the:
    a. Cell wall
    b. Biofilm
    c. Matrix layer
    d. Bio layer

402. The mechanism of action of beta-lactams is interference with:
    a. Cell wall synthesis
    b. Protein synthesis
    c. The uptake of nutrients
    d. DNA synthesis

403. The doctor would like to start a patient on a drug that increases gastrointestinal motility. He would like to be able to add it to the intravenous fluids and also to send the dog home with an oral dose on discharge. Which drug fulfills these criteria?
    a. Diphenhydramine
    b. Dolasetron
    c. Maropitant
    d. Metoclopramide

404. One method of resistance to sulfonamides is through the bacteria's ability to:
    a. Survive without folic acid
    b. Use the host's folic acid
    c. Produce a substitute for folic acid
    d. Turn the antibiotic into folic acid

405. Macrolides inhibit bacterial ribosomal action by binding which subunit?
    a. 30s
    b. 40s
    c. 50s
    d. 60s

406. A drug that requires biotransformation before it becomes active is called a:
    a. Pretransformed drug
    b. Nonactive drug
    c. Predrug
    d. Prodrug

407. When discharging a cat, you would explain to the owner that the buprenorphine should be given:
    a. po
    b. SQ
    c. TM
    d. IM

408. Which of the following drugs minimally crosses the placental barrier and is safe to use in pregnant dogs?
    a. Acepromazine
    b. Atropine
    c. Fentanyl
    d. Glycopyrrolate

409. In geriatric patients, drug doses are generally:
    a. The same as in puppies
    b. Decreased
    c. Increased
    d. The same as in adults

410. Which of the following can increase the risk of digoxin toxicity?
    a. Hypokalemia
    b. Hypochloremia
    c. Hyponatremia
    d. Hypocalcemia

411. While drawing up injectable Amikacin for a patient, you note that it has developed a pale yellow color. What should you do?
    a. Discard the rest of the bottle
    b. Don't be concerned because you know this can be normal
    c. Dilute it with saline
    d. Dilute it with sterile water

412. When applying nitroglycerin ointment, it is important to wear gloves and:
    a. Wash it off after it has had contact with the patient for 5 minutes
    b. Avoid placing it directly on the skin
    c. Make a note where it was placed
    d. Make sure it is placed thickly in a small area

413. Low molecular weight heparin is different from unfractionated heparin in that it:
    a. Is less pure than unfractionated heparin
    b. Does not block the activity of thrombin whereas unfractionated heparin does
    c. Is less expensive than unfractionated heparin
    d. Is more likely to cause hemorrhage than unfractionated heparin

414. Plavix is the brand name for:
    a. Clopidogrel
    b. Nitroprusside
    c. Sildenafil
    d. Tadalafil

415. An oral antiarrhythmic that includes an action similar to injectable propranolol is:
    a. Hydralazine
    b. Pimobendan
    c. Prazosin
    d. Sotalol

416. Which of the following drugs can be used for atrial fibrillation?
    a. Digoxin
    b. Hydralazine
    c. Lidocaine
    d. Pimobendan

417. What can be used in the hospital, given IV, to increase a patient's phosphorus?
    a. Amphojel
    b. Dexamethasone sodium phosphate
    c. Potassium phosphate
    d. Tums

418. Feline asthma can be treated with:
    a. Amphotericin B
    b. Digoxin
    c. Hydralazine
    d. Terbutaline

419. Aminophylline is known as a:
    a. Bronchodilator
    b. Decongestant
    c. Expectorant
    d. Mucolytic

420. Which of the following is not absorbed systemically?
    a. Diphenhydramine
    b. Dolasetron
    c. Sucralfate
    d. Tramadol

421. Tums can be administered to supplement:
    a. Calcium
    b. Vitamin B
    c. Vitamin C
    d. Vitamin E

422. Vitamin B_1 is:
    a. Ascorbic acid
    b. Cyanocobalamin
    c. Riboflavin
    d. Thiamine

423. Which of the following is used to increase calcium uptake from the gastrointestinal tract, mobilize calcium from the bone, and conserve calcium from the kidneys?
    a. Alendronate
    b. Calcitonin
    c. Calcitriol
    d. Calcimimetics

424. What species should receive prednisolone instead of prednisone?
    a. Cats
    b. Cows
    c. Dogs
    d. Swine

425. The doctor would like to place a patient on a metoclopramide CRI at 2 mg/kg/day. He would like this added to a 1-L bag of fluids that will last 24 hr. The patient weighs 20 kg. How many mL of 5-mg/mL metoclopramide should be added to the bag?
    a. 2 mL
    b. 8 mL
    c. 20 mL
    d. 40 mL

426. Which of the following can be used to decrease intraocular volume (via dehydration of the vitreous humor) as treatment for glaucoma?
    a. Mannitol
    b. Methazolamide
    c. Pilocarpine
    d. Timolol

427. Because administration of medications via this route has more potential for adverse effects, what type of injection should be given slowly?
    a. IP
    b. IV
    c. IM
    d. SQ

428. What is the maximum rate at which you can administer IV potassium?
    a. 0.9 mEq/kg/hr
    b. 1.0 mEq/kg/hr
    c. 0.5 mEq/kg/hr
    d. 0.7 mEq/kg/hr

429. When a patient has received a spinal epidural, which of the following must be monitored closely?
    a. Appetite
    b. Attitude
    c. Urination
    d. Walking

430. Which of the following is primarily used as a sedative that can also be used to increase the duration of an epidural?
    a. Bupivacaine
    b. Dexmedetomidine
    c. Hydromorphone
    d. Morphine

431. What can be used to decrease the damage caused by reperfusion injury?
    a. Bupivacaine
    b. Lidocaine
    c. Marcaine
    d. Procaine

432. Glucosamine/Chondroitin is a nutraceutical that is used to treat:
    a. Anemia
    b. Arthritis
    c. Pruritus
    d. Urinary incontinence

433. What antibiotic also has anti-inflammatory actions in the gastrointestinal tract?
    a. Ciprofloxacin
    b. Enrofloxacin
    c. Metronidazole
    d. Tetracycline

434. Because sucralfate is more effective in an acidic environment, it should be administered before:
    a. Cisapride
    b. Famotidine
    c. Lactulose
    d. Metoclopramide

435. The doctor asks you to perform a local block on a patient in preparation for a laceration repair. You know you should not exceed a dose of:
    a. 2–4 mg/kg
    b. 4–6 mg/kg
    c. 6–8 mg/kg
    d. 8–10 mg/kg

436. Which of the following cannot be phoned in to the pharmacy and will require a written prescription?
    a. Buprenorphine
    b. Diazepam
    c. Morphine
    d. Phenobarbital

437. Vetmedin is the brand name for:
    a. Atenolol
    b. Pimobendan
    c. Procainamide
    d. Quinidine

438. Lidocaine can be diluted with sodium bicarbonate to decrease pain associated with injection. What should this dilution be (sodium bicarbonate: lidocaine)?
    a. 1:1
    b. 1:4
    c. 1:5
    d. 1:9

439. Which of the following will have the longest duration of action when used as an epidural?
    a. Bupivacaine
    b. Butorphanol
    c. Ketamine
    d. Morphine

440. Alpha-tocopherol is also known as:
    a. Vitamin E
    b. Vitamin D_2
    c. Vitamin D_3
    d. Vitamin B_2

441. DMSO should not be used in patients with:
    a. Hemangiosarcoma
    b. Lymphoma
    c. Mast cell tumors
    d. Osteosarcoma

442. A vaccine that produces immunity to a toxin is called a:
    a. Live
    b. Modified live
    c. Recombinant
    d. Toxoid

443. An example of a semisolid dosage form is:
    a. Implant
    b. Injectable
    c. Ointment
    d. Syrup

444. Which of the following can affect drug absorption, distribution, metabolism, and elimination?
a. Cardiac disease
b. Kidney disease
c. Liver disease
d. Pancreatic disease

445. Idiosyncratic drug reactions are those that are:
a. Predictable
b. Unpredictable
c. Synchronized with other reactions
d. Unsynchronized with other reactions

446. Regarding the storage of drugs, room temperature (in Fahrenheit) falls in the range of:
a. Less than 46°
b. 46°–59°
c. 60°–68°
d. 87°–104°

447. Which of the following drugs can become inactivated by shaking?
a. Amoxicillin
b. Clavamox
c. Insulin
d. Metronidazole

448. Which drug is preferred over Atropine for use in rabbits, because Atropine is less predictable in this species?
a. Acepromazine
b. Glycopyrrolate
c. Diazepam
d. a and b

449. Midazolam can be administered to rabbits in all of the following methods, *except:*
a. Intraperitoneal
b. Intramuscular
c. Intravenous
d. Subcutaneous

450. Yohimbine can be used to reverse all of the following alpha-2 adrenoreceptor agonists, *except:*
a. Xylazine
b. Medetomidine
c. Midazolam
d. Dexmedetomidine

451. Atipamezole, when administered SC to rabbits, can reverse the effects of medetomidine within:
a. 2–5 minutes
b. 5–10 minutes
c. 10–25 minutes
d. 25–30 minutes

452. Anticholinergic drugs are used for:
a. Tachycardia
b. Tachypenia
c. Bradycardia
d. Bradypnea

ⓔ *Answers and rationales available on Evolve*
http://evolve.elsevier.com/Prendergast/QAvettech/

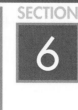
Surgical Nursing

Marianne Tear, MS, LVT

QUESTIONS

1. If during surgery you notice an item at the edge of a sterile field, you should:
   a. Ask others to find out whether it was contaminated
   b. Consider it unsterile if you are not absolutely certain
   c. Consider it sterile
   d. Move it further into the sterile field

2. What type of instrument is a Kelly?
   a. Needle holder
   b. Scissors
   c. Towel clamp
   d. Hemostatic forceps

3. Which of the following suffixes is used to describe the surgical alteration of a shape or form?
   a. *-pexy*
   b. *-plasty*
   c. *-ostomy*
   d. *-rrhapy*

4. What agent, method, or device is most appropriate for sterilizing a needle holder to be used in a surgical procedure?
   a. Autoclave
   b. Dry heat
   c. Ethylene oxide gas
   d. Liquid chemical disinfectant

5. What is the significance of an autoclave that will not properly seal, but still has steam rising from it?
   a. Because it is the sterilizing agent, it will work fine, but you must be more cautious to prevent burns to personnel
   b. The pressure is what kills the microbes, and thus the autoclave will not work
   c. It will continue to sterilize but will require more water as the steam escapes
   d. The pressure will not increase, which is required to meet the minimum temperature for sterilization

6. When attaching an ECG, which leg should have the red lead attached to it?
   a. Right foreleg
   b. Left foreleg
   c. Right hind leg
   d. Left hind leg

7. Preparing a patient's skin for surgery:
   a. Renders the skin sterile
   b. Does nothing to affect the outcome of the surgery
   c. Reduces the bacterial flora to a level that can be controlled by the patient's immune system
   d. Is not necessary if antibiotics are administered

8. During a surgical procedure, which of the following does not have to be sterile to maintain aseptic technique?
   a. Mask
   b. Drapes
   c. Instruments
   d. Gloves

9. The effectiveness of a surgical scrub on the hands and arms with an antibacterial soap depends on the:
   a. Combination of contact time and scrubbing action
   b. Amount of soap used throughout the scrub
   c. Scrubbing action of the brush
   d. Temperature of the water

10. Which statement regarding first-intention wound healing is false?
    a. It occurs without infection
    b. It occurs when the skin edges are held together in apposition
    c. It usually has some degree of suppuration
    d. It occurs with minimal scar formation

11. Which of the following statements about electrocautery is false?
    a. If the patient is not properly grounded, the surgeon may receive a shock
    b. The intensity of the current passed through the unit is adjustable
    c. Small bleeding blood vessels are sealed with a controlled electrical current that burns the bleeding end
    d. All portions of the electrocautery unit can and should be sterilized

12. What is the size of a scalpel blade used for making an abdominal skin incision in a dog?
    a. No. 10
    b. No. 11
    c. No. 12
    d. No. 15

13. Before starting the surgical procedure, the technician who has scrubbed in with the surgeon should do all of the following, *except:*
    a. Count the gauze sponges in the pack
    b. Arrange the instruments to be located quickly and easily
    c. Place the scalpel blade on the handle
    d. Open the suture material

14. An ovariohysterectomy might be performed for all of the following reasons, *except:*
    a. Prevention of prostate cancer
    b. Prevention of pyometra
    c. Sterilization of the animal
    d. Prevention of estrus

15. Place the following surgeries in the order in which they should be scheduled, from first to last:
    a. Cruciate repair, OHE, compound fracture repair, intestinal resection
    b. Intestinal resection, cruciate repair, compound fracture repair, OHE
    c. Compound fracture repair, cruciate repair, OHE, intestinal resection
    d. Cruciate repair, compound fracture repair, OHE, intestinal resection.

16. If an animal goes home with a bandage, the client should observe the bandage daily and remove it if any of the following are observed, *except:*
    a. Skin irritation at the edge of the bandage
    b. All bandages should be removed 24 hours after being applied
    c. The bandage is wet
    d. The position of the bandage has shifted

17. Which of the following is *not* true about dogs that are spayed before their first estrous cycle?
    a. The hair coat will change and become easier to manage with less shedding
    b. The surgery is generally considered easier to perform if the bitch has not been through an estrous cycle
    c. Mammary cancer is less likely to occur in a bitch that has been spayed before her first estrous cycle
    d. The uterus and ovaries enlarge after the first estrous cycle. This necessitates a larger abdominal incision when the bitch is spayed

18. Which of the following statements regarding pyometra is false?
    a. The bitch that goes to surgery will have the ovaries and uterus removed.
    b. The bitch that goes to surgery will have only her uterus removed.
    c. The uterus might have ruptured before surgery begins.
    d. The patient represents a high-risk anesthesia case, because other organs in the body might be compromised.

19. All of the following statements regarding cesarean sections are true, *except:*
    a. After the newborns are removed, the mother is out of danger, and most of the technician's attention should be on the newborns.
    b. A cesarean section is also known as a *hysterotomy.*
    c. For some breeds of dogs, such as the English bulldog, it is expected that a cesarean section will need to be performed.
    d. Wait to place the mother with the newborns until after she has adequately recovered from anesthesia.

20. Which of the following statements regarding cesarean sections is false?
    a. Bloody vaginal discharge is expected following surgery.
    b. The newborns delivered by cesarean section are under the effects of anesthesia.
    c. The client should observe the surgical incision starting after 1 week, because the newborns don't start moving around the mammary area until then.
    d. The newborn should be immediately removed from the membranous sac that covers its body when it is removed from the uterus.

21. When a male dog is presented to the hospital for a castration procedure, the technician should do all of the following, *except:*
    a. Ensure that the dog is a male.
    b. Ensure that there are two testicles in the scrotum.
    c. Ensure that the dog is not in heat.
    d. Ensure that there is a telephone number to reach the client.

22. All of the following are benefits to having a peripheral IV catheter placed in advance of surgery, *except* for:
    a. Administering anesthesia
    b. Administering emergency drugs in case of anesthetic complications
    c. Administering intravenous fluids
    d. Administering enteral nutrition

23. When a bitch is presented to the hospital for an ovariohysterectomy, the technician should do all of the following *except:*
    a. Ensure the dog is a female
    b. Obtain a telephone number where the client can be reached that day
    c. Ensure that the bitch does not have an abdominal scar
    d. Give the dog aspirin, because the surgical procedure will be painful

24. Clipper burn can cause all of the following adverse effects *except:*
    a. Excessive licking of the area
    b. Follicular damage preventing hair regrowth
    c. Inhibition of wound healing
    d. Promotion of bacteria growth

25. When a dog is presented for castration, and both testicles are descended, the veterinary technician will prepare the surgical site. In which area is the incision most commonly made?
    a. Flank
    b. Scrotum
    c. Prescrotal prepuce
    d. Midabdomen

26. Which of the following suffixes is used to describe the surgical creation of an artificial opening?
    a. *-ectomy*
    b. *-otomy*
    c. *-ostomy*
    d. *-rrhapy*

27. When a cat is presented for castration, and both testicles are descended, the veterinary technician will prepare the surgical site. In which area is the incision most commonly made?
    a. Flank
    b. Scrotum
    c. Prescrotal prepuce
    d. Midabdomen

28. When a dog is presented to the hospital to be spayed, the veterinary technician should prepare the surgical site. In which area is the incision most commonly made?
    a. Inguinal
    b. Scrotum
    c. Prescrotal prepuce
    d. Abdominal ventral midline

29. What is the primary function of a Brown-Adson?
    a. Retractor
    b. Rongeur
    c. Periosteal elevator
    d. Thumb forceps

30. The hair coat can be most efficiently and gently removed when preparing a dog for spaying by which of the following methods?
    a. Plucking
    b. Clipping with sharp scissors
    c. Clipping against the grain of the hair with electrical clippers using a No. 40 blade
    d. Clipping against the grain of the hair with electrical clippers using a No. 10 blade

31. Which of the following statements is false after serious oral surgery, such as mandibular fracture repair or oral-nasal tumor resection?
    a. The patient might refuse to eat
    b. The patient might need a gastrotomy tube
    c. The patient might refuse to drink
    d. The patient will no longer be in pain

32. When feeding the patient through a gastrostomy tube, the technician should:
    a. Rapidly inject the fluids and food
    b. Flush the tube with water
    c. Flush the tube with air
    d. Feed a full day's caloric requirement immediately after placement

33. Postoperative physical therapy can help the patient in each of the following ways, *except* in:
    a. Enhancing patient comfort
    b. Preventing complications from disuse
    c. Slowing the healing process
    d. Decreasing edema

34. A semipermanent feeding tube may be placed in all of the following ways, *except:*
    a. Through the nose
    b. Through a pharyngostomy site
    c. Through a gastrostomy site
    d. Through the mouth

35. All of the following statements are true regarding gastrointestinal (GI) surgery, *except:*
    a. It is absolutely essential that all patients fast before GI surgery. The GI tract must be empty before surgery.
    b. At no point is the GI tract sterile; therefore, it is important to guard against contamination.
    c. Irrigation of the peritoneal cavity with a sterile isotonic solution after GI surgery helps reduce the number of microorganisms that remain free in the peritoneum following the procedure.
    d. The surgical assistant must be alert to the possibility of intestinal contents contaminating the abdominal cavity and must help the surgeon prevent this from happening.

36. It is important that the nursing care provided to paralyzed patients focuses on patient comfort. The prevention of decubital ulcers can be accomplished by all of the following procedures, *except:*
    a. Frequent turning or repositioning of the patient
    b. Adequate padding in the cage or bed
    c. Appropriate analgesic therapy
    d. Massage

37. A proptosed globe:
    a. Can be caused by overzealous restraint of the animal
    b. Is not considered an emergency
    c. Can most easily occur in dolichocephalic breeds, such as collies
    d. Is commonly a consequence of conjunctivitis

38. An abscess is:
    a. Usually lanced, drained, flushed, and sutured closed
    b. A solid infiltration of inflammatory cells
    c. A rare consequence of bite wounds
    d. A "walled-off" or circumscribed accumulation of pus

39. All of the following are instructions provided to a client when the patient has had a Penrose drain placed, *except:*
    a. An Elizabethan collar may be needed
    b. Clean the skin around the drain with warm water or dilute chlorhexidine
    c. The drain will fall out, and there is no need to return for removal
    d. Carefully watch the animal and prevent it from licking or chewing at the drain

40. The client should be instructed to contact the veterinary hospital if any of the following occur with a splint or cast, *except:*
    a. The animal chews at the splint or cast
    b. The splint or cast is wet
    c. The leg looks swollen above or below the cast
    d. The animal is walking on or using the splinted or casted leg

41. Proper splint and bandage care includes all of the following, *except:*
    a. Washing the splint or bandage daily
    b. Preventing the bandage or splint from becoming wet
    c. Inspecting the bandage or splint daily for any change, such as swelling above or below the splint or bandage
    d. Inspecting the bandage or splint for any shifting or change in position on the limb

42. Which of the following is not true of an aural hematoma?
    a. An aural hematoma must be drained
    b. Trimming back the pinna repairs it
    c. It is painful and bothersome to the animal
    d. An aural hematoma may be drained and bandaged by wrapping the head with the ear folded back across the top of the head

43. Which of the following instruments should be available for use during abdominal exploratory surgery?
    a. Balfour retractor
    b. Weitlaner retractor
    c. Gelpi retractor
    d. Senn retractor

44. Suture materials are:
    a. Absorbable
    b. Nonabsorbable only
    c. Braided or monofilament
    d. Only supplied with a needle attached

45. When passing surgical instruments to the surgeon, the technician should do all of the following *except:*
    a. Gently but firmly slap the palm of the surgeon with the instrument
    b. Pass the instrument in the open position
    c. Pass the instrument with the handle placed into the surgeon's hand
    d. Pass the curved instrument so that it is oriented in the surgeon's hand with the concave side up

46. When assisting the surgeon, the technician should:
    a. Always cut sutures on top of the knot
    b. Cut sutures with the middle tip part of the scissors blade
    c. Blot the surgical site with a gauze square to clear the site of blood
    d. Attach the scalpel blade to the handle using a pair of hemostats

47. Staples and other metal clips can:
    a. Resist infection
    b. Cause little scarring
    c. Be removed easily using scissors
    d. Be applied by hand without any special application device

48. Surgical instruments should be:
    a. Lubricated with oil between uses
    b. Cleaned without water to avoid the possibility of rusting
    c. Placed on surfaces and never dropped or thrown
    d. Cleaned with abrasive cleaners

49. External fixation devices include all of the following, *except:*
    a. Cast
    b. Splint
    c. Bone plate
    d. Kirschner-Ehmer (K-E) apparatus

50. Overinflation or underinflation of the endotracheal tube cuff can result in all of the following *except:*
    a. Prevention of fluid aspiration into the lungs
    b. Pressure necrosis of the cells lining the trachea
    c. Inability to keep the patient under anesthesia with the expected concentration of gas anesthetic
    d. Increased levels of waste gas anesthesia in the surgical room

51. A chest tube is placed when an animal has:
    a. Subcutaneous emphysema
    b. Pulmonary edema
    c. Ascites
    d. Pneumothorax

52. There is more concern about pulling out the endotracheal tube too soon in the _____, versus an English mastiff:
    a. English bulldog
    b. German shepherd
    c. Jack Russell terrier
    d. Greyhound

53. Dystocia is:
    a. Difficulty in breathing
    b. A side effect of opioid drugs
    c. A difficult or abnormal birth
    d. Difficulty in urinating

54. Surgical procedures of the ear include all of the following *except:*
    a. Otoplasty
    b. Bulla osteotomy
    c. Aural hematoma drainage
    d. Enucleation

55. Surgical procedures of the eye and adnexal structures include all of the following, *except:*
    a. Entropion repair
    b. Keratectomy
    c. Onychectomy
    d. Enucleation

56. A patient is to be prepared for a cystotomy. What part of the body is prepped?
    a. Ventral abdomen
    b. Lumbar spine
    c. Ventral cervical area
    d. Top of the head

57. A patient is to be prepared for an ovariohysterectomy. What part of the body is prepped?
    a. Paw
    b. Ventral chest wall
    c. Ventral abdomen
    d. Ear

58. A patient is to be prepared for a femoral head ostectomy. What part of the body is prepped?
    a. Top of the head
    b. Hip
    c. Shoulder
    d. Lumbar spine

59. A patient is to be prepared for an orchidectomy. What part of the body is prepped?
    a. Ventral abdomen
    b. Scrotal/prescrotal area
    c. Paw
    d. Ear

60. The patient is to be prepared for a popliteal lymph node biopsy. What part of the body is prepped?
    a. Caudal aspect of the stifle
    b. Cranial aspect of the elbow
    c. Medial aspect of the thigh
    d. Area cranial to the shoulder

61. A declaw is also known as an:
   a. Orchidectomy
   b. Onychectomy
   c. Ovariohysterectomy
   d. Onychotomy

62. Which structure is *not* part of the spermatic cord?
   a. Pampiniform plexus
   b. Vas deferens
   c. Testicular artery
   d. Epididymis

63. Which of the following is *not* completely removed in an ovariohysterectomy?
   a. Broad ligament
   b. Ovaries
   c. Uterine horns
   d. Oviducts

64. An enucleation may be required to correct a/an:
   a. Third eyelid prolapse
   b. Penile prolapse
   c. Proptosis of the eye
   d. Aural hematoma

65. Which of the following is a needle driver that is also able to cut suture material?
   a. Olsen-Hegar
   b. Mayo-Hegar
   c. Adson-Brown
   d. Rochester-Pean

66. Which of the following forceps has the best crushing action?
   a. Rochester-Carmalt
   b. Adson-Brown
   c. Ochsner
   d. Crile

67. Which of the following is a nondesirable characteristic of ethylene oxide?
   a. Carcinogenic
   b. Teratogenic
   c. Mutagenic
   d. Mitogenic

68. Which of the following suture materials remains in the body for the longest period?
   a. Polydioxanone
   b. Prolene
   c. Chromic catgut
   d. Vicryl

69. Scrotal swelling after orchidectomy is most likely caused by a:
   a. Hematoma
   b. Seroma
   c. Hemangioma
   d. Lipoma

70. Which of the following instruments is the only one appropriate for handling tissues during surgery?
   a. Dressing forceps
   b. Standard surgical scissors
   c. Sponge forceps
   d. Rat-tooth forceps

71. What suture pattern is commonly used to close the skin of cattle following a rumenotomy?
   a. Simple interrupted
   b. Simple continuous
   c. Continuous Ford interlocking pattern
   d. a and c

72. Which of the following suture materials is most appropriate to close the muscle layers of a cow following a left-displaced abomasum surgery?
   a. 3-0 catgut
   b. 3-0 polydioxanone
   c. 3 chromic catgut
   d. 3 polydioxanone

73. Which of the following statements regarding pyometra is incorrect?
   a. Onychectomies are usually curative
   b. A purulent vaginal discharge is always present
   c. Affected females usually have polyuria and polydipsia
   d. It often occurs soon after a heat cycle

74. Which of the following procedures is *not* considered elective?
   a. Orchidectomy
   b. Ovariohysterectomy
   c. Onychectomy
   d. Enucleation of a proptosed eye

75. Nephrectomy refers to:
   a. An incision into the kidney
   b. The removal of a kidney
   c. The removal of a tumor from the kidney
   d. The biopsy of a kidney

76. When preparing for an orthopedic surgery, shaving the surgical site should be performed:
   a. The previous night to shorten the anesthesia time
   b. The first thing in the morning to help the procedures run more smoothly
   c. Immediately before the induction of anesthesia
   d. Just after the induction of anesthesia

77. Fracture apposition reduction refers to:
    a. Placing bones back in their normal positions
    b. Keeping bones still until healing has occurred
    c. Removing small fragments from around the fracture
    d. Placing pins through the marrow cavity

78. Which of the following suffixes is used to describe the removal of an organ?
    a. *-ectomy*
    b. *-otomy*
    c. *-ostomy*
    d. *-rrhapy*

79. A Caslick operation is performed in horses to:
    a. Stop roaring
    b. Prevent uterine infection
    c. Treat navicular disease
    d. Clean out the guttural pouches

80. Which of the following agents can be used as both an antiseptic as well as a disinfectant?
    a. Quaternary ammonium compounds
    b. Mercurial chloride compounds
    c. Isopropyl alcohol
    d. Formaldehyde

81. For which of the following surgeries are stay sutures *not* normally necessary?
    a. Cystotomy
    b. Gastrotomy
    c. Intestinal anastomosis
    d. Hepatic biopsy

82. What is the minimum number of throws required when making a surgical knot?
    a. One
    b. Two
    c. Three
    d. Four

83. When would it be considered an advantage to use a hand tie versus an instrument tie?
    a. When suturing very tough tissue
    b. When suturing the linea alba or areas that are difficult to reach
    c. When suturing the skin
    d. When suturing hollow organs

84. The chemical or mechanical destruction of pathogens is known as:
    a. Disinfection
    b. Decontamination
    c. Barrier
    d. Aseptic technique

85. Which of the following is an advantage of monofilament material over multifilament material?
    a. Greater knot security
    b. Greater suture strength
    c. Less likely to cause suture reactions
    d. Passes through tissue more easily

86. What type of instrument is a Mayo-Hegar?
    a. Needle holder
    b. Scissors
    c. Towel clamp
    d. Hemostatic forceps

87. Which of the following suture sizes is most appropriate for eye surgeries?
    a. 0
    b. 3-0
    c. 6-0
    d. 10-0

88. All of the following are important reasons to reduce the amount of dead space with drains in a wound, *except:*
    a. To decrease the chance of infection
    b. To decrease the chance of seroma formation
    c. To decrease hemostasis
    d. To minimize necrosis

89. Which of the following is an absorbable suture material?
    a. Polydioxanone
    b. Prolene
    c. Silk
    d. Cotton

90. What factor will *not* influence how rapidly the body absorbs suture materials?
    a. Age of the patient
    b. Presence of infection
    c. The location of the suture
    d. The composition of the suture material

91. Which of the following is *not* considered a contaminated surgery and would be considered the cleanest?
    a. Cruciate repair
    b. Dental extractions
    c. Intestinal anastomosis
    d. Gastrotomy

92. Which of the following forceps should *not* be used to hold the edges of the incision open?
    a. Rat-tooth
    b. Brown-Adson
    c. Crile
    d. Allis tissue

93. Which of the following does *not* describe a type of surgical scissors?
    a. Mayo
    b. Metzenbaum
    c. Iris
    d. Lembert

94. A sponge count should be done:
    a. At the beginning of the surgery and before closure
    b. Several times during the surgery
    c. Before surgery only
    d. Before closure only

95. To maintain sterility throughout the surgical procedure, the method by which contamination with microorganisms is prevented is known as:
    a. Sterile technique
    b. Sterile field
    c. Sterility
    d. Terminal sterilization

96. Which of the following clinical signs would *not* normally be seen if a dog were suffering from hemorrhage after an ovariohysterectomy?
    a. Decreased respiratory rate
    b. Pale mucous membranes
    c. Slow recovery from anesthesia
    d. Slow capillary refill time

97. You are monitoring a cat during an exploratory surgery and notice the pupils are central and dilated. The cat is:
    a. Too light
    b. Too deep
    c. Under the influence of atropine
    d. In a state impossible to determine without more information

98. Which of the following does *not* cause an increase in respiratory rate (RR) in an anesthetized animal?
    a. Increased blood CO_2
    b. Anesthesia is too light
    c. Increased PaO_2
    d. Hyperthermia

99. What is the proper term for trimming the edges of a jagged tear before suturing?
    a. Debridement
    b. Decoupage
    c. Curettage
    d. Cauterization

100. Which of the following is *not* a factor influencing the formation of exuberant granulation tissue?
    a. Presence of infection
    b. Amount of missing tissue
    c. Depth of the wound
    d. Location of the wound

101. If a surgical incision is dehiscing, the discharge, if present, is most likely:
    a. Mucopurulent
    b. Serosanguineous
    c. Serous
    d. Purulent

102. Which of the following agents has been associated with causing neurological disorders in cats?
    a. Chlorhexidine
    b. Povidone iodine
    c. Quaternary ammonium compounds
    d. Hexachlorophene

103. If a nonsterile person must move to the other side of a sterile person, the nonsterile person should pass:
    a. Back to back
    b. Front to front
    c. Facing the back of the surgeon
    d. With his or her side facing the back of the surgeon

104. When opening a double-wrapped gown pack, nonscrubbed surgical personnel may touch the:
    a. Autoclave tape
    b. Indicator
    c. Towel
    d. Gown

105. Which of the following suture materials is most likely to cause stitch granulomas if left in too long?
    a. Silk
    b. Cotton
    c. Nylon
    d. Prolene

106. When the surgeon and surgical technician are scrubbing for surgery, the hands should be held:
    a. Below the elbows
    b. Parallel to the elbows
    c. Above the elbows
    d. Above the head

107. When cleaning instruments, the instruments should first be soaked in a surgical soap solution (e.g., Asepti-Zyme) to:
    a. Remove bacteria
    b. Remove blood
    c. Sterilize them
    d. Enhance the effect of the ultrasonic cleaner

108. Which of the following patterns is *not* suitable for the closure of an intestinal biopsy incision?
    a. Simple continuous
    b. Simple interrupted
    c. Everting
    d. Inverting

109. Which of the following does *not* need to be included when labeling a surgical pack?
    a. Contents of the pack
    b. Date the pack was made up
    c. Initials or name of the person making up the pack
    d. Date by which the pack must be used

110. Which of the following hemostatic forceps has striations different from the others?
    a. Halstead mosquitoes
    b. Crile
    c. Rochester-Pean
    d. Rochester-Carmalt

111. Which of the following is *not* the formal name of a retractor?
    a. Finochietto
    b. Gelpi
    c. Lembert
    d. Balfour

112. Which of the following is *not* a requirement for fracture healing?
    a. Apposition
    b. Shearing
    c. Fixation
    d. Reduction

113. Using the dissection method, which parts of the distal forelimb are removed in an onychectomy?
    a. Nail and proximal phalanx
    b. Proximal and distal phalanges
    c. Middle and distal phalanges
    d. Distal phalanx and nail

114. What type of instrument is an Adson?
    a. Retractor
    b. Rongeur
    c. Periosteal elevator
    d. Thumb forceps

115. Anterior drawer movement detects a problem with the:
    a. Elbow
    b. Stifle
    c. Hip
    d. Hock

116. An incision into the bladder is known as a:
    a. Cystotomy
    b. Cystectomy
    c. Cystocentesis
    d. Cystostomy

117. Which of the following conditions does *not* require surgical repair?
    a. Gastric dilatation and volvulus (GDV)
    b. Intussusception
    c. Mesenteric torsion
    d. Ileus

118. A laminectomy is used to treat:
    a. Intervertebral disk disease
    b. Fractures of spinous processes
    c. Hip dysplasia
    d. Foot disorders in horses

119. If a fracture is found on the proximal part of the tibia, it is:
    a. Distal to the femur
    b. Proximal to the femur
    c. In the middle of the bone
    d. Distal to the metatarsals

120. If the testicles are not palpable, and a cryptorchidectomy is performed, the incision would most likely be:
    a. Prescrotal
    b. Inguinal
    c. Ventral midline
    d. Perineal

121. In dogs, the most common location for a thoracotomy incision is:
    a. Through the sternum
    b. Through the diaphragm
    c. Along the linea alba
    d. Between the ribs

122. What is the minimum number of air changes per hour required for adequate ventilation in a surgical suite?
    a. 2
    b. 5
    c. 10
    d. 15

123. Which of the following disinfectants includes the weakest virucidal activity?
    a. Glutaraldehyde (2%)
    b. Quaternary ammonium compounds at standard concentrations
    c. Formalin (37%)
    d. Isopropyl alcohol (70%)

124. Which of the following instruments is *not* considered surgical scissors?
    a. Iris
    b. Metzenbaum
    c. Wire-cutting
    d. Mayo-Hegar

125. Which of the following instruments is most suitable for the removal of bone to perform spinal surgery?
    a. Rongeur
    b. Curette
    c. Periosteal elevator
    d. Trephine

126. Clear fluid removed from thoracic cavity is known as:
    a. Pleural effusion
    b. Pulmonary edema
    c. Ascites
    d. Pyothorax

127. Where is the most likely place for a rumenotomy incision in a dairy cow?
    a. Right paralumbar fossa
    b. Left paralumbar fossa
    c. Linea alba
    d. Paramedian

128. What does a change in color in autoclave tape indicate to a surgical nurse?
    a. The surgical instruments in the pack have been adequately sterilized
    b. During the autoclaving process, steam has reached the tape
    c. Adequate temperature and pressures have been achieved
    d. The pack has been exposed to adequate pressures

129. Assuming 15 psi, the minimum conditions that must be met to ensure that a pack has been adequately sterilized by autoclaving are:
    a. 121° C for 15 minutes
    b. 131° F for 15 minutes
    c. 121° C for 25 minutes
    d. 131° F for 30 minutes

130. Which of the following is *not* a common concern when assisting a surgeon with canine cesarean section surgery?
    a. Minimizing anesthetic drugs that may pass on to the puppies
    b. Minimizing the time the bitch is in dorsal recumbency because of the weight of the uterus on the aorta
    c. Suctioning fluid from the puppies' nasal cavities and mouths to stimulate breathing
    d. Intubating the puppies

131. Which of the following is *not* a primary concern when assisting a surgeon performing a pyometra surgery?
    a. Providing preoperative and intraoperative antibiotics for the patient
    b. Gentle handling of the friable tissue to prevent rupture and drainage of the contents of the uterus into the abdominal cavity
    c. Fluid therapy to diurese the kidneys
    d. Lidocaine infusion to prevent ventricular arrhythmias

132. When assisting a surgeon in a gastric dilatation and volvulus surgery, which of the following is *not* your immediate concern?
    a. Establishing intravenous access to deliver shock doses of fluids
    b. Calculating lidocaine dose for constant rate infusion
    c. Monitoring for cardiac arrhythmias intraoperatively and postoperatively
    d. Preparing the ultrasound unit to confirm gastric dilatation and volvulus status of animal

133. What size scalpel blade fits on a No. 3 scalpel handle?
    a. No. 10
    b. No. 20
    c. No. 21
    d. No. 30

134. What size scalpel blade fits on a No. 4 scalpel handle?
    a. No. 10
    b. No. 12
    c. No. 15
    d. No. 20

135. Which of the following suffixes is used to describe the surgical repair by suturing?
    a. *-ectomy*
    b. *-otomy*
    c. *-ostomy*
    d. *-rrhapy*

136. Pathogenic bacteria is defined as bacteria that:
    a. Produce toxins
    b. Cause disease
    c. Live off and gain nutrients from the host
    d. Multiply in the host

137. Which of the following need *not* be considered in the timing of the autoclave cycle?
    a. Time required to heat up the interior of the chamber
    b. Time required to allow the steam to penetrate the interior of the packs
    c. Time required to seal the chamber
    d. Time required to sterilize those items in contact with the steam

138. The definition of sterile is:
    a. Without microbes or living spores
    b. Without pathogenic microbes
    c. With the presence of commensal organisms only
    d. Without bacteria or their byproducts

139. What items should all personnel wear when entering the operating room?
    a. Cap and mask
    b. Cap, mask, and booties
    c. Cap, mask, booties, and clean scrubs or gown
    d. Cap, mask, and sterile gown

140. Which of the following surgical packs would *not* be considered contaminated and would *not* need to be reautoclaved?
    a. Single-wrapped crepe paper pack stored on an open shelf for 8 weeks
    b. Pack that was opened for a procedure but was not used and was needed for the next day's procedure
    c. Double-wrapped paper pack stored in a closed cabinet for 6 weeks
    d. Instrument in an autoclave pouch that has a very small tear near the top of the pack

141. Instruments are autoclaved:
    a. With the ratchets closed to prevent tearing the wrap material
    b. With the ratchets open to allow steam exposure to the entire surface
    c. Always in a surgical tray to prevent the instruments from shifting
    d. Without touching any other instruments to prevent corrosion

142. An advantage of using a Gelpi retractor over a Senn retractor is:
    a. The Gelpi is much less expensive to purchase
    b. The Gelpi is smaller overall than the Senn
    c. The Senn must be molded to fit the position required
    d. The Gelpi is self-retaining

143. Which of the following suffixes is used to describe the surgical fixation?
    a. *-pexy*
    b. *-otomy*
    c. *-ostomy*
    d. *-rrhapy*

144. All of the following are true regarding aseptic technique, *except:*
    a. It provides a clean surgical environment
    b. It prevents pathogenic microbes from entering the surgical suite
    c. It provides a sterile surgical environment
    d. It reduces the likelihood of fatal infections

145. What specifically does the strip on the autoclave tape indicate when it turns dark?
    a. The correct temperature has been reached.
    b. The correct pressure has been reached.
    c. The correct temperature for the proper amount of time has been reached.
    d. The correct temperature, pressure, and time have been reached.

146. Metzenbaum scissors are used only for:
    a. Cutting suture
    b. Cutting paper drape
    c. Ophthalmic surgery
    d. Cutting tissue

147. Where is the sterile zone located on scrubbed personnel?
    a. Front and sides, from the neck below the neckline to the bottom of the gown, including the arms
    b. Front, from below the neckline to the bottom of the gown, including the arms
    c. Front, sides, and back, from the neck to the waist
    d. Front, from below the neckline to the waist, including the arms

148. Rank the following from greatest tensile strength to least:
    a. 00 gut, 3-0 Vicryl, 1 chromic gut, 6-0 silk
    b. 1 chromic gut, 00 gut, 3-0 Vicryl, 6-0 silk
    c. 6-0 silk, 3-0 Vicryl, 00 gut, 1 chromic gut
    d. 6-0 silk, 3-0 Vicryl, 1 chromic gut, 00 gut

149. Why must instrument milk be used after ultrasonic cleaning?
    a. To complete the sterilization process
    b. To provide further cleaning and sanitizing of the instruments
    c. To replace lubrication removed by the ultrasonic cleaner
    d. To prevent rust spots from forming on the instruments

150. What type of needle is reusable?
    a. Swaged-on
    b. Taper point
    c. Trocar tip
    d. Eyed

151. Which of the following operating room personnel should face the sterile field during a procedure?
    a. The surgeon only
    b. The scrubbed-in technicians and surgeon only
    c. All personnel, both scrubbed in and nonsterile
    d. Only the surgeon and nonsterile personnel; the scrubbed-in technician should face the instrument field.

152. All of the following sutures have a degree of capillarity, *except:*
    a. Polyglycolic acid
    b. Silk
    c. Surgical gut
    d. Polypropylene

153. An advantage of the braided suture over the monofilament is:
    a. Knot security
    b. Tensile strength
    c. It does not hide bacteria in contaminated wounds
    d. Tissue reactivity

154. When attaching an animal to an ECG, which lead is hooked up to the right foreleg?
    a. Red
    b. Black
    c. White
    d. Green

155. A disinfectant labeled as a virucidal:
    a. Prevents bacteria from growing
    b. Kills all spores
    c. Kills viruses
    d. Prevents viruses from growing

156. What is the purpose of the surgical drape?
    a. To keep the animal warm
    b. To keep the surgeon focused on the surgical area
    c. To establish a sterile field
    d. To protect the table and mayo stand from contamination

157. When autoclaving, the minimum temperature and exposure times for the center of the surgical packs are:
    a. 121.5° F for 10 minutes
    b. 250° F for 13 minutes
    c. 250° F for 20 minutes
    d. 300° F for 30 minutes

158. In general, the difference between a disinfectant and an antiseptic is:
    a. Disinfectants are agents used on inanimate objects, and antiseptic agents are used on living tissue
    b. Disinfectants are used on living tissues, and antiseptics are used on inanimate objects
    c. Disinfectants are bacteriostatic, and antiseptics are bacteriocidal
    d. Disinfectants kill microbes, whereas antiseptics inhibit their growth only

159. How can you help prevent "strike through" during surgery?
    a. Make sure sharp instruments are protected so they do not puncture the wrap and cause contamination
    b. Assist in keeping the surgical drapes and gown from becoming wet during surgery
    c. Make sure the drape is properly placed and opened so the fenestration is not over a contaminated area
    d. Have reverse cutting needles available so the suture does not pull through the tissue

160. The agent used in gas sterilization is:
    a. Glutaraldehyde
    b. Chlorhexidine
    c. Ethylene oxide
    d. Formaldehyde

161. Needle holders that do not have scissors, but have a needle-holding surface, are called:
    a. Mayo-Hegar
    b. Olsen-Hegar
    c. Metzenbaum
    d. Crile-Wood

162. Rochester-Carmalt Pean forceps:
    a. Are generally smaller than a Kelly forceps
    b. Have longitudinal serrations with interdigitating teeth at the tips
    c. Have longitudinal serrations with a crosshatched pattern at the tips
    d. Have transverse longitudinal serrations along the entire length

163. A Buhner needle is used in:
    a. The repair of bovine vaginal and uterine prolapses
    b. Eye enucleations in dogs
    c. Intestinal anastomosis surgeries
    d. Orthopedic surgeries

164. A Snook hook is typically used during:
    a. A castration
    b. An ovariohysterectomy
    c. A diaphragmatic hernia repair
    d. Declawing

165. What does the medical term ovariohysterectomy mean?
    a. Removal of the ovaries only
    b. Removal of the uterus only
    c. Removal of the ovaries and uterus only
    d. Removal of the entire reproductive tract, including ovaries, uterus, cervix, and vagina

166. An accumulation of purulent discharge within the uterus is called:
    a. Pyometritis
    b. Mastitis
    c. Peritonitis
    d. Vaginitis

167. A pack double wrapped in muslin and kept in a closed cabinet is good for how long?
    a. 1 week
    b. 3 to 4 weeks
    c. 6 to 7 weeks
    d. 6 months

168. Instruments suitable for cutting sutures include:
    a. Scissors on Mayo-Hegar needle holders, operating scissors, and Mayo scissors
    b. Operating scissors, scissors on Olsen-Hegar needle holders, and Metzenbaum scissors
    c. Operating scissors, scissors on Olsen-Hegar needle holders, and Mayo scissors
    d. Suture (stitch) scissors, Mayo scissors, and Metzenbaum scissors

169. What is a Steinmann IM pin?
    a. An intramedullary pin used in orthopedics
    b. An intramuscular pin used in orthopedics
    c. A type of screw used in orthopedics
    d. A staple used to hold muscle or bone fragments together

170. You are checking on a recent surgical wound and find that the tissue is slightly warmer and redder than the surrounding tissue. What is the significance of this?
    a. It is an indication that the wound is contaminated and requires an emergency intervention
    b. The wound will likely dehisce and should be checked immediately by the veterinarian
    c. It is normal, because the first stage of wound healing is inflammation
    d. It is an indication that the sutures are interfering with blood flow, and necrosis is likely

171. What is the correct order of tasks when preparing an animal for routine surgery?
    a. Premedicate, place IV catheter, clip and prep, move into surgery, final prep
    b. Place IV catheter, premedicate, clip and prep, move into surgery, final prep
    c. Premedicate, IV catheter, move into surgery, clip and prep, final prep
    d. Place IV catheter, premedicate, clip and prep, move into surgery, final prep

172. What should you wear when working as a nonsterile surgical assistant?
    a. Mask and clean scrubs
    b. Mask, cap, and clean scrubs
    c. Mask, cap, shoe covers, and clean scrubs
    d. Mask, cap, shoe covers, and sterile gown

173. While you are working as a sterile surgical assistant, your mask slips down below your nose. What should you do?
    a. The nonsterile assistant may stand in front of you and secure the mask in its proper position
    b. The nonsterile assistant may secure the mask in position while standing behind you
    c. You may take a nonsterile piece of gauze and place it over the mask to allow you to adjust it into position
    d. You are completely contaminated and must leave surgery

174. Which of the following is not a recommended agent for patient surgical preparation?
    a. Chlorhexidine
    b. Roccal
    c. Alcohol
    d. Povidone iodine

175. Abscesses are generally allowed to heal open to provide continuous drainage. This type of wound healing is considered:
    a. Primary intention
    b. Second intention
    c. Third intention
    d. Fourth intention

176. Which of the following best describes the location of an incision through the skin and linea alba, extending from the xiphoid process to the umbilicus?
    a. Flank
    b. Paracostal
    c. Paramedian
    d. Ventral midline

177. Cesarean sections in cattle are most commonly performed via what surgical approach?
    a. Through a right paracostal incision
    b. Through a right paravertebral approach
    c. Through the left paralumbar fossa
    d. Through the ventral midline approach

178. Emasculators are used:
    a. In large-animal castrations
    b. During surgical ovariectomies in heifers and mares
    c. During enucleations in large-breed dogs
    d. To remove dewclaws in dogs

179. You are to assist with a rumenotomy. Where on the patient would you prep for the surgery?
    a. Ventral midline from xiphoid to pubic bone
    b. Left paralumbar fossa
    c. Right paralumbar fossa
    d. Right paramedian region

180. A *disadvantage* of tilting the surgical table so the patient's head is lower than its tail is:
    a. The increased pressure on the diaphragm, which can interfere with respiration
    b. The tension on the large bowel, which may initiate defecation
    c. It interferes with visualization of the caudal abdomen
    d. It can cause a gastric volvulus

181. A visiting relief veterinarian whom you are assisting in surgery asks you to provide a nonabsorbable suture that is less than 2-0 in size. Which of the following would meet the request?
    a. 3-0 chromic gut
    b. 4-0 silk
    c. 00 Dermalon nylon
    d. 0 polydioxanone

182. A surgical prep for feline castration:
    a. Involves clipping the prescrotal region from the umbilicus to the scrotum
    b. Involves clipping the scrotum with a No. 40 clipper blade
    c. Does not involve hair removal, because the entire scrotal area is prepped with Nolvasan and alcohol
    d. Includes plucking or pulling the hair from the scrotum before the surgical scrub

183. Which of these is not a common surgical site for the correction of a left-displaced abomasum in cattle?
    a. Right paralumbar
    b. Left paralumbar
    c. Ventral midline
    d. Right paramedian

184. Postoperative care for horses following castration:
    a. Includes strict confinement to the stall for at least 1 week to prevent hemorrhage
    b. Includes suture removal at 10 to 14 days
    c. Involves antibiotic administration for 5 days following surgery
    d. Involves exercise twice daily to promote drainage

185. The term that means *surgically opening the abdominal cavity* is:
    a. Laparotomy
    b. Pleurotomy
    c. Thoracotomy
    d. Cystotomy

186. What parameter(s) does the pulse oximeter measure?
    a. Heart rate only
    b. Respiration rate and depth
    c. Oxygen saturation of hemoglobin and heart rate
    d. Respiration rate and heart rate

187. Which of the following is false regarding the ECG?
    a. It measures the electrical impulses of the heart
    b. There can be a normal ECG tracing when there is no cardiac output
    c. There is always a pulse beat with each QRS complex
    d. Alcohol and sterile lubricant will enhance the connection of the skin leads

188. What orthopedic fixation consists of pins that penetrate fractured bones and skin from the outside and are held in place externally by bolts attached to another cross pin?
    a. Rush pinning
    b. External fixators
    c. Steinmann fixation
    d. Bone plating

189. What is a nosocomial infection?
    a. Infection arising from bacteria in the gastrointestinal tract
    b. Infection originating from the respiratory tract, especially the nose
    c. Hospital-acquired infection
    d. Resistant infection

190. Which of the following should *not* be used to help prevent hypothermia in surgical patients?
    a. Electric heating pad set on low
    b. Warm-water circulating pad
    c. Warm rice pads
    d. Towel placed between the surgery table and patient

191. In what type of surgical procedure would you make sure that the Jacob's bone chuck is sterilized and available?
    a. Onychectomy
    b. Celiotomy
    c. Thoracotomy
    d. Orthopedic

192. Which of the following is *not* an advantage to neutering a male dog?
    a. Decreased risk for perineal hernias
    b. Decreased roaming
    c. It will prevent it from lifting its leg to urinate
    d. Decreased aggression toward other dogs

193. Which of the following can be used as a surgical scrub on a patient?
    a. Povidone iodine solution
    b. Chlorhexidine scrub
    c. Alcohol
    d. Nolvasan solution

194. Which of the following need not be done before moving a horse into surgery for a general anesthesia procedure?
    a. Remove the shoes
    b. Rinse the mouth
    c. Clip as much of the surgical area as possible
    d. Perform a complete tail wrap

195. What is an important measure that can help prevent myositis during equine surgery?
    a. Providing proper padding
    b. Ensuring that the horse does not experience hypothermia
    c. Not overinflating the endotracheal tube cuff
    d. Withholding food for 12 hours

196. If a single technician is responsible for setting the patient up in surgery, what task should be performed first?
    a. Tying the animal to the table
    b. Applying the final prep
    c. Attaching the monitoring devices
    d. Opening the surgery pack

197. Which of the following statements regarding compartment syndrome in the equine surgical patient is correct?
    a. Compartment syndrome only affects the surgery compartment
    b. The "up" side of the patient can be affected
    c. Following all proper precautions can prevent compartment syndrome
    d. Compartment syndrome rarely results in euthanasia

198. A gastrotomy refers to a surgical incision into the:
    a. Gastrocnemius muscle
    b. Peritoneal wall
    c. Stomach
    d. Small intestines

199. During a surgical scrub, you bump your hand on the faucet. What should you do?
    a. Continue the scrub, giving the bumped area double the number of brush strokes to compensate
    b. You have contaminated yourself and must start the entire scrub again
    c. Rescrub the area immediately, rinse the brush, and then continue the scrub
    d. Continue the scrub and add one more cycle on the bumped hand, because you cannot make your hands truly sterile anyway

200. Why are such elaborate measures taken to maintain aseptic technique during surgery?
    a. To protect personnel from pathogenic microbes encountered in the animals
    b. To decrease the risk of nosocomial infections spread among patients
    c. To decrease the risk of contamination into the surgical site and interference with wound healing
    d. To decrease the virulence of the microbes in the hospital

201. A fenestrated drape:
    a. Has a window opening in middle through which the surgery is performed
    b. Is folded in half in accordion style for ease of opening
    c. Is folded such that the middle of the drape can easily be found
    d. Is a cloth drape made of three doubled layers of muslin

202. What is the pressure that must be reached in a steam autoclave for the temperature to reach 121.5° C?
    a. 1 psi
    b. 10 psi
    c. 15 psi
    d. 45 psi

203. Healing of a properly sutured surgical wound is most appropriately termed:
    a. First-intention healing
    b. Granulation
    c. Second-intention healing
    d. Third-intention healing

204. Which of the following has the poorest potential for healing and return to normal function after damage and effective surgical repair?
    a. Bone
    b. Gastrointestinal tract
    c. Liver
    d. Nervous tissue

205. Which of the following best describes the location of an incision extending from the xiphoid process to the umbilicus of an animal?
    a. Flank
    b. Paracostal
    c. Paramedian
    d. Ventral midline

206. What agent, method, or device is most appropriate for sterilizing an electric drill to be used in an orthopedic surgical procedure?
    a. Autoclave
    b. Dry heat
    c. Ethylene oxide gas
    d. Liquid chemical disinfectant

207. Which of the following is the most effective and timely indicator that sterilization conditions have been met in an autoclaved surgery pack?
    a. Autoclave tape
    b. Chemical indicator
    c. Culture test
    d. Melting pellet

208. What is the proper term for microorganisms that gain entrance into an incision during a surgical procedure?
    a. Contamination
    b. Debridement
    c. Infection
    d. Septicemia

209. Which of the following do/does not have to be sterile during a surgical procedure to maintain aseptic technique?
    a. Drapes
    b. Gloves
    c. Gown
    d. Mask

210. Which of the following is the agent for autoclave sterilization?
    a. Chemical disinfectant solution
    b. Dry heat
    c. Ethylene oxide gas
    d. Steam

211. What size of electrical clipper blade is most commonly used for removing the hair from a surgical site?
    a. No. 10
    b. No. 20
    c. No. 30
    d. No. 40

212. Which of the following is *not* an effective form of surgical hemostasis?
    a. Crushing
    b. Curettage
    c. Ligation
    d. Pressure

213. Which of the following is *not* a likely cause of dehiscence of an abdominal incision?
    a. Excessive physical activity
    b. Stormy recovery from anesthesia
    c. Surgical wound infection
    d. Suture material larger than needed

214. Which of the following is *not* an effective aseptic surgical technique?
    a. Considering a sterile item to be nonsterile if it touches a nonsterile item
    b. Considering an item sterile if its sterility is in doubt
    c. Allowing nonscrubbed personnel to touch nonsterile items only
    d. Allowing sterile items to touch only other sterile items

215. Which of the following does *not* enhance the healing of an open wound?
    a. Debridement
    b. Exuberant granulation tissue
    c. Granulation tissue
    d. Wound flushing

216. Which of the following is *not* a characteristic of first-intention wound healing?
    a. Minimal contamination
    b. Minimal tissue damage
    c. No continuous movement of wound edges resulting from body movement
    d. Wound edges not approximated

217. What incision is the most appropriate for exploratory surgery of the abdomen of a dog in which the precise location of the problem is *not* known?
    a. Flank
    b. Paracostal
    c. Paramedian
    d. Ventral midline

218. Which of the following is *not* an early sign of wound dehiscence during the first 24 hours after abdominal surgery?
     a. Body temperature elevation of 1° to 2°
     b. Serosanguineous discharge from the incision
     c. Swollen incision
     d. Very warm incision

219. The main goal of aseptic surgical technique is to prevent contamination of the:
     a. Sterile fields
     b. Sterile zones
     c. Surgical instruments
     d. Surgical wound

220. What factor relating to the infection of a surgical wound can an aseptic technique reasonably be expected to influence significantly?
     a. Number of microorganisms entering the wound
     b. Pathogenicity of microorganisms entering the wound
     c. Route of exposure to infectious microorganisms
     d. Susceptibility of the patient to infection

221. The effectiveness of a surgical scrub of the hands and arms with a bactericidal soap depends on the:
     a. Combination of contact time and scrubbing action
     b. Time the soap is in contact with the skin
     c. Scrubbing action of the brush
     d. Temperature of the water

222. Which of the following is a surgical scrub soap that forms a bacteriostatic film on the skin when it is used exclusively?
     a. Chlorhexidine
     b. Chlorpheniramine
     c. Hexachlorophene
     d. Povidone-iodine

223. Which of the following does *not* normally need to be sterilized as a part of good aseptic surgical technique?
     a. Cap
     b. Drapes
     c. Gown
     d. Scrub brush

224. Liquid chemical sterilization is used primarily for:
     a. Electrical equipment
     b. Endoscopic equipment
     c. Orthopedic equipment
     d. Surgical drapes

225. The time necessary to disinfect surgical instruments with liquid chemicals can be shortened by:
     a. Cooling the solution
     b. Making the solution less concentrated than recommended
     c. Making the solution more concentrated than recommended
     d. Warming the solution

226. What surgical drape material prevents bacteria from penetrating the drape by capillary action when the top surface of the drape becomes wet?
     a. Polyester
     b. Muslin
     c. Paper
     d. Plastic

227. The best surgical monitoring device is:
     a. An esophageal stethoscope
     b. A pulse oximeter
     c. A capnograph with ECG capability
     d. A skilled veterinary technician

228. What is the most appropriate wound-flushing solution?
     a. Hydrogen peroxide
     b. Isotonic saline
     c. Povidone-iodine solution
     d. Tap water

229. How should one handle a ventral midline surgical wound dehiscence of the muscle, subcutaneous tissue, and skin layers?
     a. As an emergency
     b. It would be for cosmetic purposes only, so surgery could be scheduled
     c. As of minor significance
     d. As serious but not as an emergency

230. Why is a recent surgical wound usually slightly warmer than surrounding normal tissues?
     a. Contamination
     b. Debridement
     c. Infection
     d. Inflammation

231. When does a sutured surgical wound begin to gain significant strength from the production of collagen strands so that the wound edges are held together not only by the sutures?
     a. Immediately
     b. In 5 days
     c. In 14 days
     d. In 35 days

232. Wound contraction is produced by:
    a. Reproduction of the dermis
    b. Movement of the epidermis only
    c. Movement of the whole thickness of skin
    d. Reproduction of epidermal cells

233. As a part of effective aseptic technique, surgical gowns:
    a. Are commonly made of cloth, paper, or plastic
    b. Are folded so that the inside of the gown faces outward
    c. Are routinely sterilized by ethylene oxide gas
    d. Do not need to be sterile, only clean

234. Which of the following is *not* a sign of hemorrhagic shock in a postsurgical patient?
    a. Deep, slow breathing
    b. Slow capillary refill
    c. Tachycardia
    d. Weakness

235. The usual significance of a small seroma beneath a suture line in the skin is:
    a. Emergency
    b. Cosmetic only
    c. Major problem
    d. Serious but not an emergency

236. The healing potential for a fractured bone that is properly aligned and kept immobile is:
    a. Excellent
    b. Fair
    c. Good
    d. Poor

237. All of the following are methods of microorganism transmission in the veterinary hospital, *except:*
    a. Team members
    b. Contaminated instruments
    c. Equipment contamination
    d. Uterus

238. What abdominal incision is most appropriate for a standing cesarean section on a heifer?
    a. Ventral midline
    b. Flank
    c. Paracostal
    d. Ventral paramedian

239. What portion of a surgical gown is considered sterile during surgery?
    a. Front and sides, from the neck to the bottom, including the arms
    b. Front, from the neck to the bottom, including the arms
    c. Front and sides, from the waist to the neck
    d. Front, from the waist up, including the arms

240. The first phase of the wound-healing process involves:
    a. Endothelial cell proliferation
    b. Fibroblast proliferation
    c. Inflammation
    d. Equilibrium of collagen synthesis

241. In the first 24 hours of primary union wound healing, most of the resistance to the opening of the wound is provided by:
    a. Collagen strands
    b. Fibrin strands
    c. Granulation tissue
    d. Sutures

242. In what type of abdominal incision can the muscle wall be most effectively closed with one layer of sutures?
    a. Flank
    b. Paracostal
    c. Paramedian
    d. Ventral midline

243. Scrubbed surgical personnel become contaminated if they touch:
    a. Objects in sterile fields
    b. Objects outside of the sterile zone
    c. Properly sterilized surgical instruments
    d. Freshly exposed tissues of the patient

244. Nonscrubbed surgical personnel may properly touch anything that is:
    a. Contaminated
    b. Inside the patient's body
    c. Inside the sterile zone
    d. Part of a sterile field

245. When *not* otherwise occupied, scrubbed surgical personnel should stand with:
    a. Arms folded
    b. Hands above shoulder level
    c. Hands clasped between waist and shoulder level
    d. Hands down at their sides

246. When is it permissible for nonscrubbed surgical personnel to pass between scrubbed personnel and the patient during surgery?
    a. Never
    b. When opening suture material
    c. When adjusting the anesthesia machine
    d. When adjusting the intravenous drip

247. When aseptically opening a sterile surgical pack on an instrument stand, it is *not* proper for nonscrubbed surgical personnel to touch:
     a. Autoclave tape
     b. Contents of the pack
     c. Corners of the wrap
     d. Instrument stand

248. What characteristic is true of ethylene oxide gas?
     a. It is flammable
     b. Exposure to it is not considered a health hazard
     c. It is noncombustible
     d. It is nontoxic to tissues

249. Which of the following is *not* a likely contributor to postoperative wound dehiscence?
     a. Chronic postoperative vomiting
     b. Internal suture ends cut too short
     c. Infection
     d. Skin sutures left in too long

250. What type of dressing best helps debride a wound with extensive tissue damage?
     a. Dry gauze
     b. Gauze dressing with an oily antiseptic
     c. Gauze dressing with a water-soluble antiseptic
     d. Wet saline dressing

251. Most of the clinical signs seen in an animal in shock from excessive blood loss are attributable to:
     a. Acidosis
     b. Alkalosis
     c. Cell death
     d. Redistribution of blood flow

252. The main goal of surgery to remove a pus-filled uterus (pyometra) is:
     a. A prophylactic measure
     b. To make a diagnosis
     c. To restore the animal to a normal reproductive state
     d. To return the animal to health without restoring normal reproductive function

253. What tissue must form in a wound that is healing by second intention before wound contraction or epithelial regeneration can occur?
     a. Collagen fibers
     b. Fibrin clot
     c. Granulation tissue
     d. Scar tissue

254. When gloving for surgery, which of the following is *not* permitted?
     a. One gloved thumb touches the other gloved thumb
     b. The scrubbed fingers touch the outside of the glove
     c. The outside of the gown cuff is touched by inside of the glove cuff
     d. The scrubbed fingers touch the inside of the glove cuff

255. How should a pack be placed in an autoclave for sterilization?
     a. Diagonally
     b. Horizontally
     c. Upside down
     d. Vertically

256. Metzenbaum scissors are used for:
     a. Cutting sutures
     b. Soft-tissue dissection
     c. Cutting the linea alba
     d. Cutting skin

257. What retractors are *not* handheld?
     a. Deaver
     b. Senn
     c. Rake
     d. Gelpi

258. What is the appropriate time to soak an instrument in a cold sterilization solution before adequate sterilization is achieved?
     a. 30 minutes
     b. 15 minutes
     c. 45 minutes
     d. 10 hours

259. How long does an instrument that is sterilized and wrapped in paper remain sterile?
     a. 6 months
     b. 1 week
     c. 1 month
     d. 1 year

260. Instrument milk is used for all of the following *except:*
     a. Lubrication
     b. Rust inhibition
     c. Extending the life of the instrument
     d. Cleaning the instrument

261. What type of instrument is a Backhaus?
     a. Needle holder
     b. Scissors
     c. Towel clamp
     d. Hemostatic forceps

262. For what bovine surgical procedure are obstetric (OB) chains used?
    a. Rumenotomy
    b. Abomasopexy
    c. Cesarean section
    d. Uterine torsion correction

263. Which of the following does *not* have to be gas sterilized?
    a. Arthroscope
    b. Plastic pipette tips
    c. Polyethylene tubing
    d. Plastic spray bottles

264. Ultrasonic cleaners are used for:
    a. Removing small particles of blood and tissue from instruments
    b. Removing rust from instruments
    c. Disinfecting instruments
    d. Lubricating instruments

265. All of the following are signs of hypotension during surgery, *except:*
    a. Excessive vasodilation
    b. Hypovolemia
    c. Hypothermia
    d. Anesthetic depth

266. Which of the following is *not* a consideration when evaluating a surgical pack for sterility?
    a. Sterilization date
    b. Indicator color change
    c. Holes or moisture damage
    d. Incorrect labeling

267. Mayo-Hegar scissors are used in all of the following situations *except* for cutting:
    a. Sutures
    b. Delicate tissue
    c. Paper drapes
    d. Skin or muscle

268. All of the following are duties assigned to the sterile surgical assistant *except:*
    a. Passing instruments
    b. Draping the patient
    c. Identifying suture patterns
    d. Administering drugs intraoperatively

269. How long must instruments be aerated for (after ethylene oxide gas sterilization) before they can be used?
    a. 1 hour
    b. 15 hours
    c. 4 days
    d. 7 days

270. What size scalpel blade is generally used in an arthroscopy for making the stab incision into the joint because of its pointed, rather than rounded or hooked, end?
    a. No. 10
    b. No. 11
    c. No. 12
    d. No. 15

271. What type of sterilization technique is *not* acceptable for instruments used in canine castration?
    a. Gas sterilization
    b. Autoclaving
    c. Chemical sterilization
    d. Boiling

272. All of the following are objectives of the surgical hand scrub *except:*
    a. To remove gross dirt and oil from the hands
    b. To sterilize the hands
    c. To reduce the microorganism count on the hands to as close to zero as possible
    d. To produce a prolonged depressant effect on the number of microflora on the hands and forearms

273. What type of surgical scrub solution is most effective in reducing the number of bacteria on the skin and maintaining the longest residual activity?
    a. Hexachlorophene alcohol
    b. Povidone-iodine
    c. Chlorhexidine gluconate
    d. Polypropylene parachormeta-xylenol

274. When a surgeon encounters bleeding, all of the following can be used to control it *except:*
    a. Electrocautery
    b. A hemostat
    c. Suction
    d. Rat-tooth forceps

275. How long does a sealed item remain sterilized after being sterilized by gamma radiation?
    a. 1 year
    b. 6 months
    c. Until it is opened
    d. 1 month

276. What retractor is *not* self-retaining?
    a. Weitlaner
    b. Alms
    c. Senn
    d. Balfour

277. Sterilization is the process of killing microorganisms by physical or chemical means. What is the quickest and most reliable form of sterilization?
    a. Steam under pressure
    b. Gas
    c. Dry heat
    d. Radiation

278. Instruments wrapped in a single linen wrap can become contaminated with microbes within 2 to 3 days. How long does double wrapping an instrument extend the sterility period?
    a. 6 months
    b. 4 weeks
    c. 4 to 6 days
    d. 1 year

279. What is the best type of cleaner to use when washing surgical instruments by hand?
    a. Ordinary hand soap
    b. Abrasive compounds
    c. Low-sudsing detergents
    d. Plain hot water

280. Which of the following is an absorbable suture?
    a. Prolene
    b. Vicryl
    c. Mersilene
    d. Silk

281. All of the following are considered benefits of using skin staples *except:*
    a. Skin is more resistant to abscess formation than when sutures are used
    b. Staples provide excellent wound healing
    c. Staples are more cost effective
    d. Staples save time

282. If skin edges are under extreme tension (e.g., in a large skin wound), what is the suture pattern of choice?
    a. Simple continuous
    b. Simple interrupted
    c. Interrupted horizontal mattress
    d. Continuous horizontal mattress

283. All of the following can contribute to a prolonged recovery *except:*
    a. Breed predisposition
    b. Poor perfusion
    c. Hyperglycemia
    d. Hypothermia

284. What suture is *not* recommended for skin closure?
    a. Polydioxanone
    b. Nylon
    c. Chromic gut
    d. Stainless steel

285. What is the purpose of using a subcuticular suture pattern for final closure?
    a. To decrease the amount of suture material needed
    b. To eliminate the need for skin sutures
    c. To eliminate infection
    d. To be more cost effective

286. What suture pattern would *not* be used to close skin?
    a. Cushing
    b. Horizontal mattress
    c. Simple interrupted
    d. Ford interlocking

287. Which of the following suture patterns is an inverting stitch?
    a. Cruciate
    b. Cushing
    c. Horizontal mattress
    d. Vertical mattress

288. In what way is a surgeon's knot different from a square knot?
    a. A surgeon's knot has one throw on the first pass and two throws on the second pass; a square knot has two throws on each pass.
    b. A surgeon's knot has two throws on the first pass and one throw on the second pass; a square knot has one pass on each throw.
    c. A surgeon's knot has one throw on each pass; a square knot has two throws on each pass.
    d. A surgeon's knot has two throws on the first pass and one throw on the second pass; a square knot has one throw on each pass.

289. Why is it better to ligate many small vessels rather than one mass ligation of tissues?
    a. Mass ligation of tissues is unsightly
    b. Mass ligation of tissue might result in an infected area
    c. Mass ligation of tissue is more likely to fail
    d. Tissues included in a mass ligation may be too difficult for the body to resorb

290. What is the purpose of a transfixation ligature?
    a. To make the ligature stronger
    b. To close a hollow organ
    c. To prevent breakage of the suture
    d. To prevent slippage of the suture

291. All of the following are good reasons for using an instrument tie (with the use of a needle holder) *except:*
    a. It is economical; small pieces of suture can be used, and therefore suture material is not wasted.
    b. It saves time.
    c. It is more accurate than a one- or two-handed tie.
    d. It is readily adaptable to any type of wound closure.

292. Which of the following is *not* a consideration when choosing a needle for use in a surgical procedure?
    a. Type of tissue to be sutured
    b. Location of the tissue to be sutured
    c. Size of suture material
    d. Strength of suture material

293. When suturing skin, the needle of choice is:
    a. Blunt
    b. Reverse cutting
    c. Cutting
    d. Taper

294. What is the most significant advantage of using a swaged-on needle as opposed to a closed-eye needle?
    a. The needle never separates from the suture
    b. The suture diameter is smaller than the needle diameter
    c. Tissue is subjected to fewer traumas, because a single strand is pulled through the tissue
    d. It saves time and money

295. Suture patterns can be classified into three types: appositional, inverting, and tension. What tissue is most appropriately sutured in an appositional pattern?
    a. Tendon
    b. Hollow viscus
    c. Skin
    d. Nerve

296. Which of these sequences correctly lists suture material diameter, from largest to smallest?
    a. 3-0, 2-0, 0, 1, 2, 3
    b. 000, 00, 0, 1, 2, 3
    c. 3, 2, 1, 1-0, 2-0, 3-0
    d. 7-0, 5-0, 3-0, 1

297. Which of the following suffixes is used to describe a process of cutting into an organ?
    a. *-ectomy*
    b. *-otomy*
    c. *-ostomy*
    d. *-rrhapy*

298. All of the following are contributing factors of wound dehiscence *except:*
    a. Suture failure
    b. Infection
    c. Tissue weakness
    d. Optimal nutrition

299. Wound dehiscence is usually seen within the first:
    a. 1–2 days
    b. 3–4 days
    c. 5–6 days
    d. 10–14 days

300. When the term *eviscerates* is used, this can indicate:
    a. The wound has dehisced
    b. Abdominal contents protrude through the suture line
    c. The aseptic technique has been broken and contamination has occurred
    d. Infection has entered the body through the surgical wound

301. All of the following are factors that determine whether infection occurs, *except:*
    a. Number of microorganisms
    b. Virulence of microorganisms
    c. Susceptibility of the patient
    d. Length of exposure time

302. Increased risk of nosocomial infection may result from improper application of methods of:
    a. Sanitation
    b. Sterilization
    c. Disinfection
    d. All of the above

303. Sterile patient preparation generally consists of _____ round(s) of alternating antiseptic solution with saline rinse, and every pass with gauze moves in a circular motion from the anticipated incision site radiating outward.
    a. 1
    b. 2
    c. 3
    d. 4

304. All of the following are clinical signs of pain that a patient may exhibit when recovering from an ovariohysterectomy, *except:*
    a. Tachycardia
    b. Hyperpnea
    c. Muscle tension
    d. Hypotension

305. For suturing a uterine incision in a cow, the proper suture size is:
a. 2-0
b. 1
c. 2
d. 3-0

306. Which of the following is a disadvantage of multifilament suture material?
a. Less knot security than monofilament suture material
b. Tears tissue more easily than monofilament suture material
c. Has a greater tendency for wicking bacteria than monofilament suture material
d. Has less strength than monofilament suture material

307. Which of the following is a monofilament suture material?
a. Polyglactin 910 (Vicryl)
b. Polyester (Mersilene)
c. Polyethylene (Dermalene)
d. Cotton

308. Which of the following has the poorest handling ease?
a. Silk
b. Braided polyglycolic acid (Dexon-Plus)
c. Chromic catgut
d. Monofilament stainless steel wire

309. Characteristics of an ideal suture material include all of the following *except:*
a. Minimal tissue reaction
b. Favorability for bacterial growth
c. Comfort in working with it
d. Economical to use

310. An example of an inverting suture pattern is the:
a. Purse-string
b. Simple interrupted
c. Interrupted horizontal mattress
d. Simple continuous

311. After what amount of time does a synthetic absorbable suture lose its tensile strength?
a. 120 days
b. 60 days
c. 30 days
d. 6 months

312. What suture material is absorbed most rapidly from an infected wound through increased local phagocytic activity?
a. Vicryl (polyglactin 910)
b. PDS (polydioxanone)
c. Catgut
d. Nylon

313. Which of the following is *not* a consideration when choosing a suture material?
a. The surgeon's training and experience
b. The part of the body where it will be used
c. The size of the animal on which it will be used
d. The age of the animal on which it will be used

314. Regarding wound healing, it is better to:
a. Increase the size of the suture material rather than the number of sutures
b. Increase the number of sutures rather than the size of the suture material
c. Decrease both the size of the suture material and the number of the sutures
d. Increase both the size of the suture material and the number of the sutures

315. Which of these statements concerning surgical catgut is false?
a. It can be used for ligating superficial blood vessels.
b. It is recommended for epidermal use.
c. It is recommended for internal use.
d. It is absorbs quickly.

316. Chromic catgut is produced by exposure to basic chromium salts. How does this process affect it?
a. Increases intermolecular bonding
b. Decreases its strength
c. Increases tissue reaction to it
d. Decreases absorption time

317. Perioperative antibiotics:
a. Should never be used
b. Should always be used
c. Are indicated in surgical procedures longer than 1.5 hours
d. Are questionable in their effectiveness

318. What is the primary function of a Balfour?
a. Retractor
b. Rongeur
c. Periosteal elevator
d. Thumb forceps

319. What is the primary function of a Lempert?
a. Retractor
b. Rongeur
c. Periosteal elevator
d. Thumb forceps

320. All of the following statements regarding chlorhexidine gluconate surgical scrub are true *except:*
    a. Tends to stain the skin and hair coat
    b. Is effective against the *Pseudomonas* species
    c. Is marketed as Nolvasan
    d. Should be rinsed with alcohol

321. What if a gauze sponge that is being used for the surgical scrub inadvertently touches the patient's hair?
    a. It can continue to be used for the scrub, because the antimicrobial agents in the scrub will kill any bacteria picked up from the hair
    b. It should be thrown out and replaced with a new sponge
    c. It should now be used only for the edges of the clipped site
    d. It should not be considered contaminated unless gross contamination is visible

322. Surgical scrubs are applied to the surgically prepared site:
    a. In any pattern, just so the area is covered thoroughly
    b. In target fashion, starting with the incision site and spiraling outward toward the edge of the clipped area
    c. Starting with the edges, because they are the dirtiest areas, and working in toward the incision site
    d. Without subsequent rinsing, because dilution reduces the antimicrobial effect

323. Why is an anal purse-string suture placed before perianal surgery?
    a. To keep the tail out of the surgical field
    b. To prevent fecal contamination during surgery
    c. To close the urethra
    d. To tighten loose folds of perianal skin

324. In male dogs, the prepuce is:
    a. Sutured closed before an abdominal surgical procedure to prevent contamination
    b. Considered an uncontaminated area that is not given special consideration
    c. Flushed with alcohol while the dog is awake
    d. Flushed with a weak povidone-iodine and saline solution before abdominal surgery

325. What structure is commonly emptied before abdominal surgery?
    a. Stomach
    b. Anal sac
    c. Urinary bladder
    d. Gallbladder

326. What type of instrument is a Metzenbaum?
    a. Needle holder
    b. Scissors
    c. Towel clamp
    d. Hemostatic forceps

327. The most effective use for a rongeur is to:
    a. Pinch off a bleeding vessel
    b. Elevate soft tissue off a bony surface
    c. Remove small pieces of bone
    d. Retract soft tissue away from bone

328. Talking in the surgery room should be kept to a minimum to:
    a. Prevent unnecessary injection of bacteria into the operating theater
    b. Prevent distractions
    c. Expedite the surgery
    d. Talking does not need to be kept to a minimum

329. The instrument suitable for cutting a paper drape is:
    a. Operating scissors
    b. Metzenbaum scissors
    c. Scalpel blade
    d. Wire scissors

330. What instrument is *not* a self-retaining tissue retractor?
    a. Finochietto
    b. Army-Navy
    c. Balfour
    d. Gelpi

331. A surgical scrub with residual antibacterial activity is important because:
    a. Bacteria below the superficial dermal area are constantly rising to the surface
    b. It makes it unnecessary to worry about touching a scrubbed area with an ungloved hand
    c. It makes it unnecessary to be as fastidious in the scrubbing technique
    d. It makes it unnecessary to worry about prepping the area with alcohol, in addition to the surgical scrub.

332. The most effective sterilizing method for an object that could be damaged by heat is:
    a. Autoclaving
    b. Gas sterilization
    c. Flash flaming
    d. Alcohol scrub

333. What term best describes freedom from infection as it applies to the surgical technique?
    a. Uncontaminated
    b. Asepsis
    c. Healthy
    d. Clean

334. What surgical materials are sterilized by filtration?
    a. Nutrient solutions
    b. Irrigation solutions
    c. Surgical solutions
    d. Pharmaceutical solutions

335. What piece of equipment delivers saturated steam under pressure?
    a. Oven
    b. Crematorium
    c. Autoclave
    d. Plasma sterilizer

336. A safeguard to ensure that a pack is sterilized adequately is:
    a. Sterilization tape
    b. Sterilization indicators
    c. Feeling how hot the instrument is after the sterilization process is complete
    d. Visually inspecting the pack for microorganisms

337. An autoclave:
    a. Is not a safe method to sterilize metal implants for orthopedic procedures
    b. Must not be overloaded because this decreases its effectiveness
    c. Can be used to sterilize syringes for future vaccination clinics
    d. Is expensive and is therefore not practical for most veterinary clinics

338. Electrocautery is:
    a. An effective way to sterilize skin
    b. Used to coagulate blood flow from a cut vessel
    c. Cannot be used for most surgical procedures
    d. Atraumatic and can be used liberally

339. Peripheral catheters should be monitored frequently and changed every:
    a. 12 hours
    b. 24 hours
    c. 36 hours
    d. 72 hours

340. The main goal of the aseptic surgical technique is to prevent contamination of the:
    a. Operative personnel
    b. Surgical instruments
    c. Surgical wound
    d. Surgical drapes

341. When preparing a feline patient for a routine spay, administration of antibiotics before surgery:
    a. Should be given only if the surgeon does not wear a cap or a mask
    b. Is not indicated for short, uncomplicated procedures
    c. Should always be given as a precaution to prevent infection
    d. Is never useful in conjunction with surgery

342. The main function of bactericidal disinfectants is to:
    a. Slow bacterial proliferation
    b. Kill bacteria
    c. Remove organic debris from the site
    d. Flush bacteria from the site

343. Keeping the environment (floors, walls, counters) clean throughout the hospital is:
    a. Not important if your surgery areas are separate from other areas of the clinic
    b. Advisable because it is good for public relations
    c. Mandated by the AVMA
    d. Mandatory to prevent cross-contamination into the surgery area

344. The sterile field in the surgery room:
    a. Is the entire surgical suite
    b. Consists of the shaved and prepared area on the animal's skin
    c. Consists of the draped field and instrument table
    d. All of the above

345. The surgical nurse circulating for the scrubbed-in surgeon(s):
    a. Has the task of keeping the animal anesthetized
    b. Does not need a cap and mask because he or she is not assisting with surgery
    c. Must constantly be concerned with maintaining an aseptic technique
    d. Need not wear sterile surgical gloves

346. Perineal urethrostomies are performed only on:
    a. Pregnant cats
    b. Male cats with urethral obstruction
    c. Large-breed dogs with gastric torsion
    d. Small dogs with pyometra

347. Assuming that good aseptic technique is being followed, the most common source of contamination in a surgical wound is:
    a. The patient's skin or internal organs
    b. Your own breath
    c. Dust falling from the ceiling
    d. Dust from the floor

348. The clothing worn in a surgical room:
 a. Can be clothes worn on the street
 b. Should be clothes worn while in the clinic only
 c. Should be a scrub suit dedicated to surgery use
 d. Is required to be clean only and not torn

349. Surgical masks:
 a. Prevent unpleasant odors from reaching the surgeon's nose
 b. Lose their effectiveness when saturated with moisture
 c. Are used for orthopedic procedures only
 d. Can be tied loosely so that they are not as confining

350. When folding surgical gowns for sterilization:
 a. Tie the arms together so they do not dangle when the surgeon is gowning.
 b. Have the ends of the sleeves on top for easy grasping.
 c. Make sure the ties are on top so they can be used to pick up the gown.
 d. Place the inside of the shoulder seams on top and fold all outer areas of the gown to the inside.

351. During surgery, the back outside aspect of a surgeon's gown should be considered:
 a. Sterile
 b. Sterile as long as someone has not touched it
 c. Unsterile
 d. Neither sterile nor unsterile, because it is not likely to contact the patient

352. If a gowned and gloved person at the surgery table is *not* participating in the surgery at some point:
 a. His or her hands should be held quietly at the sides
 b. His or her hands may be held behind the back if it is still sterile
 c. His or her hands should be folded at chest level or placed on the instrument table
 d. He or she must leave the room

353. The counted brush stroke method for surgical scrubbing:
 a. Is not practical on a routine basis
 b. Is quicker than a timed scrub
 c. Refers to scrubbing the arms and hands in a methodical, consistent manner
 d. Is more thorough than a timed scrub

354. A timed scrub should last at least:
 a. 15 minutes
 b. 5 minutes
 c. 30 minutes
 d. 1 minute

355. The preferred method for gloving is:
 a. Open
 b. Closed
 c. Assisted
 d. Double

356. When scrubbing for a surgical procedure, the position of the arms:
 a. Varies with the height of the scrub sink
 b. Should always be with the hands higher than the elbows
 c. Should always be with the elbows higher than the hands
 d. Varies with the height of the scrubbing personnel

357. Iodophors, such as povidone-iodine scrub:
 a. Are the ideal surgical preparation solutions
 b. Have been replaced by newer, more effective scrubbing agents
 c. Are effective when used with alcohol only
 d. Have better residual activity than chlorhexidine

358. The number of personnel in the operating theater:
 a. Has no bearing on the outcome of the surgery
 b. Cannot be controlled in most situations
 c. Must be high to keep the temperature in the room high
 d. Should be kept to a minimum to keep airborne bacteria levels low to reduce the likelihood of contamination.

359. Cleaning instruments before sterilization:
 a. Must be performed carefully by hand
 b. Is done only if there is time
 c. Can be done exclusively with ultrasonic cleaners
 d. Is not necessary if proper sterilization practices are followed

360. Ethyl and isopropyl alcohols:
 a. Have characteristics that make them ideal for sterilizing instruments
 b. Have the ability to act both as disinfectants and as antiseptics
 c. Have excellent residual effects because of rapid evaporation
 d. Have no place in veterinary surgery

361. An effective disinfectant to clean a cage after an animal has had a *Pseudomonas*-contaminated wound is:
 a. Chlorhexidine
 b. Isopropyl alcohol
 c. Quaternary ammonium
 d. Povidone-iodine

362. A good solution to instill in the conjunctival sac before surgery is:
   a. 10% chlorhexidine gluconate
   b. 10% povidone-iodine solution
   c. 5% isopropyl alcohol
   d. Dilute soapy water

363. Clean-contaminated surgery refers to:
   a. All surgeries
   b. Incisions in sterile areas that become contaminated during surgery
   c. A clean wound in which a drain is placed
   d. Incisions in a previously contaminated area that has been rendered sterile

364. In terms of surgical contamination, endogenous organisms are those that:
   a. Originate from the patient's own body
   b. Come from the external surgical environment
   c. Rarely cause any problem in surgical wounds
   d. Come from the surgeon

365. When a break in aseptic technique occurs:
   a. The surgery must be called off immediately.
   b. The break can be ignored and surgery can continue if the surgery is nearly finished.
   c. The patient is unlikely to recover from the surgery because of infection.
   d. Steps must be taken to remedy the situation immediately to the best of everyone's ability.

366. A good time to clean the surgery room is:
   a. On the night before surgery to allow airborne dust to settle before surgery
   b. Immediately before the surgery so things can be as clean as possible
   c. Once a week
   d. Once a month

367. Lavaging (flushing) a body cavity with warm, sterile saline after completing a surgical procedure and before closing the incision:
   a. Is of minimal value in abdominal surgeries
   b. Decreases the amount of bacteria left behind and warms the patient
   c. Serves as a medium in which bacteria can multiply, so it should be avoided
   d. Is necessary only if a break in aseptic technique has occurred

368. An example of an elective procedure is:
   a. Ovariohysterectomy
   b. Nephrotomy
   c. Exploratory laparotomy
   d. Splenectomy

369. A tapered suture needle is:
   a. Best to use in skin
   b. The least traumatic and most often used in deep tissue layers
   c. Not used very often because of its relative inability to penetrate tissue
   d. Too expensive for routine surgical use

370. A thoracotomy is an incision into the:
   a. Abdomen
   b. Chest
   c. Skull
   d. Ear

371. The suffix -ectomy refers to:
   a. Surgical removal
   b. Reduction
   c. Drainage
   d. Incision into

372. Which orthopedic fixation consists of pins that penetrate fractured bones that are held in place externally by bolts?
   a. Rush pinning
   b. Steinmann fixation
   c. Stack pinning
   d. Kirschner-Ehmer fixation

373. The term arthrotomy refers to an incision into a/an:
   a. Artery
   b. Joint
   c. Muscle
   d. Long bone

374. Arresting the flow of blood from a vessel or to a part is called:
   a. Aspiration
   b. Fibrinolysis
   c. Hemostasis
   d. Hemolysis

375. Peritonitis refers to:
   a. Inflammation of the pericardial space
   b. Inflammation of the lining of the abdominal cavity
   c. Inflammation caused by parasite infection
   d. Inflammation of the perianal area

376. Cryptorchidectomy is performed on male dogs:
   a. When one or both testicles have not descended into the scrotal sac
   b. When no other treatment for cryptosporidiosis is available
   c. And is similar to the vasectomy procedure performed in people
   d. When complications from routine castration arise

377. Fenestration refers to:
- a. Cutting a part exactly in half
- b. Creating a window in tissue
- c. The draping procedure
- d. Folding back the top skin layer

378. Ovariohysterectomy is routinely performed:
- a. In excitable dogs that need immediate calming
- b. In young female dogs that the owners wish rendered sterile
- c. In male dogs with female characteristics
- d. Exclusively in female dogs who have already had litters of puppies

379. Hepatic refers to:
- a. Heparin preparations
- b. Liver
- c. Blood
- d. Stomach

380. Blood vessels are ligated:
- a. To remove them completely from the body
- b. When blood flow needs to be stopped
- c. With suture material only
- d. Rarely and in emergency situations only

381. Chemical cauterization:
- a. Releases toxic fumes, exposing team members to a potential hazard
- b. Is rarely used in veterinary medicine
- c. Is traumatic to adjacent tissues and therefore is not used in surgical cases
- d. Is a misnomer; chemicals cannot stop bleeding

382. Keeping tissues moist during a surgical procedure:
- a. Is important, because dry tissues are less resistant to bacterial infection
- b. Is undesirable, because wet tissue is an ideal medium for bacterial regeneration
- c. Is of little value
- d. Should be accomplished with 70% isopropyl alcohol

383. Plating a fractured bone:
- a. Refers to coating the bone with a rigid metallic solution to induce healing
- b. Is beyond the scope of most veterinary practices
- c. Is an internal method of fracture fixation involving stainless steel plates and screws
- d. Can be done without skin incision

384. The distal portion of a long bone is:
- a. The one closest to the trunk of the body
- b. The one farthest away from the trunk of the body
- c. The inner portion of the bone
- d. The outer layer of the bone

385. *Torsion* of an organ or part refers to:
- a. Swelling or expansion
- b. Inflation with fluid
- c. Inflation with gas
- d. Twisting or rotation

386. What surgical procedure is least likely to combat the debilitating complications of canine hip dysplasia?
- a. Triple pelvic osteotomy
- b. Total hip replacement
- c. Intramedullary pinning
- d. Pectineal myotomy

387. Ear canal ablation refers to:
- a. Irrigation of the ear canal
- b. Instilling antibiotics to correct otitis media
- c. Surgical removal and closure of the external ear canal
- d. The instrument used to examine the ear canal

388. *Perioperative* refers to:
- a. The day before surgery
- b. The day after surgery
- c. Immediately before and after surgery
- d. During surgery

389. Onychectomy:
- a. Is the procedure used to remove a cat's testicles and spermatic cord
- b. Is the procedure used to remove a cat's claws and associated phalanges
- c. Can be performed without anesthesia
- d. Can be performed on female cats only

390. Postoperative complications:
- a. Do not occur if the surgeon is skilled
- b. Should never be discussed with a client
- c. Can occur even if the surgery went well
- d. Are almost always attributable to poor assistance in surgery

391. Fracture reduction:
- a. Involves trimming the areas of bone adjacent to the fracture site
- b. Involves apposing (pulling together) the fractured bone ends
- c. Is rarely necessary for good healing
- d. Can usually be performed without anesthesia

392. A diaphragmatic hernia:
- a. Is a diaphragm that is in continuous spasm
- b. Is displacement of the heart and part of the lungs into the abdomen
- c. Cannot be corrected and is considered fatal
- d. Should be suspected if the animal is dyspneic following a traumatic experience

393. When an animal is sent home after surgery:
   a. The wound should already be completely healed
   b. The client should be given written detailed home care instructions
   c. The animal is no longer legally your patient and is no longer your concern
   d. The technician should make daily visits to ensure that the patient is given the same care as in the hospital

394. Absorbable gelatin sponges:
   a. Are typically soaked or sutured into a bleeding site
   b. Should never be left in the body after surgery
   c. Are radiopaque
   d. Are not available for veterinary surgery

395. Exteriorizing a body part or organ during surgery:
   a. Is a routine practice when the part or organ contains contaminants
   b. Is very hazardous to the patient and is not routinely done
   c. Precludes the need for lavaging
   d. Is done only if that part or organ is to be resected (surgically removed)

396. A dog presents at your clinic with a suspected intestinal foreign body. During the laparotomy the doctor removes the object and notes that a section of the intestines is necrotic. What is the name of the procedure to remove the necrotic area and rejoin the healthy intestines?
   a. Resection and intussusception
   b. Resection and enterotomy
   c. Resection and anastomosis
   d. Resection and celiotomy

397. During a cystotomy, the doctor requests a suture to close the bladder. Which suture is the most appropriate?
   a. Monofilament, absorbable with a taper point
   b. Monofilament, nonabsorbable with a taper point
   c. Multifilament, absorbable with cutting point
   d. Multifilament, nonabsorbable with a taper point

398. While monitoring a patient under anesthesia, you notice its blood pressure begins to drop. After notifying the veterinarian, what steps do you initially take to correct the situation?
   a. Decrease fluid rate and increase oxygen flow
   b. Increase fluid rate and increase oxygen flow
   c. Decrease fluid rate and increase anesthetic
   d. Increase fluid rate and decrease anesthetic

399. Which of the following situations can cause hypocarbia?
   a. Decreased respiratory rate
   b. Increased respiratory rate
   c. Exhausted soda lime
   d. Kinked endotracheal tube

400. What is considered the most painful portion of a routine spay procedure?
   a. The initial abdominal incision
   b. Applying the angiotribe
   c. The plucking/tearing of the suspensory ligament
   d. Ligation of the ovarian pedicle.

401. How soon after surgery should animals be offered food?
   a. 8 hours after recovery
   b. 12 hours after recovery
   c. 24 hours after recovery
   d. As soon as possible after recovery

402. Which of the following is used primarily to determine patient safety as opposed to anesthetic depth?
   a. Respiratory rate
   b. Palpebral reflex
   c. Eye position
   d. Muscle tone

403. If a patient is at an adequate surgical plane of anesthesia, which of the following statements would be true?
   a. The pedal reflex would be present
   b. The palpebral reflex would be present
   c. The swallowing reflex would be present
   d. The corneal reflex would be present

404. How many phases of wound healing are present in animals?
   a. 1
   b. 2
   c. 3
   d. 4

405. During the debridement phase of wound healing, all of the following are components of exudate, *except:*
   a. WBC
   b. RBC
   c. Dead tissue
   d. Wound fluid

406. Moist wound healing:
   a. Enhances wound healing
   b. Slows wound healing
   c. Has no effect on healing
   d. Increases the bacterial contamination of the wound

407. Which of the following external factors can delay wound healing?
   a. Steroids
   b. Radiation therapy
   c. Chemotherapeutic agents
   d. All of the above

408. All of the following items are removed when debriding a wound, *except:*
   a. Dead or damaged tissue
   b. Foreign bodies
   c. Microorganisms
   d. WBCs

409. How often should the surgery-room floor be cleaned?
   a. Only as needed
   b. Daily
   c. Morning and Evening
   d. Weekly

410. Regarding disinfectants, to what does "contact time" refer?
   a. The time required for disinfectants to be in contact with microorganisms to achieve the intended effect
   b. The time of day when the manufacturer can be contacted for assistance
   c. The time required for a microorganism to develop resistance to a disinfectant
   d. The latent phase of microorganisms, providing the disinfectant "a window of opportunity" to kill the microorganism

411. The surgical preparation room is located:
   a. Within the surgical suite
   b. Adjacent to the surgical suite
   c. Separated from the surgical suite by a treatment room
   d. Upstairs, above the surgical suite

ⓔ *Answers and rationales available on Evolve*
http://evolve.elsevier.com/Prendergast/QAvettech/

QUESTIONS

1. Apical means "toward the _____."
   a. Root tip
   b. Crown
   c. Cheeks
   d. Tongue

2. When assessing and quantifying gingivitis, the modified Löe and Silness index is often referred to. According to this index, a gingival index 3 indicates:
   a. Clinically healthy gingiva
   b. Mild gingivitis with slight reddening and swelling of the gingival margins
   c. Moderate gingivitis, with gentle probing resulting in bleeding
   d. Severe gingivitis, in which there is spontaneous hemorrhage and/or ulceration of the gingival margin

3. Hypodontia is defined as:
   a. Congenital absence of many, but not all, teeth
   b. Total absence of teeth
   c. Absence of only a few teeth
   d. Inflammation of the mouth

4. Abbreviations are commonly used in veterinary practice, and some abbreviations are exclusive to dental terminology. Which abbreviation best aligns with the complicated crown fracture?
   a. CCF
   b. UCF
   c. UCRF
   d. CCRF

5. When grading furcation involvement, which of the following descriptions is termed Grade 3?
   a. No furcation involvement
   b. The furcation can be felt with the probe/explorer, but horizontal tissue destruction is <⅓ of the horizontal width
   c. The furcation can be explored, but the probe cannot pass through it
   d. The probe can be passed through the furcation from buccal to palatal/lingual

6. When grading tooth mobility, which of the following grades corresponds to a Grade 3?
   a. No mobility
   b. Horizontal movement <1 mm
   c. Horizontal movement >1 mm
   d. Vertical and horizontal movement

7. Which teeth on each side of the dog's mouth have three roots?
   a. Maxillary: third and fourth premolars and first molar
   b. Maxillary: fourth premolars and first and second molars
   c. Mandibular: fourth premolars and first and second molars
   d. Mandibular and maxillary: fourth premolars and first and second molars

8. At what age do the permanent canine and premolar teeth in dogs generally erupt?
   a. 3–5 months
   b. 4–6 months
   c. 5–7 months
   d. 6–8 months

9. Using the Triadan system, the proper way to describe a dog's first maxillary left permanent premolar is:
   a. 205
   b. 105
   c. 306
   d. 502

10. Using the Triadan system, the proper way to describe a cat's first mandibular right molar is:
    a. 407
    b. 409
    c. 109
    d. 909

11. The pulp canal of a tooth contains:
    a. Nerves
    b. Blood vessels
    c. Connective tissue and blood vessels
    d. Blood vessels, nerves, and connective tissues

12. As part of normal tooth development, what part of the tooth widens?
    a. Enamel
    b. Pulp
    c. Dentin
    d. Gingiva

13. Which of the following statements regarding enamel is true?
    a. Contains living tissue
    b. Covers the tooth crown and root
    c. Continues production by the ameloblasts after eruption
    d. Is relatively nonporous and impervious

14. Dentin is covered by:
    a. Enamel and bone
    b. Bone and pulp
    c. Cementum and enamel
    d. Pulp and cementum

15. Normal scissor occlusion occurs when the maxillary fourth premolars occlude:
    a. Level with the mandibular fourth premolar
    b. Buccally to the mandibular first molar
    c. Buccally to the mandibular fourth premolar
    d. Lingually to the mandibular first molar

16. Which of the following correctly describes the adult feline dental formula?
    a. $2 \times \{$I 2/1:C 0/0:P 3/2:M 3/3$\}$
    b. $2 \times \{$I 3/3:C 1/1:P 4/4:M 2/3$\}$
    c. $2 \times \{$I 3/3:C 1/1:P 3/2:M 1/1$\}$
    d. $2 \times \{$I 3/3:C 1/1:P 3/3$\}$

17. The carnassial teeth in dogs are:
    a. ^{4}P4 and $_1$M$_1$
    b. $_4$P^4 and ^{4}P$_4$
    c. ^{1}M^1 and $_1$M$_1$
    d. ^{1}C^1 and $_1$C$_1$

18. The free or marginal gingiva:
    a. Occupies the space between the teeth
    b. Is the most apical portion of the gingiva
    c. Forms the gingival sulcus around the tooth
    d. Is tightly bound to the cementum

19. The periodontium includes the periodontal ligament and all of the following *except:*
    a. Gingiva
    b. Cementum
    c. Alveolar bone
    d. Enamel

20. A bulldog would be described as having what type of head shape?
    a. Brachycephalic
    b. Dolichocephalic
    c. Mesaticephalic/mesocephalic
    d. Prognacephalic

21. In veterinary dentistry, chlorhexidine solutions are used because they:
    a. Prevent cementoenamel erosion
    b. Have antibacterial properties
    c. Remove enamel stains and whiten teeth
    d. Are used to treat gingival hyperplasia in brachycephalic breeds

22. When using hand instruments to clean teeth:
    a. Use a modified pen grasp with a back-and-forth scraping motion.
    b. Use a modified pen grasp with overlapping pull strokes that are directed away from the gingival margin.
    c. Use the sickle scaler for subgingival curettage.
    d. The curette is best used supragingivally.

23. Pocket depth is measured from the:
    a. Cementoenamel junction to the bottom of the pocket
    b. Current free gingival margin to the bottom of the gingival sulcus
    c. Cementoenamel junction to the current free gingival margin and then adding 1–2 mm
    d. Cementoenamel junction to the apical extent of the defect

24. Between patients, it is best to maintain instruments in which following order:
    a. Use, sharpen, wash, and sterilize
    b. Use, wash, sterilize, and sharpen
    c. Use, wash, sharpen, and sterilize
    d. Wash, sterilize, use, and sharpen

25. When performing a dental prophylaxis, minimal safety equipment includes:
    a. Gloves only
    b. Gloves and mask only
    c. Safety glasses only
    d. Safety glasses, mask, and gloves

26. You have an instrument in your hand that has two sharp sides, a rounded back, and a rounded point. Which instrument are you holding?
    a. Sickle scaler
    b. Morse scaler
    c. Universal curette
    d. Sickle curette

27. When polishing teeth using an air-driven unit, at what speed should the hand piece be set?
    a. High speed
    b. Low speed
    c. Either high or low is acceptable
    d. Finishing speed

28. The term that best describes a dog with an abnormally short mandible is:
    a. Prognathism
    b. Brachygnathism
    c. Mesaticephalic
    d. Dolichocephalic

29. A malocclusion where one side of the mandible or maxilla is disproportionate to its other side is known as:
    a. Posterior crossbite
    b. Base-narrow mandibular canines
    c. Wry mouth
    d. Rostral crossbite

30. A malocclusion in which the upper fourth premolar lies palatal to the first molars is known as:
    a. Posterior crossbite
    b. Base-narrow mandibular canines
    c. Wry mouth
    d. Rostral crossbite

31. A malocclusion in which the canines erupt in an overly upright position, or the mandible is narrowed, is known as:
    a. Posterior crossbite
    b. Base-narrow mandibular canines
    c. Wry mouth
    d. Rostral crossbite

32. A malocclusion in which one or more of the upper incisor teeth are caudal to the lower incisors is known as:
    a. Posterior crossbite
    b. Base-narrow mandibular canines
    c. Wry mouth
    d. Rostral crossbite

33. To prep a patient for surgical tooth extraction, which of the following should occur?
    a. No prep is needed. It is best to extract, and then to clean the remaining teeth (this is a more efficient process, yielding a shorter anesthesia time)
    b. Rinse the mouth with chlorhexidine, then extract
    c. Scale, polish, then extract
    d. Scale, polish, rinse with chlorhexidine, then extract

34. Dry socket is more likely to occur when one:
    a. Ensures there is an increased blood supply to the area
    b. Practices good surgical technique
    c. Allows a blood clot to form so that fibroblasts are formed
    d. Overirrigates the tooth socket so that no clot can form

35. Gingivoplasty is the:
    a. Addition of more gingiva to the site
    b. Binding of the loose teeth together to stabilize them during a healing process
    c. Removal of hyperplastic gingival tissue
    d. Removal of a portion of the tooth structure

36. To protect the pulp tissue of teeth from thermal damage during ultrasonic scaling, one should:
    a. Use constant irrigation
    b. Change tips frequently
    c. Use slow rotational speed
    d. Use appropriate amounts of paste

37. Another term for neck lesions often seen on feline teeth is:
    a. Peripheral odontogenic fibroma
    b. Stomatitis
    c. Feline odontoclastic resorptive lesions
    d. Enamel fracture

38. The most common dental procedure performed on a horse is:
    a. Quidding
    b. Curettage
    c. Scaling
    d. Floating

39. Stomatitis is defined as:
    a. Bad breath that is evident when dental work must be completed
    b. Inflammation of the mouth's soft tissue
    c. Resorption of hard dental tissues by odontoclasts
    d. Inflammation and infection of some or all of the tooth's supportive tissues

40. A client would like to know what chew toy would be safest for her dog's teeth. You suggest that she is best to give "Fido" a:
a. Dried cow hoof
b. Nylon rope toy
c. Dense rubber exerciser
d. Large knucklebone

41. When taking radiographs of the canine tooth in a large breed dog, what size of dental film should be used to ensure that the whole tooth is included?
a. 0
b. 2
c. 4
d. 8″ × 10″ screen film

42. Dental film should be placed in the mouth with the dimple facing:
a. Up and pointing rostrally
b. Up and pointing caudally
c. Down and pointing rostrally
d. Down and pointing caudally

43. The flap side of the dental film should face:
a. Any direction, because it does not matter
b. Toward the tube head
c. Away from the tube head
d. The caudal side of the animal

44. The bisecting angle principle states that the plane of an x-ray beam should be 90 degrees to the:
a. Long axis of the tooth
b. Plane of the film
c. Imaginary line that bisects the angle formed by the tooth's long axis and the film plane
d. Imaginary line that bisects the angle formed by the animal's head and the film plane

45. You are looking at your dental radiograph and notice that the tooth is elongated. This happened because the beam was perpendicular to the:
a. Film
b. Tooth
c. Bisecting angle
d. Wrong tooth

46. Abbreviations are commonly used in veterinary practice, and some abbreviations are exclusive to dental terminology. Which abbreviation best aligns with a complicated crown and root fracture?
a. CCF
b. UCF
c. UCRF
d. CCRF

47. A scaler is used to:
a. Check the tooth's root surface for any irregularities
b. Measure the depth of gingival recession
c. Scale large amounts of calculus from the tooth surface
d. Scale calculus from the tooth surface located in the gingival sulcus

48. What mineralized tissue covers the root of the tooth?
a. Calculus
b. Enamel
c. Cementum
d. Dentin

49. The nerves and blood vessels of a tooth are located in the:
a. Sulcus
b. Pulp cavity
c. Marrow cavity
d. Calculus

50. When scaling gross calculus from the teeth:
a. Hold the scaler using a modified pen grasp
b. Hold the scaler using a modified screwdriver grasp
c. Use long controlled strokes toward the gums
d. Hold the curette using a modified pen grasp

51. Which of the following statements is true about ultrasonic scaling?
a. Ultrasonic scaling is the only method to clean a tooth surface fully
b. Ultrasonic scaling causes thermal damage to the tooth if the tip is kept on a tooth for < 5 seconds
c. The ultrasonic scaler works by spraying the tooth with water to wash the tooth clean
d. The purpose of the water spray on an ultrasonic scaler is to cool the tip of the instrument and cool the tooth to prevent pulp damage

52. The following statements are all true *except*:
a. Sulcus depth is measured using a probe
b. A sulcus depth ≤3 mm is normal in a cat
c. A sulcus depth >3 mm indicates periodontal disease
d. The probe is inserted gently into the gingival sulcus parallel to the root of the tooth

53. All of the following are complications that may result from extraction, *except:*
a. Hemorrhage
b. Jaw fracture
c. Stomatitis
d. Oronasal fistula

54. An older dog with dental disease is presented to the clinic with a draining tract below his right eye. What is the most likely cause?
    a. Right-sided maxillary carnassial tooth root abscess
    b. Left-sided maxillary carnassial tooth root abscess
    c. Right-sided mandibular carnassial tooth root abscess
    d. Maxillary incisor tooth root abscess

55. What members of the veterinary staff make up the oral health care team?
    a. The veterinarian
    b. The veterinary technician
    c. The receptionists
    d. All of the above

56. Why would thermal bone injury be a complication of tooth extraction?
    a. The bur will overheat and damage the soft tissue and bone
    b. Thermal injury is not a concern, as you are removing the tooth anyway
    c. Tooth elevators cause excessive heat, which could injure the soft tissue around the tooth that is being extracted
    d. Tooth extractors cause excessive heat, which could injure the remaining teeth

57. Brachygnathism is a genetic defect best characterized as:
    a. A maxilla that is longer than the mandible
    b. A mandible that is longer than the maxilla
    c. A lack of incisors
    d. Polydontia

58. Prognathism is a normal condition in brachycephalic breeds but is considered a genetic defect in other breeds. It is best characterized as:
    a. A mandible that is longer than the maxilla
    b. A maxilla that is longer than the mandible
    c. One side of the head being longer than the other
    d. An overly long soft palate

59. Malocclusions can lead to dental disease for all of the following reasons *except:*
    a. Soft-tissue trauma from teeth that are abnormally positioned
    b. Accelerated development of periodontal disease resulting from the lack of normal wear and the normal flushing of teeth with saliva
    c. Abnormal wear of teeth resulting from malposition leading to fracture and pulp exposure
    d. Presence of resorptive lesions leading to the destruction of teeth

60. Which of the following teeth are not normally present in the adult cat?
    a. P1 and P1 and P2
    b. P_1 and P^1 and P2
    c. I^2 and I_1
    d. PM3 and PM4

61. The furcation is best described as:
    a. The area between the cementum and the enamel
    b. The space between two roots where they meet the crown
    c. The space between the root and the alveolar bone
    d. The space between two teeth

62. What is the most common clinical sign of feline stomatitis?
    a. Fractured crowns and/or granulation tissue at the cementoenamel junction
    b. Thickening or bulging of the alveolar bone of the maxillary canine teeth
    c. Erythematous, ulcerative, proliferative lesions affecting the gingiva, glossopalatine arches, tongue, lips, buccal mucosa, and/or hard palate
    d. Granular, orange-colored ulcerations found on the upper lips adjacent to the philtrum

63. An oronasal fistula can often occur secondary to:
    a. Abscess of the mandibular canine tooth
    b. Incisor root abscess
    c. Abscess of the maxillary canine tooth
    d. Retained deciduous incisors

64. Which of the following statements about canine toy breeds is true?
    a. Chronic impaction of incisor teeth with hair and debris often results in a chronic osteomyelitis
    b. Malocclusions are rare in toy breeds in comparison with giant-breed dogs
    c. Enamel hypoplasia is a common finding in toy breeds
    d. Prognathism is considered a genetic defect in brachycephalic breeds

65. A biopsy report confirms that an oral mass is an acanthomatous ameloblastoma or an acanthomatous epulis. Which of the following statements is true regarding this growth?
    a. It is a nonmalignant tumor
    b. It is a malignant tumor
    c. It is very likely to metastasize
    d. It is related to the presence of a malocclusion

66. While performing a routine prophylactic dentistry, the veterinary technician notes a large, red raised lesion on the lip of her feline patient. The client noted that the lesion "comes and goes." What is a reasonable differential for this lesion?
    a. Feline resorptive lesion
    b. Trauma-related lesion
    c. Eosinophilic ulcer
    d. Tumor

67. Feline cervical line lesions/feline neck lesions/feline resorptive lesions are of great concern to veterinarians. Which of the following statements regarding these lesions is false?
    a. Feline resorptive lesions are aggressive dental caries that result in resorption of roots and subsequent tooth loss
    b. Feline resorptive lesions often present with a raspberry seed-type sign at the base of the tooth where it meets the gingival margin
    c. Feline resorptive lesions are effectively managed with steroid administration
    d. It is common to find more than one feline cervical line lesion in the oral cavity

68. Which of the following statements about the eruption of permanent teeth is false?
    a. The permanent upper canines erupt mesial to the deciduous canines
    b. The permanent lower canines erupt buccal to the deciduous canines
    c. The permanent incisors erupt distal to the deciduous incisors
    d. The permanent canine teeth erupt at 5 to 6 months of age in the dog

69. The pulp of the tooth has which of the following functions?
    a. Anchors the root to the alveolar bone with a fibrous ligament
    b. Provides the crown with a protective, hard surface
    c. Contains blood vessels and nerves that provide nutrition and sensation to the tooth
    d. Makes up the bulk of the tooth structure

70. When the pulp cavity of a tooth is exposed, what is(are) the appropriate procedure(s) that should be performed?
    a. Tooth extraction or root canal therapy
    b. No procedure is required
    c. Crown amputation with intentional root retention
    d. Prophylactic dentistry to reduce tartar and plaque buildup on the tooth

71. In patients with severe, chronic periodontal disease, medication can be administered before a dental cleaning is performed. What is the most common type of medication chosen for these animals?
    a. Corticosteroids
    b. Antimicrobials
    c. Nonsteroidal anti-inflammatories
    d. Immunostimulants

72. From birth to 9 months of age, what condition is not present in the oral cavity?
    a. Occurrence of oral masses
    b. Missing teeth
    c. Extra teeth
    d. Abnormal jaw length

73. Perioceutics refer to which of the following?
    a. Procedure to restore the periodontal ligament
    b. Application of time-released antibiotics directly within the oral cavity
    c. Use of antibiotics before dental procedure
    d. Procedure to cap the pulp cavity of the tooth

74. The bisecting angle technique is a method for radiographing the oral cavity. The description that adequately describes this technique is
    a. The central radiation beam is directed perpendicular to the line that bisects the angle formed by the film and the long axis of the tooth.
    b. The central radiation beam is directed parallel to the line that bisects the angle formed by the film and the perpendicular axis of the tooth.
    c. The central radiation beam is directed perpendicular to the tooth root.
    d. The central radiation beam is directed perpendicular to the film or sensor.

75. A curette is used to:
    a. Check the tooth's surface for any irregularities
    b. Measure the depth of gingival recession
    c. Scale large amounts of calculus from the tooth's surface
    d. Scale calculus from the tooth surface located in the gingival sulcus

76. Which of the following statements is false when performing an ultrasonic scaling during routine dental prophylaxis?
    a. The ultrasonic scaler should not be on the tooth for longer than 10–15 seconds at a time to prevent thermal damage to the pulp cavity
    b. The ultrasonic scaler should be grasped like a pencil
    c. The side of the instrument should be used against the tooth rather than the tip
    d. The ultrasonic scaler can be used for supragingival scaling only

77. Which of the following statements is false regarding patient safety during dentistry?
    a. Provide thermal support to the patient during the dental procedure as hypothermia can result, especially in cats and smaller dogs
    b. The endotracheal tube should be uncuffed so that the tube can be easily manipulated when performing dentistry
    c. Large-breed dogs should be rolled with their legs under to prevent a gastric dilatation and volvulus crisis
    d. One must monitor the patient to ensure that fluids and debris from the dentistry do not gain access to the trachea

78. A dog exposed to distemper as a puppy may develop which of the following oral conditions?
    a. Adontia
    b. Polydontia
    c. Enamel hypoplasia
    d. Enamel staining

79. Sometimes a 0.12%-chlorhexidine solution is sprayed in the patient's mouth before beginning dental prophylaxis. What is the benefit of this activity?
    a. Sterilizes the patient's mouth before the procedure
    b. Reduces the bacterial load in the mouth to reduce exposure to the technician who performs the procedure
    c. Substitutes for prophylactic antibiotic therapy
    d. Provides topical anesthetic activity

80. Which of the following statements is false with respect to polishing an animal's teeth following scaling?
    a. The polishing paste used should be of medium or fine granularity
    b. Polishing acts to remove microscopic grooves left by the scaling process
    c. The polishing instrument should be moved from tooth to tooth to prevent thermal damage to the pulp
    d. Polishing is a means for removing stubborn plaque that occurs below the gum line

81. The Triadan system is a:
    a. Tooth identification system designed to aid in dental charting
    b. Complete system that includes an ultrasonic scaler and polisher
    c. Method for performing radiographs of molars
    d. Complete home care dental system for use by clients

82. Oligodontia is defined as:
    a. Congenital absence of many, but not all, teeth
    b. Total absence of teeth
    c. Absence of only a few teeth
    d. Difficulty eating

83. When comparing the size of the upper canine tooth, how much of the tooth is exposed versus that below the gumline?
    a. $\frac{1}{3}$ of the tooth is exposed
    b. $\frac{1}{2}$ of the tooth is exposed
    c. $\frac{2}{3}$ of the tooth is exposed
    d. $\frac{3}{4}$ of the tooth is exposed

84. The upper fourth premolar communicates with what sinus?
    a. Mandibular
    b. Occipital
    c. Maxillary
    d. Orbital

85. The crown of a tooth is defined as:
    a. That portion above the gum line and covered by enamel
    b. The most terminal portion of the root
    c. That portion below the gum line
    d. The layer of bony tissue that attaches to the alveolar bone

86. The range for acceptable gingival sulcus measurements in cats is:
    a. 1–3 mm
    b. 0.5–1 mm
    c. 1.5–4.5 mm
    d. 0.005–0.007 mm

87. How does tracheal rupture occur in feline dental patients?
    a. Packing the pharyngeal area too tightly
    b. Using a cuffed endotracheal tube
    c. Overinflation of the endotracheal tube cuff
    d. Disconnecting the breathing circuit before turning the patient

88. What stage of periodontal disease shows no change to the alveolar height, but includes mild gingival inflammation?
    a. Stage I
    b. Stage II
    c. Stage III
    d. Stage IV

89. When assessing and quantifying gingivitis, the modified Löe and Silness index is often referred to. According to this index, a gingival index 0 indicates:
    a. Clinically healthy gingiva
    b. Mild gingivitis with slight reddening and swelling of the gingival margins
    c. Moderate gingivitis, with gentle probing resulting in bleeding
    d. Severe gingivitis, in which there is spontaneous hemorrhage and/or ulceration of the gingival margin

90. What drug should not be given to pregnant dogs because it may cause discoloration of the puppies' teeth?
    a. Amoxicillin
    b. Tetracycline
    c. Chloramphenicol
    d. Penicillin

91. The occlusal surface is defined as the:
    a. Surface facing the hard palate
    b. Surface nearer the cheek
    c. Chewing surface of the tooth
    d. Surface nearer the tongue

92. The normal adult canine mouth has how many permanent teeth?
    a. 40
    b. 42
    c. 48
    d. 52

93. When grading tooth mobility, which of the following grades corresponds to a Grade 2?
    a. No mobility
    b. Horizontal movement of <1 mm
    c. Horizontal movement >1 mm
    d. Vertical and horizontal movement

94. Which of the following is a complication that might develop if a curette is used improperly?
    a. Etched tooth enamel
    b. Torn epithelial attachment
    c. Overheated tooth
    d. Bitten technician

95. Which tooth has three roots?
    a. Upper canine
    b. Lower first premolar
    c. Lower first molar
    d. Upper fourth premolar

96. Which statement concerning the polishing aspect of dental prophylaxis is the least accurate?
    a. A slow speed should be used
    b. Adequate prophy paste is needed for lubrication and polishing
    c. The polisher should remain on the tooth for as long as is needed to polish the tooth
    d. If teeth are not polished, the rough enamel will promote bacterial plaque formation

97. What term identifies the wearing away of enamel by tooth-against-tooth contact during mastication?
    a. Plaque
    b. Attrition
    c. Calculus
    d. Abrasion

98. When grading furcation involvement, which of the following descriptions would be termed Grade 1?
    a. No furcation involvement
    b. The furcation can be felt with the probe/explorer, but horizontal tissue destruction is $<\frac{1}{3}$ of the horizontal width
    c. The furcation can be explored, but the probe cannot pass through it
    d. The probe can be passed through the furcation from buccal to palatal/lingual

99. What term identifies the loss of tooth structure by an outside cause?
    a. Plaque
    b. Attrition
    c. Calculus
    d. Abrasion

100. The thin film covering a tooth that is composed of bacteria, saliva, and food particles is:
    a. Plaque
    b. Attrition
    c. Calculus
    d. Abrasion

101. What is the minimum age for a cat to have all of its permanent teeth?
    a. 6 months
    b. 8 months
    c. 10 months
    d. 1 year

102. In general, most dental instruments should be held as you would hold a:
    a. Knife
    b. Pencil
    c. Hammer
    d. Toothbrush

103. What is the most common dental disease found in dogs and cats?
    a. Endodontic disease
    b. Oral tumors
    c. Jaw fractures
    d. Periodontal disease

104. Removal of calculus and necrotic cementum from the tooth roots is called:
    a. Curettage
    b. Splinting
    c. Gingivoplasty
    d. Scaling

105. Prevention of periodontal disease involves all of the following *except:*
    a. Daily teeth brushing or mouth rinsing
    b. Full mouth extractions
    c. Routine professional scaling and polishing
    d. Proper diet

106. Luxation of a tooth *cannot* be termed as:
    a. Attrition
    b. Intrusion
    c. Extrusion
    d. d. Avulsion

107. Ideally, the cutting edge of the scaler should be held at what angle to the tooth surface?
    a. 5–10 degrees
    b. 35–45 degrees
    c. 15–30 degrees
    d. 45–90 degrees

108. Which of the following correctly describes the puppy dental formula?
    a. 2 × {I 2/1:C 0/0:P 3/2:M 3/3}
    b. 2 × {I 3/3:C 1/1:P 4/4:M 2/3}
    c. 2 × {I 3/3:C 1/1:P 3/2:M 1/1}
    d. 2 × {I 3/3:C 1/1:P 3/3}

109. Mrs. Walker comes to pick up her dog after dental cleaning has been performed. Which of the following topics would be least helpful to discuss as a part of the discharge instructions?
    a. Postoperative complications
    b. Home care
    c. How to give injections
    d. Dietary concerns

110. After plaque bacteria have formed on the tooth, the bacteria will absorb calcium from the saliva to form what substance?
    a. Calculus
    b. Pellicle
    c. Biofilm
    d. Lipopolysaccharides

111. The most common dental problem found in rodents is:
    a. Tooth root abscess
    b. Malocclusion
    c. Scurvy
    d. Cheek pouch impaction

112. What tissue is not part of the periodontium?
    a. Periodontal ligament
    b. Alveolar bone
    c. Root
    d. Gingiva

113. Which of the following statements is false?
    a. Tooth brushing and avoiding treats containing sugars prevent caries in dogs
    b. Attrition, abrasion, and tooth fracture are prevented by modifying play behaviors or changing the animal's environment
    c. There is no magic bullet that we can feed our pets to prevent periodontal disease; daily tooth brushing remains the single most effective method of restoring inflamed gingivae to health and of then maintaining clinically healthy gingivae.
    d. After receiving instructions, clients will maintain a dental home care program on a daily basis

114. Which cells are responsible for destroying the hard surfaces of the root?
    a. Macrocytes
    b. Osteoclasts
    c. Chondrocytes
    d. Odontoclasts

115. What term identifies the space between the roots of the same tooth?
    a. Apical
    b. Rostral
    c. Furcation
    d. Buccal

116. What term identifies the tooth surface facing the cheeks?
    a. Apical
    b. Rostral
    c. Furcation
    d. Buccal

117. What is the directional term for "toward the root"?
    a. Apical
    b. Rostral
    c. Furcation
    d. Buccal

118. What is the directional term for "toward the front of the head"?
    a. Apical
    b. Rostral
    c. Furcation
    d. Buccal

119. Chlorhexidine contributes to dental prophylaxis by:
    a. Preventing plaque from mineralizing into calculus
    b. Bonding to the cell membrane and inhibiting bacterial growth
    c. Bleaching stained teeth
    d. Decreasing tooth sensitivity

120. In normal occlusion, the bite can also be called a:
    a. Scissor bite
    b. Straight bite
    c. Occlusal bite
    d. Razor bite

121. What is the proper dilution of chlorhexidine solution for use in the mouth?
    a. 20%
    b. 2.0%
    c. 0.2%
    d. 10%

122. Topical fluoride:
    a. Will stain the remaining calculus red
    b. Helps to desensitize teeth and to strengthen enamel against cariogenic bacteria that cause cavities
    c. Should never be used on feline teeth
    d. Enhances odontoclastic activity and helps desensitize teeth

123. What instrument is used for root planing?
    a. Periodontal probe
    b. Explorer
    c. Scaler
    d. Curette

124. What instrument is used to detect subgingival calculus?
    a. Periodontal probe
    b. Explorer
    c. Scaler
    d. Curette

125. What instrument is used for removal of supragingival calculus?
    a. Periodontal probe
    b. Explorer
    c. Scaler
    d. Curette

126. An elongation of one side of the animal's head results in:
    a. Anterior crossbite
    b. Wry mouth
    c. Brachygnathism
    d. Prognathism

127. The bulk of a tooth is composed of:
    a. Enamel
    b. Pulp
    c. Dentin
    d. Cementum

128. The most common mistake made in treating periodontal disease is:
    a. Inadequate removal of supragingival calculus
    b. Inadequate root planing
    c. Insufficient polishing
    d. Iatrogenic trauma to subgingival tissues

129. What is the purpose of a dentifrice when used in the dog and cat?
    a. Removes subgingival calculus
    b. Removes microetchants caused by scaling the teeth
    c. Removes supragingival calculus
    d. Provides a pleasant taste and improves the effectiveness of brushing

130. Applying fluoride and rinsing with diluted chlorhexidine at the same time:
    a. Is less effective, because the binding of one product may inactivate the other
    b. Results in temporary staining of the teeth
    c. Enhances the activity of both fluoride and chlorhexidine
    d. May be toxic to the patient

131. If the lower incisors seem excessively loose in a brachycephalic or miniature-breed dog,
    a. The teeth should be extracted
    b. The depth of the gingival sulcus should be tested
    c. The dog is calcium deficient
    d. The dog has advanced periodontal disease

132. Fractured deciduous teeth:
    a. Should be left in place until they are normally shed
    b. Should be repaired
    c. Are insignificant
    d. Should be extracted

133. The first dental examination should occur when:
    a. The patient is 2–3 years old
    b. The client requests it
    c. A problem such as drooling or bad breath is noticed
    d. The patient is 6–8 weeks old

134. What is *true* about deciduous incisors?
    a. They erupt at 4–12 weeks of age
    b. They have roots that are long, thin, and fragile
    c. They are the most frequently retained teeth
    d. They are not usually replaced with permanent incisors until the dog is 6 months old

135. Nerves and blood vessels enter the tooth through the:
    a. Apical delta
    b. Crown
    c. Pulp
    d. Sulcus

136. When one or more of the upper incisors rest caudally on the lower incisors, and the rest of the occlusion is normal, the condition is known as:
    a. Level bite
    b. Wry mouth
    c. Rostral crossbite
    d. Anodontia

137. The term *polydontia* refers to:
    a. Retained deciduous teeth
    b. Supernumerary teeth
    c. Supernumerary teeth and retained deciduous teeth
    d. Tooth loss as a result of periodontal disease

138. The normal sulcus depth in the dog is:
    a. 3 mm
    b. 7 mm
    c. 10 mm
    d. 8 mm

139. Excessive growth of gingival tissue is termed:
    a. Gingivitis
    b. Gingival hyperplasia
    c. Gingival recession
    d. Gingivectomy

140. The shrinkage of free gingiva in the presence of bacteria, plaque, and/or dental calculus is termed:
    a. Gingival hyperplasia
    b. Periodontitis
    c. Gingivectomy
    d. Gingival recession

141. Two tooth buds that grow together to form one larger tooth is referred to as
    a. Gemini
    b. Fusion
    c. Polydontia
    d. Oligodontia

142. The space between two roots, where they meet the crown, is called:
    a. Crook
    b. Furcation
    c. Apex
    d. Fissure

143. The term for a tooth that has one root but two crowns is:
    a. Gemini
    b. Fusion
    c. Polydontia
    d. Oligodontia

144. The surface of the tooth toward the lips is known as the:
    a. Occlusal
    b. Labial
    c. Buccal
    d. Mesial

145. Fewer teeth than normal is known as:
    a. Polydontia
    b. Oligodontia
    c. Fusion
    d. Wry mouth

146. The surface of the tooth that is toward the cheek is known as:
    a. Occlusal
    b. Labial
    c. Buccal
    d. Mesial

147. Where do tooth resorption lesions first appear clinically in the cat?
    a. On the cementum
    b. On the alveolar mucosa
    c. At the cementoenamel junction
    d. At the tip of the crown

148. The purpose of fluoride treatment is to:
    a. Prevent thermal damage and lubrication
    b. Strengthen enamel and help desensitize teeth
    c. Remove plaque and strengthen the enamel
    d. Irrigate and lubricate

149. Sometimes referred to as distemper teeth, the name for a condition in which sections of the tooth enamel are pitted or discolored is:
    a. Prognathic
    b. Enamel hypoplasia
    c. Attrition
    d. Abrasion

150. Malocclusion in which the mandible is caudal to the maxilla is termed:
    a. Class 3 mandibular mesioclusions
    b. Class 2 mandibular distoclusions
    c. Class 1 neutroclusions
    d. Dental malocclusion

151. Malocclusions in which the mandibular is rostral to the maxilla is termed:
    a. Class 3 mandibular mesioclusions
    b. Class 2 mandibular distoclusions
    c. Class 1 neutroclusions
    d. Dental malocclusion

152. The maxillary carnassial tooth in the cat is also known as the:
    a. Upper first premolar
    b. Upper first molar
    c. Upper last premolar
    d. Upper canine

153. Using the modified Triadan system, the right maxillary teeth would be in the ___ series.
    a. 100
    b. 200
    c. 300
    d. 400

154. Which dental radiographic projection images 101, 102, 103, 201, 202, 203?
    a. Rostral maxillary
    b. Parallel mandibular view
    c. Rostral mandibular view
    d. Lateral oblique view

155. Which dental radiographic projection images 301–304 and 401–404?
    a. Rostral maxillary
    b. Parallel mandibular view
    c. Rostral mandibular view
    d. Lateral oblique view

156. The only radiographic view that can be made with a true parallel technique is:
    a. Rostral maxillary
    b. Parallel mandibular view
    c. Rostral mandibular view
    d. Parallel oblique view

157. In dental radiographs, periapical disease appears as a:
    a. Radiopaque area around the apex of the tooth
    b. Radiolucent area around the apex of the tooth
    c. Radiopaque area inside the tooth pulp
    d. Radiolucent area inside the tooth pulp

158. Which discipline deals with dental conditions specific to puppies and kittens?
    a. Exodontics
    b. Orthodontics
    c. Pedodontics
    d. Prosthodontics

159. Which statement is *incorrect* regarding the importance of dental radiographs?
    a. They are used to measure sulcus depth
    b. They help to reach a diagnosis
    c. They are used in the performance of certain procedures
    d. They are considered as part of the creation of a treatment plan

160. What is the general appearance of a Class 5 feline resorptive lesion?
    a. Tooth will appear fractured with a red dot in the middle
    b. The tooth looks normal but the gums are inflamed
    c. The tooth is not visible, only gum tissue
    d. Only a little of the enamel is missing, exposing the dentin

161. Internal resorption primarily affects the:
    a. Enamel
    b. Crown
    c. Pulp
    d. Dentin

162. Horizontal bone loss occurs in cases of:
    a. Periodontal disease
    b. Fractured teeth
    c. Tooth resorption
    d. Orthodontic disease

163. Vital pulp therapy refers to:
    a. Operating outright on the pulp on a live tooth
    b. Root canal therapy
    c. Procedure to turn a live tooth into a dead tooth
    d. Generally used when the tooth has been dead for a long time

164. If a tooth is fractured and there is a black spot in the center of the cut surface, into which you can place a dental explorer, the best treatment would be:
    a. An x-ray to see if there are changes in the tooth or surrounding areas, with treatment provided according to findings
    b. Either a root canal or an extraction
    c. A discussion fees with the client and a determination of whether or not the patient experiences pain before therapy
    d. An extraction

165. Which nerve block will anesthetize all the maxillary teeth on the injected side?
    a. Infraorbital
    b. Middle mental
    c. Maxillary
    d. Mandibular

166. The goal of orthodontic care is to:
    a. Allow a dog or cat to compete better in breed shows
    b. Correct abnormalities so a puppy or kitten can sell for a better price
    c. Provide a better-looking pet
    d. Return the pet to a comfortable or functional bite

167. What is the best time to use the extraction forceps?
    a. At the end of the procedure when the tooth is very mobile
    b. In the middle of the procedure to help with the elevation process
    c. At the beginning of the procedure to chip off calculus
    d. An extraction forceps should not be used

168. The placement of an esophagostomy feeding tube benefits the dental patient after which procedure?
    a. Routine cleaning and polishing
    b. Extraction of a maxillary canine tooth
    c. Mandibulectomy or maxillectomy
    d. Excisional biopsy of a 3-mm epulis

169. What breed would be associated with a dolichocephalic head shape?
    a. German shepherd
    b. Seal point Siamese
    c. Persian
    d. Corgi

170. For what is crown reduction and restoration used?
    a. Care for the tooth affected by near pulpal exposure
    b. Care for the tooth affected by pulpal exposure
    c. Tooth affected by Stage 3 periodontal disease
    d. A palatal trauma caused by a lingually displaced mandibular canine

171. What breed is prone to lip fold dermatitis?
    a. Bulldogs
    b. Chihuahuas
    c. Labradors
    d. Miniature pinschers

172. Which of the following mm increments do periodontal probes with Williams markings have?
    a. 1, 2, 3, 4, 5, 6, 7, 8, 9, 10, 11, 12, 13, 14, 15
    b. 1, 2, 3, 4, 5, 7, 8, 9, 10
    c. 3, 6, 8
    d. 1, 2, 3, 5, 7, 8, 9, 10

173. When conducting a tooth-by tooth evaluation with dental radiographs, when is the client given the total estimate for care?
    a. On the telephone when the appointment is made
    b. In the examination room
    c. When the animal is picked up after treatment
    d. After the evaluation is completed while the patient is still anesthetized

174. Local antibiotic therapy is provided:
    a. Intravenously
    b. Into a foramen
    c. Into the periodontal pocket
    d. Subcutaneously

175. What is epinephrine's role in local anesthesia in relation to a dental procedure?
    a. Prolongs the anesthetic through vasoconstriction
    b. Prolongs the anesthetic through vasodilation
    c. Helps the heart beat regularly
    d. Has no effect in local anesthesia

176. Which disease causes a cat to start spontaneously and aggressively pawing at the face and mouth and to cry out in pain?
    a. Tooth resorption
    b. Chronic ulcerative gingivostomatitis
    c. Squamous cell carcinoma
    d. Orofacial pain syndrome

177. Which material is used to fill the pulp chamber inside the tooth during root canal therapy?
    a. Gutta percha
    b. Dental cement
    c. Calcium hydroxide
    d. Acrylic resin

178. What is the least effective method of local anesthesia in dental patients?
    a. Rostral maxillary block
    b. Rostral mandibular block
    c. Infiltration or splash block
    d. Caudal mandibular block

179. What is the most common cause for dental malocclusions?
    a. Retained deciduous teeth
    b. Overbite
    c. Skeletal defects
    d. Bad breeding

180. What inheritable oral condition, causing a non-neoplastic bone formation, is primarily seen in West Highland white terriers?
   a. Mandibular periostitis ossificans
   b. Cranial mandibular osteodystrophy
   c. Odontoma
   d. Osteomyelitis

181. When referring to dental-related conditions, staging is a way to:
   a. Classify tumors
   b. Plan periodontal care
   c. Plan surgical care for cancerous tumors
   d. Determine how large a tumor is

182. Equine cheek teeth are used primarily for:
   a. Grinding and mastication
   b. Prehension and cutting of food
   c. Defense and offence
   d. All of the above

183. In horses, the term *coronal* refers to which portion of the tooth?
   a. The area of the tooth farthest away from the occlusal surface
   b. The area closet to the tongue
   c. The crown
   d. The tooth closest to the incisors

184. Which of the following statements is true regarding the teeth of equine patients?
   a. Brachydont teeth fully erupt before maturity and are normally long and hard enough to survive for the life of the individual
   b. Brachydont teeth do not fully erupt before maturity, however they are hard enough to survive for the life of the individual
   c. Brachydont teeth fully erupt before maturity, however they are not hard enough to survive for the life of the individual
   d. Hypsodont teeth do not have a limited time of growth

185. Teeth that grow throughout an equine patient's life are termed:
   a. Brachydont
   b. Hypsodont
   c. Anelodont
   d. Elodont

186. How many deciduous teeth do horses have?
   a. 20
   b. 24
   c. 36
   d. 44

187. How many incisors are present in the adult equine patient?
   a. 6
   b. 12
   c. 24
   d. 36

188. Canine teeth are always present in which of the following patients?
   a. Donkeys
   b. Female horses
   c. Male horses
   d. All of the above

189. At what age do premolars erupt in foals?
   a. Foals are born with teeth
   b. 5–7 days after birth
   c. 3–4 weeks after birth
   d. 3–4 months after birth

190. An adult equine mouth normally contains _____ cheek teeth.
   a. 12
   b. 20
   c. 24
   d. 34

191. Which teeth are the most appropriate for determining the age of horses?
   a. Incisors
   b. Wolf teeth
   c. Premolars
   d. Molars

192. All of the following factors must be considered when aging a horse, *except:*
   a. Breed
   b. Quantity of food
   c. Environmental conditions
   d. Injury

193. Parrot mouth in foals is also known as an:
   a. Underbite
   b. Overbite
   c. Overjet
   d. Underjet

194. Dental dysplasia is the abnormal development of teeth that involve which of the following?
   a. Crown
   b. Roots
   c. The entire tooth
   d. Pulp

195. All of the following are common soft-tissue neoplasms seen in horses, *except:*
    a. Squamous cell carcinoma
    b. Sarcoid
    c. Ossifying fibroma
    d. Osteoma

196. All of the following are common non-neoplastic conditions seen in the oral cavity of horses, *except:*
    a. Cementoma
    b. Polyps
    c. Papillomas
    d. Epulis

197. Which of the following antiseptics are considered choice oral rinses for horses?
    a. Chlorhexidine gluconate
    b. Chlorhexidine acetate
    c. Dilute betadine
    d. Glutaraldehyde

198. When using motorized equipment for an equine prophylaxis, speeds should range from _____ to prevent thermal damage.
    a. 100–200 rpm
    b. 2000–3000 rpm
    c. 3000–4000 rpm
    d. 4000–5000 rpm

199. Which of the following safety items should be used when operating motorized dental instruments on the equine patient?
    a. Protective eyewear
    b. Air filter mask
    c. Ear protection
    d. All of the above

200. All of the following instruments may be used to used to remove deciduous cheek tooth remnants, *except:*
    a. Forceps
    b. Elevators
    c. Gelpi retractors
    d. Dental picks

201. Which of the following instruments should be used to reduce the crown of sharp canine teeth?
    a. Nippers
    b. Cutters
    c. Small files
    d. Elevators

202. Which of the following patients would benefit from prophylactic antibiotics?
    a. A 1-year-old Yorkshire Terrier with stage 2 periodontal disease
    b. A 10-year-old King Charles Spaniel with cardiomyopathy
    c. A 5-year-old gelding
    d. All of the listed patients would benefit from prophylactic antibiotics

203. Which of the following options are best suited for rinsing a mouth before a dental prophy?
    a. 10% dilute betadine solution
    b. Chlorhexidine gluconate
    c. 50% dilute ampicillin solution
    d. There is no need to rinse a mouth before a prophylaxis, but rinsing should be done after the procedure is completed

204. What is a common cause of pain/discomfort and severe oral pathology in dental patients?
    a. Malocclusion
    b. Periodontal disease
    c. Stomatitis
    d. Gingival recession

205. All of the following would be considered part of an oral assessment, *except:*
    a. Facial bones and zygomatic arch
    b. Temporomandibular joint
    c. Popliteal lymph nodes
    d. Salivary glands

206. When inspecting the mucous membranes during an oral assessment, one would look at:
    a. Vesicle formation and ulceration
    b. Gingival recession
    c. Tonsillary crypts
    d. Fauces

207. When inspecting the pathology of a patient during an oral assessment, one would look at:
    a. Vesicle formation and ulceration
    b. Gingival recession
    c. Tonsillary crypts
    d. Fauces

208. When assessing and quantifying gingivitis, the modified Löe and Silness index is often referred to. According to this index, a gingival index 2 indicates:
a. Clinically healthy gingiva
b. Mild gingivitis with slight reddening and swelling of the gingival margins
c. Moderate gingivitis, with gentle probing resulting in bleeding
d. Severe gingivitis, in which there is spontaneous hemorrhage and/or ulceration of the gingival margin

209. Which of the following is the correct dental term/definition describing a tooth surface?
a. Mesial—farthest from the midline
b. Mesial—nearest the front
c. Distal—nearest the midline
d. Distal—farthest from the midline

210. A curette:
a. Is used strictly as a supragingival instrument
b. Can be used either supragingivally or subgingivally
c. Is used to remove microetchants on the tooth surface after power scaling
d. Is used to irrigate the teeth with air or water

211. When grading furcation involvement, which of the following descriptions would be termed Grade 2?
a. No furcation involvement
b. The furcation can be felt with the probe/explorer, but horizontal tissue destruction is $<\frac{1}{3}$ of the horizontal width
c. The furcation can be explored, but the probe cannot pass through it
d. The probe can be passed through the furcation from buccal to palatal/lingual

212. The dental formula for the permanent teeth in the dog is 2 (I 3/3 and C 1/1), in addition to:
a. P 3/4 and M 3/2 = 40
b. P 3/4 and M 3/3 = 42
c. P 4/4 and M 2/3 = 42
d. P 4/4 and M 3/2 = 42

213. What term identifies the hard, mineralized substance on the tooth surface?
a. Plaque
b. Attrition
c. Calculus
d. Abrasion

214. When grading tooth mobility, which of the following corresponds to Grade 1?
a. No mobility
b. Horizontal movement <1 mm
c. Horizontal movement >1 mm
d. Vertical and horizontal movement

215. What is the main purpose of premolar teeth?
a. Holding and tearing
b. Cutting and breaking
c. Grinding
d. Gnawing and grooming

216. The instrument used to measure pocket depth is a periodontal _____.
a. Explorer
b. Scaler
c. Curette
d. Probe

217. Abbreviations are commonly used in veterinary practice, and some abbreviations are exclusive to dental terminology. Which abbreviation best aligns with the uncomplicated crown fracture?
a. CCF
b. UCF
c. UCRF
d. CCRF

218. Which of the following is the correct dental term/definition for describing a tooth surface?
a. Palatal
b. Labial
c. Buccal
d. Rostral

219. Fluoride accomplishes all of the following *except:*
a. Desensitizing the tooth
b. Providing antibacterial activity
c. Strengthening the enamel
d. Strengthening the periodontal ligament

220. Which statement is true?
a. Full oral examination is only possible without general anesthesia
b. Oral examination should proceed in an orderly and structured fashion, using appropriate instrumentation
c. Adequate recording should take place at the end of the prophy, preferably on published or adapted dental charting systems
d. One radiograph should be obtained to complement visual assessments, for example, gingival index, periodontal probing depth, or periodontal/clinical attachment level

221. Which of the following statements is false?
    a. Radiography is mandatory for good dental practice
    b. Intraoral technique using parallel and bisecting angle views is essential for meaningful results to be obtained
    c. Dental x-ray machines and digital software and hardware are ideal, and such equipment proves convenient and cost-effective
    d. Full mouth radiographs (1–2 views) are strongly advocated in cats to detect odontoclastic resorptive lesions

222. Anodontia is defined as:
    a. Congenital absence of many, but not all, teeth
    b. Total absence of teeth
    c. Absence of only a few teeth
    d. Cleft palate

223. How many maxillary and mandibular premolars does the cat have in one half of the mouth?
    a. 3 in the maxilla and 2 in the mandible
    b. 3 in the maxilla and 3 in the mandible
    c. 2 in the maxilla and 3 in the mandible
    d. 2 in the maxilla and 2 in the mandible

224. Which of the following species does not have continually growing teeth?
    a. Equine
    b. Rabbit
    c. Rat
    d. Cat

225. The primary difference between primary and permanent teeth is:
    a. There is no difference in size between primary and permanent teeth
    b. Primary teeth are smaller than permanent teeth, with short, stubby roots
    c. Primary teeth are larger than permanent teeth, with long slender roots
    d. Primary teeth are smaller than permanent teeth, with long, slender roots

226. Enamel hypoplasia is also referred to as:
    a. Dysplasia
    b. Odontalgia
    c. Anodontia
    d. Oligodontia

227. Which of the following systemic factors may affect enamel development?
    a. Nutritional deficiency
    b. Febrile disorders
    c. Hypocalcemia
    d. All of the above

228. Local factors that could affect enamel development include all of the following *except:*
    a. Trauma
    b. Infection
    c. Bite injury
    d. Hypocalcemia

229. Medium- and large-breed dogs are most commonly affected by dental decay, which is also known as:
    a. Trauma
    b. Enamel hypoplasia
    c. Caries
    d. Furcation

230. Which of the following statements regarding common oral conditions is false?
    a. Osteomyelitis requires differentiation from neoplasia
    b. The most common malignant oral tumors are malignant melanomas and squamous cell carcinomas
    c. Most epulides are neoplastic
    d. Odontogenic tumors are benign neoplasms arising from odontogenic tissues

231. Periodontal disease is the result of the inflammatory process to:
    a. Dental plaque
    b. Systemic bacteria
    c. Systemic lupus
    d. Chronic stomatitis

232. The inflammatory reactions in periodontitis result in the destruction of which of the following structures?
    a. Periodontal ligament
    b. Alveolar bone
    c. Tooth enamel
    d. a and b

233. How long does it take plaque to accumulate on a clean tooth surface?
    a. Minutes
    b. Hours
    c. Days
    d. Weeks

234. What is the first sign that owners see that alerts them to the fact that their pet may have dental disease?
    a. Periodontal disease
    b. Gingivitis
    c. Halitosis
    d. Visualization of plaque

235. A pseudopocket can be defined as:
    a. Deep pocket
    b. Shallow pocket
    c. False pocket
    d. Missing a pocket

236. The veterinary technician's role in treating periodontal disease includes all of the following *except:*
    a. Supragingival scaling
    b. Subgingival scaling
    c. Subgingival lavage
    d. Periodontal surgery

237. Which of the following statements is false?
    a. Gingivitis is reversible
    b. If owners brush their pet's teeth with a toothbrush and pet toothpaste, gingivitis can be prevented/reduced
    c. Dental cleanings do not need to be performed under general anesthesia to reduce the incidence of gingivitis
    d. Untreated gingivitis may lead to periodontitis

238. When scaling a tooth that has a large amount of calculus, the process should occur in which order?
    a. Remove gross dental deposits with rongeurs or extraction forceps; remove residual supragingival deposits with hand instruments; use power scaler to remove remaining deposits
    b. Remove residual supragingival deposits with hand instruments; use power scaler to remove deposits; remove gross dental deposits with rongeurs or extraction forceps
    c. Use power scaler to remove calculus buildup and deposits; remove gross dental deposits with rongeurs or extraction forceps; remove residual supragingival deposits with hand instruments
    d. A three-step process is not needed, and a power scale will remove all calculi

239. Which of the following statements regarding teeth polishing is false?
    a. Scaling, even when performed correctly, will cause minor scratches of the tooth
    b. A rough surface will impede plaque retention
    c. Polishing smooths the roughness and helps remove any remaining plaque and stained pellicle
    d. Polishing is performed by applying a mildly abrasive prophylaxis paste to the tooth surface with a prophylaxis cup mounted in a slowly rotating low-speed handpiece

240. Why would a veterinary technician lavage a pathological pocket with chlorhexidine?
    a. To remove bacteria
    b. To remove free-floating debris
    c. To prevent the formation of an abscess
    d. All of the above

241. All of the following dental conditions could be avoided with preventive care, *except:*
    a. Periodontal disease
    b. Stomatitis
    c. Excessive wear
    d. Tooth fracture

242. An owner's goal when providing oral home care is:
    a. Suprascaling
    b. To remove or reduce the accumulation of plaque
    c. Subgingival lavage
    d. All of the above

243. Which of the following is the single most effective means of removing plaque?
    a. Tooth brushing
    b. Toothpaste
    c. Dental diets
    d. All of the above

244. Why is human toothpaste not recommended for pets?
    a. The taste is different than what pets like
    b. It foams, and pets don't like that sensation in their mouths
    c. The fluoride content is too high
    d. The salt content is too high

245. When brushing a pet-patient's teeth, which angle should the brush be held at?
    a. 20-degree angle
    b. 35-degree angle
    c. 45-degree angle
    d. 65-degree angle

246. A common cause of excessive wear and attrition in teeth is:
    a. Stone chewing
    b. Playing ball
    c. Loss of teeth
    d. All of the above

247. All of the following are preventative measures that can be taken to prevent malocclusion, *except:*
    a. Extraction of persistent primary teeth
    b. Interceptive orthodontics
    c. Extraction of persistent permanent teeth
    d. A removable orthodontic device

248. Which of the following correctly describes the lagomorph dental formula?
    a. 2 × {I 2/1:C 0/0:P 3/2:M 3/3}
    b. 2 × {I 3/3:C 1/1:P 4/4:M 2/3}
    c. 2 × {I 3/3:C 1/1:P 3/2:M 1/1}
    d. 2 × {I 3/3:C 1/1:P 3/3}

249. The heaviest calculus deposition in dogs and cats is typically located on the:
    a. Lingual surfaces of the lower cheek teeth
    b. Lower canine teeth
    c. Incisor teeth
    d. Buccal surfaces of the upper cheek teeth

250. The surface of the tooth toward the tongue is:
    a. Lingual
    b. Labial
    c. Buccal
    d. Mesial

251. Most abnormal dental conditions experienced by lagomorphs and rodents are a result of:
    a. Diet
    b. Environment
    c. Husbandry
    d. All of the above

252. The purpose of polishing during the dental prophy is to:
    a. Massage the gums
    b. Smooth out the rough areas and retard plaque formation
    c. Apply fluoride
    d. Disinfect the surface of the tooth

253. The most common benign soft-tissue tumor of the oral cavity is a/an:
    a. Epulis
    b. Fibrosarcoma
    c. Malignant melanoma
    d. Squamous cell carcinoma

254. The correct dental formula for an adult dog is:
    a. 2(l 3/3 C 1/1 P 3/4 M 3/3) = 42
    b. 2(l 3/3 C 1/1 P 4/4 M 3/2) = 42
    c. 2(l 3/3 C 1/1 P 4/4 M 2/3) = 42
    d. 2(l 4/4 C 1/1 P 3/4 M 3/3) = 46

255. The correct dental formula for an adult cat is:
    a. 2(l 3/3 C 1/1 P 3/2 M 1/1) = 30
    b. 2(l 4/4 C 1/1 P 2/3 M 1/1) = 34
    c. 2(l 3/3 C 1/1 P 2/3 M 1/1) = 30
    d. 2(l 3/3 C 1/1 P 3/2 M 2/1) = 32

ⓔ *Answers and rationales available on Evolve*
http://evolve.elsevier.com/Prendergast/QAvettech/

QUESTIONS

1. What is the morphology of *Vibrio* spp. bacteria?
   a. Bacillus
   b. Coccus
   c. Spirochete
   d. Coccobacillus

2. All of the following are important functions of bacterial fimbriae, *except:*
   a. Attachment
   b. Locomotion
   c. Ion transport
   d. Antibiotic resistance

3. Bacterial endospores are:
   a. Resistant to heat and desiccation
   b. A form of asexual reproduction
   c. A consequence of mating
   d. Highly susceptible to antiseptics

4. Blood levels of total bilirubin will not be a significant finding in:
   a. Hepatocellular damage
   b. Bile duct injury or obstruction
   c. Hemolytic disorders
   d. Acute pancreatitis

5. A bacterial genus can best be described as:
   a. Composed of one or more species
   b. Composed of classes
   c. Composed of families
   d. Belonging to a species

6. An iodine scrub on skin would result in:
   a. Antisepsis
   b. Disinfection
   c. Fumigation
   d. Sterilization

7. Which of the following would be a parenteral route of pathogen transmission?
   a. Transfusion
   b. Contaminated food
   c. Droplet infection
   d. Direct contact

8. Most bacteria grow best at a pH of:
   a. 1
   b. 3
   c. 9
   d. 7

9. Which of the following is an important function of bacterial flagella?
   a. Attachment
   b. Locomotion
   c. DNA replication
   d. Ion transport

10. Which parasite only uses the cat as its definitive host?
    a. Toxoplasma gondii
    b. Giardia lamblia
    c. Isospora rivolta
    d. Balantidium coli

11. _____ is the temperature that must be reached and maintained for 13 minutes in a steam autoclave to destroy microorganisms.
    a. 110° C
    b. 121° C
    c. 170° C
    d. 240° C

12. With which of the following is the humoral immune system involved?
    a. Monocytes
    b. B cells
    c. T cells
    d. Erythrocytes

13. Which of the following is a lentivirus?
    a. Coronavirus
    b. Feline immunodeficiency virus (FIV)
    c. Herpes virus
    d. Parvovirus

14. Which of the following is not a method of culturing animal viruses?
    a. Laboratory animal inoculation
    b. Cell culture
    c. Agar plate inoculation
    d. Embryonated egg inoculation

15. What immunoglobulin is usually present in the greatest quantity?
    a. IgA
    b. IgD
    c. IgE
    d. IgG

16. Blood levels of total bilirubin are used primarily to evaluate the function of the:
    a. Kidneys
    b. Liver
    c. Pancreas
    d. Bile ducts

17. Phagocytes are a type of:
    a. Red blood cell
    b. White blood cell
    c. Platelet
    d. Antibody

18. A hospital-acquired disease is known as:
    a. Endemic
    b. Nosocomial
    c. Ergasteric
    d. Iatrogenic

19. Leukopenia is defined as:
    a. A decrease in white blood cells
    b. An increase in white blood cells
    c. A bone marrow disease
    d. A type of blood cancer

20. What laboratory test evaluates kidney function and is a breakdown product of protein?
    a. Glucose
    b. SGTP (ALT)
    c. Creatinine
    d. BUN

21. The function of hemolysins is to:
    a. Coagulate blood
    b. Break down fibrin
    c. Destroy red blood cells
    d. Indicate a viral infection

22. Nonrenal causes of increased levels of urea might include:
    a. The amount of carbohydrate ingested
    b. The amount of protein ingested
    c. Insufficient insulin
    d. Insufficient ADH

23. A decrease in albumin may occur in cases experiencing:
    a. Cardiac disease
    b. A carnivorous diet
    c. Gastroenteritis
    d. A vegetarian diet

24. To what color does "icteric serum" refer?
    a. Yellow
    b. Red
    c. Brown
    d. Green

25. What color are blood collection tubes that contain heparin?
    a. Purple
    b. Green
    c. Blue
    d. Gray

26. Which of the following substances is used to evaluate kidney filtration and function, is excreted, and then is reabsorbed?
    a. Urea
    b. Creatinine
    c. Glucose
    d. Sodium

27. With significant dehydration in an otherwise healthy patient, which of the following would likely appear on a urinalysis and CBC?
    a. Increased urine SG and increased PCV
    b. Increased urine SG and decreased PCV
    c. Decreased urine SG and decreased PCV
    d. Decreased urine SG and increased PCV

28. Water deprivation tests should never be performed on patients with:
    a. High MCV
    b. Suspected sufficient ADH
    c. Dehydration
    d. Suspected tubular malfunction

29. Glycosuria exists:
    a. When blood glucose levels exceed the renal threshold for absorption of glucose
    b. When blood glucose levels are lower than the renal threshold for absorption of glucose
    c. When urine glucose levels are lower than the renal threshold for absorption of glucose
    d. When urine glucose levels are higher than the serum threshold for absorption of glucose

30. Horses typically have higher _____ values than other species.
    a. AST
    b. ALP
    c. ALT
    d. GGT

31. What blood chemistry test should be used to measure cholangiocyte damage?
    a. ALKP
    b. AST
    c. ALT
    d. GGT

32. Electrolytes are commonly measured by what method?
    a. Ion-specific electrodes
    b. Refractometry
    c. Adsorption
    d. Enzymatic digestion

33. A test that can be performed to help diagnose hyperthyroidism is:
    a. LH
    b. Cortisol
    c. Bile acids
    d. T4

34. When performing urinalysis testing, the sample should be analyzed within ___ minutes, or refrigeration is required.
    a. 10
    b. 20
    c. 30
    d. 40

35. For cytological evaluation of urine, which of the following conditions should be observed?
    a. The specimen should be refrigerated as soon as possible.
    b. The specimen should be centrifuged as soon as possible.
    c. The specimen may sit at room temperature for ≤6 hours.
    d. The specimen may be frozen for later analysis.

36. The average urine specific gravity for a healthy adult dog is _____.
    a. 1.025
    b. 1.035
    c. 1.040
    d. 1.045

37. The average urine specific gravity for a healthy adult cat is _____.
    a. 1.025
    b. 1.030
    c. 1.035
    d. 1.040

38. Which of the following tests is not included in a routine CBC?
    a. Total WBC count
    b. Differential WBC count
    c. Total protein
    d. Reticulocyte count

39. Ketonuria is most commonly associated with what condition?
    a. Liver disease
    b. Urinary tract infection
    c. Renal failure
    d. Diabetes mellitus

40. Hoover, a canine patient, was diagnosed with a urinary tract infection 2 weeks earlier and was placed on a course of amoxicillin. The veterinarian asked that he return for a recheck to ensure the infection has resolved. The collection method of choice in this patient would be:
    a. Catheterization
    b. Free catch
    c. Cystocentesis
    d. Manual expression

41. Leukocytes in the urine sediment and a positive nitrite reaction on the urinary colorimetric strip provide presumptive evidence that the patient might have a:
    a. Neoplasm
    b. Diabetic condition
    c. Renal failure
    d. Bacterial infection

42. Aged urine samples left at room temperature and exposed to UV light may cause a false negative result in which one of the following biochemical tests?
    a. Ketones
    b. Protein
    c. Glucose
    d. Bilirubin

43. Which of the following is the best time to collect a urine sample to evaluate the specific gravity of a canine patient?
    a. First morning sample
    b. Midday sample
    c. Late afternoon sample
    d. Last sample of the day

44. Mr. Downing has brought in a urine sample from Cleo, his 6-year-old female spayed cocker spaniel. The color of the urine appears red. On centrifugation of the sample, you find that the supernatant is now clear. What was the most likely cause of the red color?
    a. Hemoglobinuria
    b. Hematuria
    c. Myoglobinuria
    d. Uroglobinuria

45. Urinary pH is not affected by the:
    a. Patient's diet
    b. Presence of bacteria in the urine
    c. Patient's acid-base status
    d. Presence of crystals in the urine

46. Squamous epithelial cells are not normally seen in urine samples obtained by:
    a. Catheterization
    b. Manual expression
    c. Free catch
    d. Cystocentesis

47. The two most common problems encountered in samples to be evaluated for clinical chemistry are:
    a. Coagulation and separation
    b. Dilution and concentration
    c. Hemolysis and lipemia
    d. EDTA and heparin

48. What biochemical tests are not considered part of a primary hepatic profile?
    a. BUN and creatinine
    b. Cholestatic enzymes
    c. Hepatocellular leakage enzymes
    d. Total protein and albumin

49. A fecal smear can be stained for fat. An increased amount of fat is indicative of:
    a. Dyschezia
    b. Dysentery
    c. Steatorrhea
    d. Tenesmus

50. Which is the correct method to use when performing a serum bile acids assay?
    a. Draw a blood sample on a fasting animal
    b. Draw a blood sample on an animal immediately after it eats a meal
    c. Draw a blood sample on a fasting animal and another sample 2 hours later
    d. Draw a blood sample on a fasting animal, feed the animal, and draw another sample 2 hours later

51. The current test of choice for evaluating liver function is:
    a. Ammonia assay
    b. Bile acids
    c. Bilirubin
    d. Alanine aminotransferase

52. Total protein levels are _____ in a dehydrated animal.
    a. Unaffected
    b. Decreased
    c. Increased
    d. Variable

53. Which of the following crystals is most likely found in the urine of an animal with ethylene glycol toxicity?
    a. Ammonium biurate
    b. Tyrosine
    c. Triple phosphate
    d. Calcium oxalate

54. What species has multiple forms of reticulocytes?
    a. Horse
    b. Cow
    c. Cat
    d. Dog

55. The etiologic agent of Lyme disease is:
    a. *Borrelia burgdorferi*
    b. Coronavirus
    c. *Lentivirus*
    d. *Pasteurella multocida*

56. Which of these tubes must never be placed on a blood rocker after being filled with blood?
    a. Blue top
    b. Green top
    c. Purple top
    d. Red top

57. Which of the following options is least likely to interfere with blood chemistry test results?
    a. Postprandial serum
    b. Icteric serum
    c. Fasting serum
    d. Hemolyzed serum

58. Where on the blood smear would you select to start your WBC differential count?
    a. Thickest area
    b. Feathered edge
    c. Monocellular layer
    d. Thinnest area

59. In which of the following species is rouleaux formation common?
    a. Rats
    b. Dogs
    c. Horses
    d. Pigs

60. Serum chemistry tests for acute pancreatitis include:
    a. Amylase and lipase
    b. Lipase and trypsin
    c. Amylase and trypsin
    d. Amylase, lipase, and trypsin

61. Pollakiuria is defined as:
    a. Frequent urination with small volume voided
    b. Complete lack of urine production
    c. Excessive drinking and urinating
    d. Excessive urination at night

62. Which of the following may an elevated hematocrit indicate?
    a. Hyperglycemia
    b. Anemia
    c. Dehydration
    d. Leukocytosis

63. Which of the following results may be found in a patient with a degenerative left shift?
    a. Leukocytosis
    b. No bands are present
    c. Lymphocytes outnumber neutrophils
    d. Bands outnumber mature neutrophils

64. Which of the following options is another term for *icterus*?
    a. Jaundice
    b. Xanthochromia
    c. Ketonemia
    d. Hemoglobinuria

65. Bile acids aid in the digestion of
    a. Proteins
    b. Carbohydrates
    c. Fats
    d. Globulins

66. When considering hematology tests, clots in an EDTA sample are:
    a. Acceptable if they are microscopic
    b. Acceptable if they are detected on a wooden stick only
    c. Acceptable if they are run through an automatic analyzer
    d. Never acceptable

67. Which is *least* likely to be a clinical sign of a patient experiencing allergies?
    a. Face rubbing
    b. Ear problems
    c. Loss of appetite
    d. Skin rashes

68. On a complete blood count (CBC), all of the following findings could be expected in a patient with an infection, *except:*
    a. Neutrophilia
    b. Leukocytosis
    c. Narrow buffy coat
    d. A left shift

69. To make a smear with anemic blood,
    a. Increase the angle of the pusher slide
    b. Decrease the angle of the pusher slide
    c. Use a larger drop of blood
    d. Wait for the drop of blood to dry partially

70. Which of the red blood cell indices indicates cell size?
    a. MCH
    b. MCHC
    c. MCV
    d. MPV

71. A correction for nucleated red blood cells (nRBC) is done to avoid a falsely:
    a. Elevated PCV
    b. Elevated WBC count
    c. Decreased PCV
    d. Decreased WBC count

72. RBCs with multiple, irregularly spaced projections are known as:
    a. Crenated cells
    b. Schistocytes
    c. Acanthocytes
    d. Anisocytes

73. Reticulocytes on a modified Wright stain (e.g., Diff-Quik) appear
    a. Polychromatic
    b. Hypochromic
    c. Hyperchromic
    d. Crenated

74. What is the most useful way to report WBC differential results?
    a. As percentages
    b. As relative numbers
    c. As absolute numbers
    d. As decimal numbers

75. Determination of which of the following is useful in the detection of inflammatory processes?
    a. Total protein
    b. Hematocrit
    c. RBC morphology
    d. Fibrinogen

76. The buffy coat in a spun hematocrit tube consists of:
    a. WBCs
    b. WBCs and platelets
    c. WBCs and NRBCs
    d. Platelets and NRBCs

77. Postrenal azotemia refers to:
    a. An increase in BUN resulting from severe liver disease
    b. An increase in BUN resulting from the inability to urinate
    c. A decrease in BUN resulting from severe renal disease
    d. An increase in BUN resulting from dehydration

78. What cells are phagocytic?
    a. Granulocytes
    b. Lymphocytes
    c. Neutrophils and macrophages
    d. Macrophages and lymphocytes

79. Monocytes typically have:
    a. Segmented nuclei
    b. Band-shaped nuclei
    c. Lobular nuclei
    d. No nuclei

80. Which one of the following options would not affect a manual WBC count?
    a. Condenser in the farthest "up" position
    b. Length of time that the hemocytometer has been loaded
    c. Objective lens used
    d. Mini clots in the blood

81. Which of the following options is not a sign of RBC regeneration?
    a. Polychromasia
    b. Nuclear remnants
    c. Spherocytes
    d. Anisocytosis with macrocytosis

82. A left shift refers to increased numbers of:
    a. Immature neutrophils
    b. Immature RBCs
    c. Immature platelets
    d. Immature lymphocytes

83. What special stain would be used in assessing anemia?
    a. Lactophenol cotton blue
    b. New methylene blue
    c. Gram
    d. Acridine orange

84. Which of the following is the most immature erythrocyte?
    a. Rubricyte
    b. Metarubricyte
    c. Rubriblast
    d. Reticulocyte

85. The intermediate host for heartworms is the:
    a. Flea
    b. Rodent
    c. Mosquito
    d. Snail

86. Serology tests can detect heartworms in a dog's blood:
    a. Immediately after becoming infected
    b. Several days after becoming infected
    c. Several weeks after becoming infected
    d. Several months after becoming infected

87. What are the two diagnostic forms of *Giardia*?
    a. Cysts and trophozoites
    b. Merozoites and schizonts
    c. Oocysts and sporocysts
    d. Ova and L3 larvae

88. Compared to roundworm ova, coccidia appear:
    a. Smaller
    b. The same size
    c. Twice as large
    d. Three times as large

89. In a healthy animal, diminished water intake or loss of water would result in ___ urine specific gravity.
    a. Increased
    b. Decreased
    c. Isosthenuric
    d. Isotonic

90. What urine sediment component would be of the most significant concern?
    a. Sperm
    b. Fat droplets
    c. Squamous epithelial cells
    d. Blood cells

91. *Struvite crystals* are also known as:
    a. Calcium carbonate crystals
    b. Calcium oxalate crystals
    c. Triple phosphate crystals
    d. Amorphous phosphate crystals

92. Crystals in urine sediment often indicate:
    a. Uroliths
    b. Nothing
    c. Inflammation
    d. Urethral blockage

93. Which of the following test results are not determined by a urine dipstick?
    a. Glucose
    b. Blood
    c. Total protein
    d. BUN

94. Casts that are seen in urine sediment are:
    a. Mucous threads filled with amorphous sediment
    b. Always significant
    c. Formed in the renal tubules
    d. Artifacts

95. The presence of protein in the urine may indicate:
    a. Acid-base imbalance
    b. Hemolytic anemia
    c. Kidney disease
    d. Diabetes mellitus

96. Which of these would not be associated with ketones in the urine?
    a. Diabetes mellitus
    b. Lactating cows
    c. Starvation
    d. Hemolysis

97. Mucus is normally seen in _____ urine.
    a. Canine
    b. Equine
    c. Feline
    d. Bovine

98. The appearance of calcium oxalate crystals are described as:
    a. Hexagonal
    b. Dark, needlelike rods
    c. Brown spheres with long spicules
    d. Small squares that contain an X

99. A common laboratory test for chronic pancreatitis is a fecal test for:
    a. Amylase
    b. Lipase
    c. Trypsin
    d. Bilirubin

100. Fat droplets in urine samples are most commonly seen in:
    a. Dogs
    b. Cats
    c. Horses
    d. Cows

101. Gram-negative bacteria retain what component of the Gram stain?
    a. Crystal violet
    b. Iodine solution
    c. Decolorizer
    d. Safranin

102. What gram-negative bacteria may "swarm" a blood agar plate, leaving a film over the entire surface?
    a. *Pseudomonas* sp.
    b. *Staphylococcus* sp.
    c. *Proteus* sp.
    d. *Escherichia coli*

103. What microorganism is frequently recovered from the ears of dogs with chronic otitis externa?
    a. *Candida* sp.
    b. *Cryptococcus* sp.
    c. *Microsporum* sp.
    d. *Malassezia* sp.

104. What microorganism is an etiologic agent of ringworm?
    a. *Microsporum* sp.
    b. *Mycobacterium* sp.
    c. *Micrococcus* sp.
    d. *Moraxella* sp.

105. Which species includes common contaminants and is the causative agent of anthrax?
    a. *Escherichia*
    b. *Corynebacterium*
    c. *Bacillus*
    d. *Enterobacter*

106. What is a common pathogen in mastitis, skin wounds, and abscesses, which is also found in the environment?
    a. *Proteus vulgaris*
    b. *Escherichia coli*
    c. *Streptococcus* spp.
    d. *Staphylococcus aureus*

107. Stress and epinephrine release in cats might cause an increase in:
    a. BUN
    b. Total protein
    c. ALT
    d. Glucose

108. A kidney function test that has been found useful in birds and dalmatians is:
    a. BUN
    b. Creatinine
    c. Uric acid
    d. AST

109. What serum component can be used as a screening test for hypothyroidism?
    a. ALT
    b. Cholesterol
    c. Total protein
    d. Creatine kinase

110. During a glucose tolerance test, glucose levels in a diabetic animal will:
    a. Show an initial peak and then diminish to normal
    b. Remain high throughout the test
    c. Show a delayed peak at the end of the test period
    d. Show below normal levels throughout the test

111. What organ conserves nutrients, removes waste products, maintains blood pH, and controls blood pressure?
    a. Kidney
    b. Liver
    c. Pancreas
    d. Spleen

112. The small intestine receives digestive enzymes from the:
    a. Kidney
    b. Pancreas
    c. Liver
    d. Spleen

113. Bile acids aid in the absorption of:
    a. Proteins
    b. Carbohydrates
    c. Fats
    d. Globulins

114. Fibrinogen is produced in the:
    a. Pancreas
    b. Bone marrow
    c. Liver
    d. Spleen

115. Which of the following samples can be frozen and successfully thawed for performing an analytic test at a later time?
    a. Feces for a fecal float test
    b. Whole blood for chemistry testing
    c. Serum for chemistry testing
    d. Whole blood for a CBC

116. If there is only a small amount of serum separated after centrifuging a tube of whole blood (and you need more for testing), what should you do?
    a. Invert the tube several times and respin it
    b. Assume the patient is dehydrated and draw off all of the serum you can
    c. Spin the tube again at a faster speed and a longer time
    d. Rim/ring the clot and spin again at a normal speed and time

117. Arterial blood is most commonly used to analyze:
    a. Hematology
    b. Blood gases
    c. Blood chemistry
    d. Organ function tests

118. All of the following cells are produced in the bone marrow, *except:*
    a. Erythrocytes
    b. Lymphocytes
    c. Neutrophils
    d. Eosinophils

119. Looking under a microscope at a blood smear, you see erythrocytes that are elliptical, not nucleated, and lacking central pallor. From which species was this sample most likely collected?
    a. Bird
    b. Horse
    c. Llama
    d. Snake

120. Under the microscope you observe a leukocyte that you identify as an eosinophil. The eosinophil cytoplasm contains numerous rod-shaped granules. From which species was this sample most likely collected?
    a. Dog
    b. Cat
    c. Horse
    d. Cow

121. Which of the following is a common finding on a blood smear from an animal with autoimmune hemolytic anemia?
    a. Heinz bodies
    b. Howell-Jolly bodies
    c. Spherocytes
    d. Target cells

122. Serum electrolyte levels should be determined when evaluating the function of the:
    a. Liver
    b. Pancreas
    c. Kidneys
    d. Heart

123. Kidney disease leads to the accumulation of metabolic waste in the blood, a condition known as:
    a. Hypernaturia
    b. Hypernatremia
    c. Azotemia
    d. Azoturia

124. For which of the following diagnostics is low-power magnification on the microscope not used?
    a. To detect the presence of rouleaux
    b. To detect RBC agglutination
    c. To detect clumping of platelets
    d. To estimate platelet numbers

125. What characteristic is not found in toxic neutrophils?
    a. Howell-Jolly bodies
    b. Vacuolated cytoplasm
    c. Döhle bodies
    d. Basophilic cytoplasm

126. What laboratory test evaluates primary hemostasis?
    a. Activated clotting time
    b. Activated partial thromboplastin time
    c. Buccal mucosal bleeding time
    d. One-step prothrombin time

127. Secondary hemostasis refers to:
    a. The coagulation cascade
    b. Vascular spasm
    c. Clot lysis
    d. Platelet plug formation

128. A good presurgical screening test for von Willebrand disease is a(n):
    a. Total platelet count
    b. Buccal mucosal bleeding time
    c. Activated clotting time
    d. Activated partial thromboplastin time

129. When collecting blood for a coagulation profile, it is especially important to:
    a. Use a gray-top Vacutainer
    b. Analyze the sample immediately
    c. Use EDTA as the anticoagulant
    d. Minimize vascular trauma during venipuncture

130. Physical signs of hypocoagulation include all of the following, *except:*
    a. Petechiae or ecchymoses
    b. Epistaxis
    c. Hematuria
    d. Thromboembolism

131. An animal that tested positive for heartworm infection might also have an elevation of which of the following blood cells?
    a. Leukocytes
    b. Lymphocytes
    c. Eosinophils
    d. Monocytes

132. When using Diff-Quik to stain bone marrow smears, it is especially important to:
    a. Use freshly filtered stain
    b. Dip the smear twice as long as blood smears
    c. Rinse thoroughly with distilled water
    d. Let the smear dry for 30 minutes before staining

133. The ability of the renal tubules to concentrate or dilute a urine sample is assessed by what component of the urinalysis?
    a. pH
    b. Volume
    c. Specific gravity
    d. Examination of the sediment

134. Which epithelial cell is the largest of the cells found in urine?
    a. Squamous epithelial cells
    b. Caudate epithelial cells
    c. Transitional epithelial cells
    d. Renal epithelial cells

135. The most common uroliths found in feline and canine urine are:
    a. Struvite
    b. Calcium oxalate
    c. Urate
    d. Cystine

136. The best urine collection method to assess the patency of the urethra is:
    a. Catheterization
    b. Manual expression
    c. Free catch
    d. Cystocentesis

137. Which of the following statements regarding casts is incorrect?
   a. A few hyaline or granular casts may be seen in normal urine
   b. All casts are cylindric with parallel sides
   c. Casts dissolve in acidic urine
   d. Casts may be disrupted with high-speed centrifugation and rough sample handling

138. Puddin, a 2-year-old castrated male domestic shorthair cat, was missing for 5 days before coming home. His owners were very concerned that he appeared weak and tired, so they brought him to the clinic. You find on initial physical examination that he is significantly dehydrated. You are not at all surprised when you find that his urine specific gravity is
   a. 1.002
   b. 1.012
   c. 1.030
   d. 1.060

139. Bilirubinuria is considered a normal finding in what species?
   a. Dogs
   b. Cats
   c. Horses
   d. Sheep

140. Sadie, a 17-year-old spayed female domestic shorthair cat, is in the final stages of chronic renal failure. On presentation, you anticipate that her urine specific gravity will probably be
   a. 1.012
   b. 1.030
   c. 1.040
   d. 1.060

141. What method of urine sample collection would not be associated with traumatic hematuria?
   a. Catheterization
   b. Manual expression
   c. Free catch
   d. Cystocentesis

142. Sasha, an 11-year-old spayed female domestic shorthair cat, was accidentally overhydrated with IV fluids. What would you expect her urine specific gravity to be?
   a. 1.002
   b. 1.012
   c. 1.030
   d. 1.060

143. In a diabetic animal, blood chemistry analysis is commonly performed to monitor insulin therapy by measuring blood levels of:
   a. Sodium
   b. Potassium
   c. Glucose
   d. Insulin

144. Leukocytes in the urine sediment and a positive nitrite reaction on the urinary colorimetric strip provide presumptive evidence that the patient may have a:
   a. Neoplasm
   b. Diabetic condition
   c. Renal failure
   d. Bacterial infection

145. What gland is the most active producer of corticosteroids?
   a. Thyroid gland
   b. Pancreas
   c. Pituitary gland
   d. Adrenal glands

146. In an animal with a history of bone resorption or convulsions, blood chemistry analysis is commonly performed to measure blood levels of:
   a. Calcium and phosphorus
   b. Urea nitrogen and creatinine
   c. Aspartate aminotransferase and alanine transaminase
   d. Sodium and potassium

147. The gland function that is evaluated by measuring blood cortisol levels before and after administration of adrenocorticotropic hormone (ACTH) is the:
   a. Thyroid gland
   b. Pancreas
   c. Liver
   d. Adrenal glands

148. Struvite crystals are composed of:
   a. Calcium potassium carbonates
   b. Magnesium ammonium phosphates
   c. Oxalates
   d. Urates

149. The gland that is evaluated by measuring blood levels of T3 and T4 is the:
   a. Thyroid gland
   b. Pancreas
   c. Pituitary gland
   d. Thymus

150. Measurement of blood levels of thyroid-stimulating hormone (TSH) and ACTH is used to evaluate the function of the:
    a. Thyroid gland
    b. Pancreas
    c. Pituitary gland
    d. Adrenal glands

151. Blood chemistry analysis is commonly performed to evaluate function of the _____ in an animal showing lethargy, obesity, mild anemia, infertility, and alopecia.
    a. Thyroid gland
    b. Pancreas
    c. Thymus
    d. Adrenal glands

152. Which of the following statements regarding creatinine is false?
    a. It is an indicator of the glomerular filtration rate.
    b. It is produced as a result of normal muscle metabolism.
    c. It is a less reliable indicator of renal function than BUN.
    d. It is usually evaluated in conjunction with the BUN and urine specific gravity.

153. A good initial urinary screening test for suspected Cushing's disease is:
    a. Endogenous ACTH
    b. Low-dose dexamethasone suppression test
    c. ACTH stimulation
    d. Cortisol/creatinine ratio

154. Chemistry evaluation of the kidney includes measurement of metabolic wastes in the blood in the form of:
    a. Aspartate aminotransferase and alanine transaminase
    b. Urea nitrogen and creatinine
    c. Ammonia and pyruvic acid
    d. Bilirubin and urobilinogen

155. Measurement of blood levels of amylase and lipase is used to evaluate the function of the:
    a. Kidneys
    b. Liver
    c. Pancreas
    d. Adrenal glands

156. Ammonia is metabolized by the liver and eliminated by the kidneys. Levels of which metabolic byproduct of ammonia are measured to assess kidney function?
    a. Phosphorus
    b. Creatinine
    c. Aspartate aminotransferase
    d. Urea nitrogen

157. The main function of bicarbonate is to:
    a. Maintain the proper osmotic pressure of fluids in the body
    b. Maintain normal muscular function
    c. Maintain normal cardiac rhythm and contractility
    d. Maintain balanced body pH levels

158. Kidney disease results in accumulation of metabolic waste in the blood, a condition known as:
    a. Azotemia
    b. Bilirubinemia
    c. Hypernatremia
    d. Hyperkalemia

159. Prerenal azotemia refers to:
    a. An increase in BUN resulting from severe liver disease
    b. A decrease in BUN resulting from severe renal disease
    c. An increase in BUN resulting from dehydration, shock, and/or decreased blood flow to the kidneys
    d. An increase in BUN resulting from the inability to urinate

160. A glucose tolerance test is used to help diagnose:
    a. Cushing's disease
    b. Hypothyroidism
    c. Addison's disease
    d. Diabetes mellitus

161. Which white blood cell is known as "the first line of defense" after a microorganism has entered the body?
    a. Eosinophil
    b. Lymphocyte
    c. Monocyte
    d. Neutrophil

162. The red-top Vacutainer tube should sit at room temperature for ___ before centrifugation, allowing a clot to form.
    a. 5 minutes
    b. 30 minutes
    c. 1 hour
    d. 0 minutes (No clot will form)

163. *Dioctophyma renale* is often found in the ___ of dogs.
    a. Right kidney
    b. Left kidney
    c. Urinary bladder
    d. Ureters

164. Which of the following is the best method of preservation if you are unable to perform a CBC within 1 hour of blood collection?
    a. Freeze the sample
    b. Spin down the sample, refrigerate cells, and freeze serum
    c. Add formalin to the sample
    d. Refrigerate the sample

165. The mucin clot test is performed on:
    a. Joint fluid
    b. Plasma
    c. Serum
    d. Urine

166. Which of the following is associated with clotting disorders?
    a. Anemia
    b. Leukopenia
    c. Thrombocytopenia
    d. Reticulocytosis

167. When preparing cytology samples for microscopic evaluation, what is the best technique to use?
    a. Wet prep
    b. Squash prep
    c. Modified Knott prep
    d. Willis prep

168. Which of the following would be considered an abnormal finding on healthy canine external ear canal cytology?
    a. Cerumen
    b. Epithelial cells
    c. *Malassezia*
    d. Debris

169. The main function of the neutrophil is:
    a. Phagocytosis
    b. Hypersensitivity reaction
    c. Allergic reaction
    d. Immune response

170. What is the primary function of eosinophils?
    a. Phagocytosis
    b. Respond to autoimmune reactions
    c. Respond to allergic reaction
    d. Initiate an immune reaction

171. How long must the typical microhematocrit tube be centrifuged for packed cell volume determination?
    a. 1 minute
    b. 5 minutes
    c. 10 minutes
    d. 15 minutes

172. What measure determines the average size of an erythrocyte?
    a. Mean corpuscular volume
    b. Packed cell volume (PCV)
    c. Mean corpuscular hemoglobin concentration (MCHC)
    d. Mean corpuscular hemoglobin

173. In what type of blood cell can Döhle bodies be found?
    a. Erythrocytes
    b. Neutrophils
    c. Platelets
    d. Nucleated RBCs

174. In what species are the platelets normally larger than the red blood cells?
    a. Bovine
    b. Canine
    c. Equine
    d. Feline

175. The term for red blood cell formation is:
    a. Erythropoietin
    b. Erythropoiesis
    c. Hematopoietin
    d. Leukopoiesis

176. What is the sequence of cells listed from most immature to most mature?
    a. Rubricyte, reticulocyte, rubriblast, erythrocyte
    b. Rubriblast, reticulocyte, rubricyte, erythrocyte
    c. Rubriblast, rubricyte, reticulocyte, erythrocyte
    d. Reticulocyte, rubriblast, rubricyte, erythrocyte

177. What test is used to diagnose autoimmune hemolytic anemia?
    a. Red cell fragility test
    b. Modified Knott
    c. Coombs
    d. Coggins

178. What term indicates an abnormally high lymphocyte count?
    a. Lymphocytosis
    b. Leukosis
    c. Lymphocytopenia
    d. Lymphosarcoma

179. It is important to keep cytology samples and unstained slides away from _____ so that the samples can be stained properly later.
    a. Acetone
    b. Ether
    c. Formalin
    d. Saline

180. Which of the following is considered a tick-borne organism found in dogs?
    a. *Toxoplasma*
    b. *Isospora*
    c. *Ehrlichia*
    d. *Cryptosporidium*

181. Which of the following terms refers to an infestation with lice?
    a. Myiasis
    b. Acariasis
    c. Paraphimosis
    d. Pediculosis

182. A skin scraping will diagnose which parasite?
    a. Bovicola
    b. Notoedres
    c. Otodectes
    d. Ctenocephalides

183. Which of the following is the largest intermediate form of a tapeworm?
    a. Cysticercus
    b. Hydatid cyst
    c. Coenurus
    d. Cysticercoid

184. What canine parasite causes nodules in the esophagus, which may then become neoplastic?
    a. *Physaloptera*
    b. *Filaroides*
    c. *Spirocerca*
    d. *Neosporum*

185. Which of the following options is not zoonotic?
    a. *Toxoplasma*
    b. *Parvovirus*
    c. *Dipylidium*
    d. *Giardia*

186. Observing a "zippy" motility in fresh feces is used to help diagnose the presence of what parasite?
    a. *Toxoplasma*
    b. *Mycoplasma (Haemobartonella)*
    c. *Tritrichomonas*
    d. *Ehrlichia canis*

187. Which parasite causes blood loss, especially in young animals?
    a. Roundworm
    b. Tapeworm
    c. Heartworm
    d. Hookworm

188. What parasite causes a very pruritic disease in dogs?
    a. *Cheyletiella*
    b. *Sarcoptes*
    c. *Demodex*
    d. *Dermacentor*

189. What causes the sensitivity of the occult heartworm test to decrease?
    a. No microfilariae present
    b. Female worms only
    c. Male worms only
    d. No clinical signs

190. Which statement is true about *Dirofilaria* infection in the cat?
    a. The life span of heartworms in cats is shorter than in dogs
    b. Microfilariae are commonly seen in cat infections
    c. Adult worm burden in cats is similar in numbers to that in dogs
    d. *Dirofilaria* causes a severe anemia in cats

191. What is the function of a megakaryocyte?
    a. Phagocytosis
    b. Produces granulocytes
    c. Produces thrombocytes
    d. Produces plasma cells

192. Which of the following is not associated with a responsive anemia?
    a. Poikilocytosis
    b. Reticulocytosis
    c. Anisocytosis
    d. Polychromasia

193. What erythrocyte index provides an indication of the average size of a red blood cell?
    a. MCHC
    b. MCV
    c. M/E ratio
    d. Reticulocyte count

194. What is the most immature cell in the granulocyte series?
    a. Megakaryoblast
    b. Leukoblast
    c. Myeloblast
    d. Progranuloblast

195. What large cell with multiple separate nuclei is found in bone marrow?
    a. Osteoclast
    b. Megakaryocyte
    c. Osteoblast
    d. Monoblast

196. What marrow finding is consistent with a responsive anemia?
    a. Myeloid hypoplasia
    b. Erythroid hyperplasia
    c. Erythroid hypoplasia
    d. Myeloid metaplasia

197. Which test is used to confirm a diagnosis of warfarin (rodenticide) toxicity?
    a. Thrombocyte count
    b. Calcium level
    c. One-step prothrombin time
    d. Partial thromboplastin time (PTT)

198. Which of the following are not observed when a patient is in DIC?
    a. Icterus
    b. Hemorrhage
    c. Thrombocytopenia
    d. Prolonged activated clotting time

199. Which clotting disorder is stimulated by hypothyroidism?
    a. Hemophilia A
    b. Von Willebrand disease
    c. Disseminated intravascular coagulation
    d. Coumarin toxicity

200. In what species is ketonuria most commonly found?
    a. Canine
    b. Feline
    c. Equine
    d. Bovine

201. What is the smallest epithelial cell seen on a urine sediment examination?
    a. Leukocyte
    b. Transitional cell
    c. Renal cell
    d. Squamous cell

202. For glucosuria to occur, which of the following must also be present?
    a. Uremia
    b. Hyperglycemia
    c. Ketonemia
    d. Azoturia

203. Which urolith is becoming quite common in cats?
    a. Oxalate
    b. Silica
    c. Urate
    d. Cystine

204. What test on the urine dipstick is the least useful in animals?
    a. Glucose
    b. Urobilinogen
    c. Protein
    d. Ketones

205. What substance increases in the urine during glomerular disease?
    a. Glucose
    b. Ketones
    c. Bilirubin
    d. Protein

206. Which breed of dog has the most problems with uric acid stones?
    a. Basenji
    b. German shepherd
    c. Dalmatian
    d. Shetland sheepdog

207. Keeping the urine _____ will keep struvite crystals dissolved in solution.
    a. Acidic
    b. Basic
    c. Isosthenuric
    d. Dilute

208. Which of the following is a disadvantage of an enzyme-linked immunosorbent assay?
    a. Sensitivity
    b. Specificity
    c. Rapid results
    d. Titer detection

209. Which of the following clinical tests may be influenced when a toxic dose of acetaminophen has been ingested?
    a. Alanine aminotransferase
    b. Ammonia
    c. Blood pH
    d. Calcium

210. Chemical neutropenia may result from the ingestion of which drugs in dogs?
    a. Chloramphenicol
    b. Estrogen
    c. Phenylbutazone
    d. All of the above

211. Xylitol ingestion may result in which of the following conditions?
    a. Hypophosphatemia
    b. Hypobilirubinemia
    c. Hypoglycemia
    d. Hyper and hypophosphatemia

212. Which fluid sample is the major vehicle for the transporting of toxicants within the body?
    a. Blood/plasma
    b. Feces
    c. Hair
    d. Urine

213. All of the following samples should be submitted when acetaminophen is suspected to have been ingested, *except:*
    a. Plasma (EDTA or heparin preserved)
    b. Liver biopsy
    c. Urine
    d. Blood Smear

214. What is the main constituent of a struvite crystal?
    a. Calcium carbonate
    b. Calcium oxalate
    c. Magnesium phosphate
    d. Silica

215. Which of the following is not considered an electrolyte?
    a. Calcium
    b. Sodium
    c. Potassium
    d. Chloride

216. Hyperkalemia is commonly associated with which endocrine disorder?
    a. Diabetes insipidus
    b. Hyperthyroidism
    c. Hyperparathyroidism
    d. Hypoadrenocorticism

217. A false positive test result is one in which the:
    a. Animal is affected and the test is negative
    b. Animal is not affected and the test is positive
    c. Animal is not affected and the test is negative
    d. Animal is affected and the test is positive

218. Polyuria and polydipsia are not commonly seen in what endocrine disorder?
    a. Hyperadrenocorticism
    b. Diabetes insipidus
    c. Hyperparathyroidism
    d. Diabetes mellitus

219. What cat blood type is considered the universal donor?
    a. A
    b. O
    c. AB
    d. None exists in the cat

220. How do transfusion reactions in the cat differ from transfusion reactions in the dog?
    a. Transfusions are more severe in the cat
    b. Transfusions are more acute in the dog
    c. Cats suffer from severe pruritus
    d. Transfusions are more severe in the dog

221. When the spun hematocrit test is completed, which of the following can be evaluated?
    a. PCV
    b. Plasma color and PCV
    c. Total protein, buffy coat, plasma color, and PCV
    d. Total protein, buffy coat, plasma color, fibrin, and PCV

222. A monolayer of cells on a blood smear is best described as:
    a. A feathered edge
    b. Cells with no overlapping or touching
    c. Cells touching each other very closely with some overlapping
    d. The body of the blood smear

223. An example of capillary action is:
    a. The blood coursing through smaller veins
    b. The perfusion of mucous membranes
    c. The action of blood filling a hematocrit tube
    d. Removing serum from a clot with a pipette

224. Which of these is not a random laboratory error?
    a. Variation in glassware
    b. Electronic or optical inconsistency
    c. Anisocytosis
    d. Contamination

225. Prolonged exposure of serum to the blood cells before the serum is removed from the clot can result in:
    a. Increased serum glucose
    b. Increased serum phosphorus
    c. Increased serum enzyme activity
    d. Increased serum sodium

226. Phagocytes include all of the following, *except:*
    a. Neutrophils
    b. Lymphocytes
    c. Monocytes
    d. Macrophages

227. Before beginning other diagnostics of the urine, a ___ examination of urine is recommended.
    a. Darkfield
    b. Gross
    c. Taste
    d. Microscopic

228. *Paragonimus kellicotti* is a:
    a. Tapeworm
    b. Tick
    c. Mite
    d. Fluke

229. Which of these is not a function of the lymphatic system?
    a. Transport of waste materials
    b. Leukocyte production
    c. Removal of excess tissue fluid
    d. Protein transport

230. What organ has both lymphatic and hematologic functions?
    a. Spleen
    b. Pancreas
    c. Tonsil
    d. Liver

231. What organ has storage sinuses that hold blood and release it into circulation when the need for oxygen is increased?
    a. Spleen
    b. Pancreas
    c. Parathyroid
    d. Liver

232. What organ releases T cells?
    a. Thyroid
    b. Thymus
    c. Splenic trabeculae
    d. Tonsils

233. What tissue processes B cells before they are sent to peripheral lymphoid tissue?
    a. GLNB
    b. GALB
    c. GALT
    d. GLAN

234. What would not cause shifts or trends in quality-control data?
    a. New lot numbers of reagents
    b. Change in calibration of the instrument
    c. Outdated reagents
    d. Change in laboratory personnel

235. What error is not detectable through the use of a quality-control program?
    a. Poor technique
    b. Sample quality
    c. Equipment malfunctions
    d. Reagent contamination or degeneration

236. For proper calibration, what solution should be used to calibrate a refractometer?
    a. Tap water
    b. Distilled water
    c. Plasma
    d. Urine

237. To separate serum, whole blood should be spun down in a centrifuge at:
    a. 4500 rpm for 30 minutes
    b. 10,000 rpm for 10 minutes
    c. 8500 rpm for 30 minutes
    d. 2500 rpm for 10 minutes

238. When using a centrifuge, it is important to do all of the following each time it is used, *except:*
    a. Balance the tubes
    b. Open the lid as the centrifuge is in the process of stopping
    c. Set the timer
    d. Check tube holders for leaked liquid

239. As a general rule, enough blood should be collected to run any test at least three times. This compensates for all of the following, *except:*
    a. Instrument error
    b. Technician error
    c. Transcription error
    d. Improper dilution of a sample

240. False decreases in serum glucose levels can be caused by:
    a. Prolonged contact with red blood cells before separating the serum
    b. Refrigerating the serum sample before analysis
    c. Freezing the serum sample before analysis
    d. A lipemic sample

241. Drawing a blood sample from an animal that has recently eaten may result in a sample that is:
    a. Hemolyzed
    b. Lipemic
    c. Icteric
    d. Anemic

242. Centrifuging a blood sample at high speed for a prolonged period may result in:
    a. Lipemia
    b. Icterus
    c. Hemolysis
    d. Bacterial contamination

243. Improper handling of a blood sample after it has been collected may result in:
a. Lipemia
b. Icterus
c. Hemolysis
d. Leukocytosis

244. A serum sample that is extremely icteric generally derives its color from an increased level of:
a. Lipids
b. Total bilirubin
c. Electrolytes
d. Glucose

245. What color is icteric plasma?
a. Brown
b. Red
c. Green
d. Yellow

246. Which statement is false concerning the collection of a plasma sample for a blood chemistry analysis?
a. If a needle and syringe are used, hemolysis can be minimized by removing the needle from the syringe before discharging the blood into a sample tube.
b. Volume changes caused by evaporation can be minimized by keeping the cap on the blood collection tube as much as possible.
c. To separate, allow the sample to clot for approximately 30 minutes; gently remove the clot from the sides of the tube, centrifuge, and then remove the plasma.
d. Avoid lipemia by fasting the animal before collecting the sample.

247. What sample condition cannot be minimized by proper animal preparation or proper sample collection and handling?
a. Hemolysis
b. Icterus
c. Lipemia
d. Evaporation

248. An allergic response that is frequently life threatening is the result of:
a. Agglutination
b. Hemolysis
c. DIC
d. Anaphylaxis

249. A total of 99% of the domestic shorthair cats in the United States have which blood type?
a. A
b. B
c. AB
d. O

250. Canine blood types are preceded by the letters "DEA." What do these letters stand for?
a. Detectable Erythrocyte Antibody
b. Detectable Erythrocyte Antigen
c. Dog Erythrocyte Antibody
d. Dog Erythrocyte Antigen

251. Coagulation tests would be useful for diagnosing:
a. Rodenticide poisoning
b. Thyroid function
c. Adrenal function
d. Ethylene glycol poisoning

252. The calibrated device used to deliver a specified volume of patient sample when performing a blood chemistry analysis is known as a:
a. Cuvette
b. Pipette
c. Graduated flask
d. Graduated cylinder

253. Laser-flow technology is used in:
a. Hematology analyzers
b. Chemistry analyzers
c. Coagulation analyzers
d. Electrolyte analyzers

254. In dogs and cats, the blood chemistry tests most commonly used to evaluate liver function are:
a. Alanine transaminase and aspartate aminotransferase
b. Electrolytes and blood urea nitrogen
c. Gamma-glutamyl transferase and sorbitol dehydrogenase
d. Amylase and lipase

255. In horses, the blood chemistry tests most commonly used to evaluate liver function are:
a. Alanine transaminase and aspartate aminotransferase
b. Electrolytes and blood urea nitrogen
c. Gamma-glutamyl transferase and sorbitol dehydrogenase
d. Amylase and lipase

256. Blood chemistry assays, including dye excretion, ammonia tolerance, and bile acid concentrations, are used to evaluate the function of the:
a. Pancreas
b. Kidneys
c. Heart
d. Liver

257. Impedance is:
     a. Used in analytic instruments to stop a test
     b. Blockage of light or electric current in analytic instruments
     c. Lack of synchronicity between the jugular pulse and the heartbeat
     d. Inability to feel pedal pulses

258. Which of the following is not a disadvantage of using the PCR testing in equine medicine?
     a. False positive reactions
     b. Lack of viable virus isolates
     c. Inability to detect new viruses
     d. Sensitivity of the test

259. The adult form of the parasite _____ is a fly, and the larval stage is an endoparasite.
     a. *Otobius*
     b. *Capillaria*
     c. *Thelazia*
     d. *Gasterophilus*

260. Bots are:
     a. Lice eggs
     b. Fly larvae
     c. Flea feces
     d. Seed ticks

261. Nits are considered:
     a. Lice eggs
     b. Fly larvae
     c. Flea feces
     d. Seed ticks

262. Which parasite could cause anemia in horses through blood sucking?
     a. *Strongylus vulgaris*
     b. *Parascaris equorum*
     c. *Anoplocephala perfoliata*
     d. *Dictyocaulus arnfieldi*

263. Which product stains fat?
     a. New methylene blue
     b. Sudan III or IV
     c. Diff-Quik
     d. Giemsa

264. Which stain is referred to as a *supravital stain*?
     a. New methylene blue
     b. Camco Quik
     c. Eosin
     d. Sudan III or IV

265. Eosinophilia is commonly seen with a:
     a. Bacterial infection
     b. Parasitic infection
     c. Viral infection
     d. Hormonal disorder

266. What is the underlying cause of icterus?
     a. Anemia
     b. Hyperbilirubinemia
     c. Ketonuria
     d. Hyperhemoglobinemia

267. Basophilic stippling is often associated with:
     a. Lead poisoning
     b. Autoimmune disease
     c. Anemia
     d. Neoplasia

268. A common finding on a stained blood smear from an animal with autoimmune hemolytic anemia is:
     a. Lymphocytosis
     b. Basophilic stippling
     c. Spherocytosis
     d. Leukemia

269. Denatured hemoglobin found in erythrocytes is referred to as a/an:
     a. Heinz body
     b. Howell-Jolly body
     c. *Anaplasma* body
     d. Spherocyte

270. Fresh frozen plasma can be stored up to _____ and still contain clotting factors.
     a. 1 month
     b. 12 months
     c. 36 months
     d. 60 months

271. What cell produces antibodies?
     a. Hepatocyte
     b. Plasma cell
     c. Thymocyte
     d. T cell

272. What appears as a blue spherical nuclear remnant seen in some Wright-stained erythrocytes?
     a. Reticulocyte
     b. Howell-Jolly body
     c. Heinz body
     d. Leptocyte

273. Frozen fresh plasma (FFP) must be separated and frozen within ____ hours to maintain all coagulation factors in normal concentrations.
    a. 2
    b. 8
    c. 12
    d. 6

274. Which of the following stimulates antibody production?
    a. Immunoglobulin
    b. Antigen
    c. T cell
    d. Plasma cell

275. A normal leukocyte count with an increase in immature neutrophils that outnumber mature neutrophils is:
    a. Leukocytosis
    b. Leukopenia
    c. A regenerative left shift
    d. A degenerative left shift

276. A variation in erythrocyte size is known as:
    a. Polycytosis
    b. Anisocytosis
    c. Poikilocytosis
    d. Erythrocytosis

277. What is the name for a nonnucleated, immature erythrocyte found in small numbers in the peripheral blood of dogs?
    a. Reticulocyte
    b. Metarubricyte
    c. Rubriblast
    d. Rubricyte

278. What sample is recommended for hemoglobin testing?
    a. Serum
    b. Plasma
    c. Whole blood
    d. Blood smear

279. What part of the CBC is the most accurate procedure?
    a. Erythrocyte count
    b. Hemoglobin determination
    c. Leukocyte count
    d. Hematocrit

280. What part of the CBC cannot be done manually with adequate accuracy?
    a. Erythrocyte count
    b. Leukocyte count
    c. Packed cell volume
    d. WBC differential

281. What would you expect to see on a Diff-Quik stained blood smear from an animal with regenerative anemia?
    a. Schistocytosis
    b. Reticulocytosis
    c. Eosinophilia
    d. Polychromasia

282. What cell is described as a central rounded area of hemoglobin surrounded by a clear zone, with a dense ring of hemoglobin around the periphery?
    a. Plasma cell
    b. Target cell
    c. Spherocyte
    d. Reticulocyte

283. Where is the buffy coat found on the refractometer?
    a. Beneath the packed red cells
    b. Above the packed red cells
    c. Above the plasma
    d. Buffy coats are not seen on refractometers.

284. What is the major difference between serum and plasma?
    a. Plasma has higher protein levels.
    b. Serum has higher electrolyte levels.
    c. Plasma has a darker color.
    d. Serum will clot.

285. What is the term used to describe plasma that appears white or milky?
    a. Leukemia
    b. Lipemia
    c. Chylemia
    d. Lactemia

286. What is the term used to describe the situation in which many of the erythrocytes stain varying shades of lavender?
    a. Anemia
    b. Anisocytosis
    c. Polychromasia
    d. Poikilocytosis

287. Which of the following is a breakdown product of hemoglobin?
    a. Bilirubin
    b. Erythropoietin
    c. Urea
    d. Carotene

288. What type of anemia is associated with icterus?
    a. Responsive
    b. Nonresponsive
    c. Hemolytic
    d. Megaloblastic

289. What is the most immature erythrocyte that can be identified in bone marrow?
    a. Prorubricyte
    b. Rubriblast
    c. Erythrocytoblast
    d. Multipotent stem cell

290. Rouleaux formation is most commonly seen on blood smears from:
    a. Horses
    b. Goats
    c. Dogs
    d. Cats

291. An MCV value below the normal reference range suggests:
    a. Hyperchromasia
    b. Hypochromasia
    c. Macrocytosis
    d. Microcytosis

292. If you count 40 reticulocytes per 1000 erythrocytes, what is the observed reticulocyte count?
    a. 2%
    b. 4%
    c. 20%
    d. 40%

293. What is indicated by a neutrophil that includes a nucleus with six lobes?
    a. Toxemia
    b. Female animal
    c. Old cell
    d. Normal cell

294. What causes dark granules called *Döhle bodies* in the cytoplasm of canine neutrophils?
    a. Leukemia
    b. Parasitic infection
    c. Immaturity
    d. Toxemia

295. What is normally the largest mature blood cell in the peripheral blood of domestic species?
    a. Monocyte
    b. Neutrophil
    c. Eosinophil
    d. Lymphocyte

296. When preparing a direct smear from feces, all of the following liquids can be mixed with the feces, *except:*
    a. Tap water
    b. Distilled water
    c. Hydrogen peroxide
    d. Saline

297. With the exception of cats, most animals have a total blood volume equivalent to ___ of their body weight.
    a. 7%
    b. 15%
    c. 25%
    d. 40%

298. What is tested in a minor crossmatch?
    a. T-cell production
    b. Recipient serum against donor erythrocytes
    c. Recipient erythrocytes against donor serum
    d. Recipient urine against donor erythrocytes

299. What anticoagulant is used most commonly in animal-blood collection for CBCs?
    a. Sodium heparin
    b. Potassium oxalate
    c. Potassium ethylenediamine tetraacetic acid
    d. Sodium citrate

300. What anticoagulant is used to determine activated partial thromboplastin time and one-stage prothrombin time?
    a. Heparin
    b. Citrate
    c. Fluoride
    d. EDTA

301. What structure is normally found in the nuclei of immature blood cells?
    a. Nucleolus
    b. Golgi apparatus
    c. Heinz body
    d. Döhle body

302. Certain oxidant drugs can denature hemoglobin and cause the production of round structures in erythrocytes that are called:
    a. Howell-Jolly bodies
    b. Russell bodies
    c. Döhle bodies
    d. Heinz bodies

303. What is the most common cause of hypochromia in erythrocytes?
    a. Hypertonic drugs
    b. Decreased hemoglobin
    c. Iron toxicity
    d. Increased erythrocyte production

304. What is the primary function of fibrinogen?
    a. Antibody production
    b. Phagocytosis
    c. Hemostasis
    d. Complement fixation

305. *Haemobartonella felis* is seen most commonly in the erythrocytes of:
    a. Cats
    b. Cattle
    c. Dogs
    d. Horses

306. An increased number of bands in the peripheral blood indicate:
    a. Leukemia
    b. Autoimmune hemolytic anemia
    c. Left shift
    d. Neutropenia

307. The first line of defense that the body has against foreign invaders is the:
    a. Hair
    b. Neutrophils
    c. Primary lymphoid tissue
    d. Skin

308. Which of these white blood cells migrate through tissue as macrophages and function to remove and destroy bacteria, damaged cells, and neoplastic cells?
    a. Lymphocytes
    b. Neutrophils
    c. Monocytes
    d. Eosinophils

309. Which immunoglobulin is most abundant in the serum and plays the major role in humoral immunity?
    a. IgG
    b. IgM
    c. IgA
    d. IgD

310. Immunity that is generated by an animal's immune system following exposure to a foreign antigen is referred to as:
    a. Passive immunity
    b. Active immunity
    c. Responsive immunity
    d. Colostral immunity

311. Which immunoglobulin is the only one that can cross the placenta?
    a. IgG
    b. IgM
    c. IgA
    d. IgD

312. Which of the following correctly lists the progressive stages of phagocytosis?
    a. Adherence, chemotaxis, ingestion, digestion
    b. Ingestion, adherence, chemotaxis, digestion
    c. Chemotaxis, adherence, ingestion, digestion
    d. Ingestion, digestion, chemotaxis, adherence

313. An attenuated vaccine is one in which:
    a. Microorganisms are killed
    b. Microorganisms are weakened but are still alive
    c. Microorganisms are 100% virulent
    d. No microorganisms are found

314. Which statement concerning passive immunity is least accurate?
    a. It involves antibodies that have been produced in a donor animal
    b. It provides immediate but short-lived immunity
    c. It may be natural or artificial
    d. It develops after exposure to a pathogen

315. Myasthenia gravis is commonly associated with:
    a. Megaesophagus
    b. Exercise intolerance
    c. Aspiration pneumonia
    d. All of the above

316. Anaphylactic shock is:
    a. A mild reaction that causes destruction of erythrocytes
    b. A moderate reaction that causes hives
    c. A severe, life-threatening reaction that occurs seconds after an antigen enters the circulation
    d. A severe reaction caused by rapid loss of large volumes of blood or other bodily fluid

317. Combined immunodeficiency is a condition in which the animal fails to produce functioning:
    a. Plasma cells
    b. B cells
    c. T cells
    d. B and T cells

318. Which of the following is not a malfunction of the immune system?
    a. Allergy
    b. Immunodeficiency
    c. Autoimmune disease
    d. Immunity by vaccination

319. What cells are chiefly concerned with the production and secretion of antibodies?
    a. B lymphocytes
    b. T lymphocytes
    c. Neutrophils
    d. Monocytes

320. What cells respond more quickly to a second antigen exposure than to the initial exposure?
    a. Thymocytes
    b. Monocytes
    c. Memory B cells
    d. Neutrophils

321. Serology is the branch of science involved with detection of:
    a. Bacteria or fungi
    b. Viruses or prions
    c. Antibodies or antigens
    d. Endoparasites and ectoparasites

322. ELISA is an acronym for:
    a. Electro-linked immunosorbent assay
    b. Enzyme-linked immunosorbent assay
    c. Enzyme-linked immunoassay
    d. Electrolytic isoantibody assay

323. Which statement concerning ELISA testing is true?
    a. The test specificity is very low
    b. Washing is a critical step in the methodology
    c. It may be used to detect only antibodies in the serum
    d. It is not available in kit form

324. What serologic test is used for the diagnosis of autoimmune hemolytic anemia?
    a. Coombs test
    b. Coggins test
    c. Intradermal testing
    d. Latex agglutination test

325. Which of these parasites sucks blood from its host?
    a. *Macracanthorhynchus hirudinaceus*
    b. *Onchocerca cervicalis*
    c. *Metastrongylus apri*
    d. *Ctenocephalides felis*

326. Which of these pig parasites can be diagnosed by muscle biopsy?
    a. *Trichinella spiralis*
    b. *Oesophagostomum dentatum*
    c. *Eimeria suis*
    d. *Fasciola hepatica*

327. Vaccines may be administered by any of the following routes, *except:*
    a. Subcutaneously
    b. Intramuscularly
    c. Intranasally
    d. Intraperitoneally

328. Which of the following is least likely to cause vaccine failure?
    a. Improper storage
    b. Administration during anesthesia
    c. Interference by maternal antibodies
    d. Improper route of administration

329. Which of these parasites is a tapeworm?
    a. *Strongyloides westeri*
    b. *Paranoplocephala mamillana*
    c. *Parascaris equorum*
    d. *Oxyuris equi*

330. Which of these parasites is classified as coccidia?
    a. *Cryptosporidium parvum*
    b. *Bunostomum phlebotomum*
    c. *Moniezia expansa*
    d. *Haemonchus contortus*

331. Pemphigus is a group of autoimmune disorders that affect the:
    a. Blood and lymph systems
    b. Skin and oral mucosa
    c. Eyes
    d. Hooves and claws

332. Signs of immune-mediated thrombocytopenia (ITP) include all of these conditions, *except:*
    a. Petechiae
    b. Ecchymoses
    c. Thrombocytosis
    d. Anemia

333. Which of these cells is the most immature?
    a. Rubricyte
    b. Metarubricyte
    c. Prorubricyte
    d. Reticulocyte

334. What is one possible site of extramedullary hematopoiesis in times of increased blood cell production?
    a. Spleen
    b. Kidney
    c. Umbilicus
    d. Bone cortex

335. *Baylisascaris procyonis* larvae have been shown to cause _____ in humans.
    a. Pneumonia
    b. Hemolytic anemia
    c. Brain damage
    d. Bloody diarrhea

336. Hemagglutination is:
    a. Clumping of erythrocytes
    b. Lysing of erythrocytes
    c. Crenation of erythrocytes
    d. Swelling of erythrocytes

337. What test is routinely used to diagnose equine infectious anemia?
    a. Indirect fluorescent antibody test
    b. Coggins test
    c. Coombs test
    d. Hemoglobin electrophoresis

338. When reviewing a blood smear, you come across an erythrocyte that does not contain its full amount of hemoglobin. What is this known as?
    a. Polychromasia
    b. Hypochromasia
    c. Basophilia
    d. Hyperchromasia

339. A neutrophil with a four-segmented nucleus would be classified as a:
    a. Hypersegmented neutrophil
    b. Immature neutrophil
    c. Normal neutrophil
    d. Aged neutrophil

340. During an allergic response, what do sensitized cells produce in abnormal quantities when an allergen reappears after an initial exposure?
    a. Antihistamines
    b. Histamine
    c. Toxins
    d. Lysins

341. Gram-positive microorganisms stain _____ using a Gram stain.
    a. Purple
    b. Red
    c. Orange
    d. Lavender

342. Acid-fast stains are used to identify:
    a. Coccidia
    b. Yeast
    c. Fungi
    d. Mycobacteria

343. What cells are sensitized by IgE to produce large quantities of histamines?
    a. Mast cells and basophils
    b. Eosinophils and basophils
    c. Monocytes and lymphocytes
    d. Neutrophils and eosinophils

344. T killer cells function to:
    a. Release histamine
    b. Recognize cancer cells as abnormal cells and eliminate them
    c. Coat cancer cells with antibody
    d. Release endorphin

345. Cats exposed to feline leukemia virus typically respond in any of the following ways, *except:*
    a. Not becoming infected at all
    b. Becoming temporarily infected, developing immunity, and overcoming the infection
    c. Becoming infected and continuing to shed the virus indefinitely without becoming ill
    d. Becoming infected, becoming ill within 3 days, and dying within a week

346. Acid-fast positive organisms stain _____ when using an acid-fast stain.
    a. Yellow
    b. Blue
    c. Pink
    d. Brown

347. What is the predominant method for the transmission of feline immunodeficiency virus in cats?
    a. Grooming
    b. Bite wounds
    c. Urine
    d. Feces

348. In assessing titers, how long after the first serum sample is collected should the second sample be collected?
    a. 7 days
    b. 3 days
    c. 2 to 6 weeks
    d. 14 weeks

349. What microorganisms are not free living?
    a. Algae
    b. Fungi
    c. Bacteria
    d. Viruses

350. What is the correct way to write the genus and species of bacteria?
    a. *Streptococcus Pyogenes*
    b. Streptococcus pyogenes
    c. S. pyogenes
    d. *Streptococcus pyogenes*

351. The acid-fast stain is used to identify the organism that causes:
    a. Anaplasmosis
    b. Colibacillosis
    c. Ringworm
    d. Tuberculosis

352. What color do gram-negative organisms appear when they are stained with Gram stain?
    a. Purple
    b. Pink
    c. Green
    d. Clear

353. Viruses are best described as:
    a. Free-living organisms
    b. Obligatory interstitial parasites
    c. Obligatory intracellular parasites
    d. Eukaryotic cells

354. A positive catalase test will be indicated by the presence of:
    a. A color change
    b. Gel formation
    c. Bubbles
    d. Fibrin

355. A nosocomial infection is always:
    a. Present but not apparent at the time of hospitalization
    b. Acquired during the course of hospitalization
    c. Caused by medical personnel
    d. Acquired during surgery

356. Generally, endotoxins are products of:
    a. Viruses
    b. Gram-negative bacteria
    c. Gram-positive bacteria
    d. Fungi

357. What organism will most likely grow on mannitol salt agar?
    a. *Streptococcus pyogenes*
    b. *Bacillus subtilis*
    c. *Clostridium perfringens*
    d. *Staphylococcus aureus*

358. Which virus causes warts?
    a. Papilloma
    b. Variola
    c. Herpes
    d. Pox

359. What organism exhibits fluorescence under ultraviolet light?
    a. *Microsporum gypseum*
    b. *Trichophyton mentagrophytes*
    c. *Microsporum canis*
    d. *Epidermophyton floccosum*

360. Pinkeye or contagious conjunctivitis in cattle is caused by:
    a. *Haemophilus aegypti*
    b. *Moraxella bovis*
    c. *Streptococcus pyogenes*
    d. *Staphylococcus aureus*

361. On a blood agar plate, an area of complete hemolysis is classified as:
    a. Alpha
    b. Beta
    c. Gamma
    d. Delta

362. *Dipylidium caninum* is a:
    a. Trematode
    b. Nematode
    c. Arthropod
    d. Cestode

363. *Fasciola hepatica* is a:
    a. Nematode
    b. Cestode
    c. Trematode
    d. Protozoan

364. A puppy infected with *Dirofilaria immitis* the day it is born will not test positive for heartworm microfilariae until it is _____ old.
    a. 12 months
    b. 6 to 7 months
    c. 3 to 4 months
    d. 1 month

365. The ELISA heartworm test kit detects the antigens of:
    a. Heartworm microfilariae
    b. Female adult heartworms
    c. Adult heartworms and microfilariae
    d. Toxins produced by adult heartworms

366. *Dirofilaria immitis* is a:
    a. Cestode
    b. Arthropod
    c. Nematode
    d. Trematode

367. *Otodectes cynotis* is a:
    a. Cestode
    b. Arthropod
    c. Nematode
    d. Trematode

368. A dog becomes infected with *Dipylidium caninum* by ingestion of:
    a. Saliva from an infected dog
    b. Feces from an infected dog
    c. Tissues of an infected rabbit
    d. Infected fleas

369. The most common intermediate host of *Taenia pisiformis* is a:
    a. Ruminant
    b. Flea
    c. Fly
    d. Rabbit

370. The parasite whose adult resembles a whip and whose eggs have bipolar plugs is:
    a. *Strongyloides stercoralis*
    b. *Trichuris vulpis*
    c. *Toxocara canis*
    d. *Toxascaris leonina*

371. In most areas of the world, rats are the reservoir host of the plague organism. However, in the Western United States, the most common species harboring this organism is:
    a. Dogs
    b. Cats
    c. Beavers
    d. Prairie dogs

372. The kennel cough syndrome in dogs is often caused by a combination of boarding at a kennel, a viral infection, and infection with:
    a. *Pasteurella multocida*
    b. *Staphylococcus aureus*
    c. *Corynebacterium diphtheriae*
    d. *Bordetella bronchiseptica*

373. What organism is a spirochete?
    a. *Corynebacterium pyogenes*
    b. *Streptococcus pyogenes*
    c. *Mycobacterium tuberculosis*
    d. *Leptospira grippotyphosa*

374. What organism causes strangles in horses?
    a. *Staphylococcus aureus*
    b. *Streptococcus equi*
    c. *Corynebacterium equi*
    d. *Strongylus vulgaris*

375. What characteristic is unique to *Mycobacterium*?
    a. It is a spore former
    b. It is anaerobic
    c. It is easily killed by antibiotics
    d. It survives phagocytosis

376. Which of the following is not a simple stain?
    a. Methylene blue
    b. Crystal violet
    c. Safranin
    d. Gram stain

377. Acquired active immunity results from:
    a. Vaccination
    b. Antitoxin administration
    c. Ingestion of colostrum
    d. Administration of gamma globulin

378. *Escherichia coli* is normally found:
    a. On the skin
    b. In the intestinal tract
    c. In the respiratory tract
    d. In the stomach

379. Pediculosis is an infestation of:
    a. Ticks
    b. Flies
    c. Lice
    d. Mites

380. In people, *Toxocara canis* is the causative agent of:
    a. Creeping eruption
    b. Scabies
    c. Hydatidosis
    d. Visceral larva migrans

381. A large ciliate protozoa that may be found in swine feces is:
    a. *Balantidium* species
    b. *Trichomonas* species
    c. *Giardia* species
    d. *Histomonas* species

382. The parasite diagnosed by vaginal washing is:
    a. *Tritrichomonas* species
    b. *Dictyocaulus* species
    c. *Dioctophyma* species
    d. *Anaplasma* species

383. The parasite diagnosed by tracheal wash is:
    a. *Tritrichomonas* species
    b. *Dictyocaulus* species
    c. *Dioctophyma* species
    d. *Anaplasma* species

384. The parasite diagnosed by examining urine is:
    a. *Tritrichomonas* species
    b. *Dictyocaulus* species
    c. *Dioctophyma* species
    d. *Anaplasma* species

385. The parasite diagnosed by examining blood is:
    a. *Tritrichomonas* species
    b. *Dictyocaulus* species
    c. *Dioctophyma* species
    d. *Anaplasma* species

386. The parasite also known as a *brown dog tick* is:
    a. *Rhipicephalus sanguineus*
    b. *Ixodes dammini*
    c. *Dermacentor variabilis*
    d. *Dermacentor albipictus*

387. The parasite also known as a *winter tick* is:
    a. *Rhipicephalus sanguineus*
    b. *Ixodes dammini*
    c. *Dermacentor variabilis*
    d. *Dermacentor albipictus*

388. The parasite also known as the *American dog tick* is:
    a. *Rhipicephalus sanguineus*
    b. *Ixodes dammini*
    c. *Dermacentor variabilis*
    d. *Dermacentor albipictus*

389. The parasite also known as a *deer tick* is:
    a. *Rhipicephalus sanguineus*
    b. *Ixodes dammini*
    c. *Dermacentor variabilis*
    d. *Dermacentor albipictus*

390. The parasite that lives in ears is:
    a. *Sarcoptes* species
    b. *Demodex* species
    c. *Chorioptes* species
    d. *Otodectes* species

391. The parasite that lives on the skin's surface is:
    a. *Sarcoptes* species
    b. *Demodex* species
    c. *Chorioptes* species
    d. *Otodectes* species

392. The parasite that burrows into the skin is:
    a. *Sarcoptes* species
    b. *Demodex* species
    c. *Chorioptes* species
    d. *Otodectes* species

393. The parasite that lives in hair follicles is:
    a. *Sarcoptes* species
    b. *Demodex* species
    c. *Chorioptes* species
    d. *Otodectes* species

394. Which of the following ticks is considered a single host tick?
    a. *Boophilus annulatus*
    b. *Otobius megnini*
    c. *Ixodid sp.*
    d. *Argasidae sp.*

395. *Cheyletiella* mites use ___ as their hosts.
    a. Dogs, cats, and rabbits
    b. Dogs, rabbits, and birds
    c. Cats, birds, and rodents
    d. Cats, dogs, and rodents

396. Infection of this parasite is via skin penetration.
    a. *Trichuris vulpis*
    b. *Taenia pisiformis*
    c. *Dipylidium caninum*
    d. *Strongyloides stercoralis*

397. People may serve as the intermediate hosts of:
    a. *Echinococcus granulosus*
    b. *Anoplocephala magna*
    c. *Taenia pisiformis*
    d. *Moniezia benedeni*

398. What parasite ova have three pairs of hooklets?
    a. *Trichuris* species
    b. *Taenia* species
    c. *Alaria* species
    d. *Moniezia* species

399. What parasite ova have bipolar plugs?
    a. *Trichuris* species
    b. *Taenia* species
    c. *Alaria* species
    d. *Moniezia* species

400. The double-pore tapeworm is:
    a. *Paragonimus kellicotti*
    b. *Moniezia expansa*
    c. *Dipylidium caninum*
    d. *Echinococcus granulosus*

401. The parasite that infects the liver of its host is:
    a. *Diphyllobothrium* species
    b. *Hymenolepis* species
    c. *Paragonimus* species
    d. *Fasciola* species

402. The parasite whose larvae encyst in the subcutaneous tissue of rabbits is:
    a. *Gasterophilus* species
    b. *Hypoderma* species
    c. *Oestrus* species
    d. *Cuterebra* species

403. The parasite whose eggs are cemented to the hair of horses is:
    a. *Gasterophilus* species
    b. *Hypoderma* species
    c. *Oestrus* species
    d. *Cuterebra* species

404. The parasite whose larvae form warbles in subcutaneous tissue along the backs of cattle is:
    a. *Gasterophilus* species
    b. *Hypoderma* species
    c. *Oestrus* species
    d. *Cuterebra* species

405. The parasite whose larvae enter the nasal cavity of sheep is:
    a. *Gasterophilus* species
    b. *Hypoderma* species
    c. *Oestrus* species
    d. *Cuterebra* species

406. What parasite completes its life cycle on or in its host?
    a. *Ctenocephalides* species
    b. *Otodectes* species
    c. *Hypoderma* species
    d. *Dermacentor* species

407. What species causes a disease known as walking dandruff?
    a. *Trombicula* species
    b. *Sarcoptes* species
    c. *Demodex* species
    d. *Cheyletiella* species

408. Scabies is caused by:
    a. *Trombicula* species
    b. *Otodectes* species
    c. *Melophagus* species
    d. *Sarcoptes* species

409. In which stage of the tick life cycle does it have six legs?
    a. Nymphal
    b. Larval
    c. Adult female
    d. Adult male

410. What is the definition of hematopoiesis?
    a. The destruction of platelets
    b. The production of blood cells and platelets
    c. The creation of fibrinogen
    d. The decrease of red blood cells

411. What urinary stone is most associated with a urinary tract infection?
    a. Calcium oxalate crystal
    b. Struvite crystal
    c. Calcium carbonite crystal
    d. Cystine crystal

412. A urine specimen collected by free catch at 8 AM and left at room temperature until the afternoon could be expected to have:
    a. Decreased numbers of bacteria
    b. Increased numbers of bacteria
    c. Decreased numbers of epithelial cells
    d. Increased numbers of epithelial cells

413. An intestinal fluke is of the:
    a. *Alaria* species
    b. *Fascioloides* species
    c. *Stephanurus* species
    d. *Metastrongylus* species

414. The parasite also known as a lungworm is of the:
    a. *Alaria* species
    b. *Fascioloides* species
    c. *Stephanurus* species
    d. *Metastrongylus* species

415. The parasite also known as a kidney worm is of the:
    a. *Alaria* species
    b. *Fascioloides* species
    c. *Stephanurus* species
    d. *Metastrongylus* species

416. The parasite also known as the large American liver fluke is of the:
    a. *Alaria* species
    b. *Fascioloides* species
    c. *Stephanurus* species
    d. *Metastrongylus* species

417. Which statement concerning fleas is true?
    a. "Flea dirt" is flea feces
    b. Fleas are host specific
    c. Adults cannot survive for long periods without feeding
    d. Flea eggs are not sticky and they fall off into the environment

418. The parasite that causes generalized pruritus is of the:
a. *Ancylostoma* species
b. *Melophagus* species
c. *Notoedres* species
d. *Echinococcus* species

419. The urine of an animal with hematuria is likely to be:
a. Cloudy and red
b. Clear and brown
c. Red and clear
d. Brown and cloudy

420. Calcium carbonate crystals are often seen in ___ urine.
a. Dog
b. Horse
c. Cat
d. Cattle

421. What crystal is commonly described as having a coffin-lid appearance?
a. Bilirubin crystal
b. Calcium oxalate crystal
c. Cystine crystal
d. Triple phosphate crystal (Struvite)

422. An ammonium biurate crystal is sometimes described as:
a. Shaped like an envelope
b. Shaped like a pyramid
c. Like a thorny apple in appearance
d. Like a bicycle wheel in appearance

423. The best urine sample from a housebroken dog is collected in:
a. Late evening
b. Afternoon
c. Midmorning
d. Early morning

424. Urine samples collected in the morning from housebroken dogs tend to be:
a. Unacceptable for sediment analysis
b. The most concentrated samples
c. Bright orange
d. The least concentrated samples

425. What are the two preferred methods of collecting a urine sample for culture?
a. Catheterization and voiding
b. Expressing the bladder and cystocentesis
c. Cystocentesis and catheterization
d. Cystocentesis and voiding

426. Polyuria is:
a. Lack of urine production
b. Production of excessive amounts of urine
c. Lack of water intake
d. Excessive protein in the urine

427. Oliguria is:
a. Excessive eating
b. Green urine
c. Excessive bilirubin in the urine
d. Decreased urine output

428. Anuria is:
a. Decreased urine output
b. Decreased drinking
c. Complete lack of urine production
d. Excessive drinking

429. An alkaline urine pH can be the result of:
a. Urinary tract obstruction
b. Uncontrolled diabetes
c. Prolonged diarrhea
d. Starvation

430. Blood in the urine is reported as:
a. Dysuria
b. Hematuria
c. Pyuria
d. Proteinuria

431. An excessive number of WBCs in the urine is reported as:
a. Dysuria
b. Hematuria
c. Pyuria
d. Proteinuria

432. Painful urination is recorded as:
a. Dysuria
b. Hematuria
c. Pyuria
d. Proteinuria

433. Pancytopenia is characterized by:
a. Decreased numbers of white blood cells
b. Decreased numbers of all blood cells
c. Decreased numbers of red blood cells
d. Decreased numbers of granulocytes and monocytes

434. Erythropoietin is produced in the:
a. Bone marrow
b. Kidney
c. Liver
d. Pituitary gland

435. What is the appropriate amount of time needed for antibiotics to dissolve struvite crystals?
    a. 3–5 days
    b. 10–14 days
    c. 2–3 months
    d. 6 months

436. Prerenal azotemia is:
    a. Dehydration without true impaired kidney function
    b. Stage 1 renal disease
    c. Urinary tract infection that is affecting kidney function
    d. Dehydration with true impaired kidney function

437. What is an example of enteral nutrition?
    a. ITP given through an IV catheter
    b. Fasting or NPO
    c. Coaxing: warming the food, feeding by hand, etc.
    d. Water only

438. What are two examples of anticholinergic drugs?
    a. Propofol and ketamine
    b. Atropine and glycopyrrolate
    c. Cyclosporine and mycophenolate
    d. Dexdomitor and antisedan

439. What does the term MAC stand for?
    a. Maximum arterial concentration
    b. A sandwich at McDonalds
    c. Minimum alveolar concentration
    d. Mild acid concentration

440. What does an iohexol clearance test determine?
    a. Estimated GFR in dogs and cats
    b. Liver function
    c. Blood glucose values
    d. Food sensitivity

441. What is fructosamine?
    a. Another term for blood glucose
    b. A type of insulin
    c. A carbohydrate molecule to which glucose binds
    d. A protein to which glucose binds

442. What is the half-life of fructosamine?
    a. 3–5 days
    b. 1–2 weeks
    c. 3–5 months
    d. more than 6 months

443. How quickly must slides evaluating bone marrow samples be made if EDTA is used?
    a. 1 hour
    b. Immediately
    c. 15 minutes
    d. EDTA cannot be used for bone marrow samples

444. What does the buccal mucosa bleeding time test assess?
    a. Platelet function
    b. Prothrombin time (PT)
    c. Partial thromboplastin time (PTT)
    d. Fibrinogen

445. A canine patient experiencing high triglycerides may have serum that is colored:
    a. Milky
    b. Yellow
    c. Red
    d. Clear

446. Which of the following specific gravity concentrations would be expected in a healthy, hydrated, 4-year-old Labrador patient?
    a. 1.000
    b. 1.005
    c. 1.010
    d. 1.040

447. To avoid serum lipemia, animals should be fasted for:
    a. 2 hours
    b. 4 hours
    c. 8 hours
    d. 12 hours

ⓔ *Answers and rationales available on Evolve*
http://evolve.elsevier.com/Prendergast/QAvettech/

Animal Nursing

Ed Carlson, CVT, VTS (Nutrition), Kenichiro Yagi, BS, RVT, VTS (ECC, SAIM), and Heather Prendergast, RVT, CVPM

QUESTIONS

1. Which of the following animals are strict omnivores?
   a. Dogs
   b. Ferrets
   c. Prairie dogs
   d. Rabbits

2. Which of the following is a true effect of pain?
   a. It prevents further patient harm by preventing movement
   b. It places the animal in an anabolic state, leading to weight gain
   c. It suppresses the immune system, leading to an increased chance of infection
   d. It promotes inflammation and increases the healing rate

3. Taking a complete and accurate patient history:
   a. Is an important task that may be performed by veterinary technicians
   b. Should only be performed by a veterinarian
   c. Is only necessary if the patient has never been to the hospital
   d. Is not necessary for wellness exams in healthy patients

4. Which of the following animals are herbivores?
   a. Dogs
   b. Ferrets
   c. Prairie dogs
   d. Iguanas

5. Serum centrifuged in a microhematocrit tube characterized by varying degrees of redness is likely a result of:
   a. Hemolysis
   b. Hyperproteinemia
   c. Icterus
   d. Lipemia

6. Which of the following agencies regulates pet food labels and research facilities?
   a. AAFCO—Association of American Feed Control Officials
   b. FDA—Food and Drug Administration
   c. FTC—Federal Trade Commission
   d. USDA—United States Department of Agriculture

7. To fill prescriptions or administer a medication, technicians must be familiar with medical abbreviations. Which of the following abbreviations indicates a medication that is to be applied to both eyes?
   a. AU
   b. OD
   c. OS
   d. OU

8. Which of the following is a characteristic commonly seen in rabbits, in which the stool is ingested for nutritional purposes?
   a. Coprophagy
   b. Dysbiosis
   c. Dystrophic calcification
   d. Vitamin A deficiency

9. Which of the following is an example of a standardized method in assessing the effectiveness of analgesia in a patient?
   a. ASA Score
   b. Glasgow Coma Scale
   c. Colorado Pain Score
   d. Shock Index

10. When obtaining a patient history it is important to:
    a. Ask leading questions to save time and keep on schedule
    b. Ask open-ended questions
    c. Always use medical terms
    d. Ask leading questions when you already know what the problem is

11. When performing a physical exam on a patient:
    a. It is only necessary to exam the body part that is of concern to the client
    b. Always start at the rear of the patient
    c. Always start at with the patient's head
    d. All aspects of the exam should be examined in the same order whenever possible

12. Which of the following is commonly seen in rabbits, in which the intestinal flora is disrupted?
    a. Coprophagy
    b. Dysbiosis
    c. Dystrophic calcification
    d. Vitamin A deficiency

13. The proper pathway in which an animal perceives pain is:
    a. Transduction, transmission, modulation, perception
    b. Transmission, modulation, transduction, perception
    c. Perception, transmission, modulation, transduction
    d. Transduction, transmission, perception, modulation

14. Which of the following results in infertility and neonatal mortality in rabbits?
    a. Coprophagy
    b. Dysbiosis
    c. Dystrophic calcification
    d. Vitamin A deficiency

15. Which of the following is the most commonly seen cardiovascular disease in the dog?
    a. Boxer right ventricular cardiomyopathy
    b. Dilated cardiomyopathy
    c. Hypertrophic cardiomyopathy
    d. Ventricular septal defect

16. Which of the following endocrine diseases results in hyponatremia and hyperkalemia in a dog?
    a. Hyperadrenocorticism
    b. Hypoadrenocorticism
    c. Hyperthyroidism
    d. Hypothyroidism

17. Halitosis is an indication of a problem with which of the following body systems?
    a. Cardiovascular
    b. Digestive
    c. Nervous
    d. Hematologic

18. When performing a TPR on a patient, you should:
    a. Always auscult the heart while palpating the pulse
    b. Palpate the patient's pulse while taking its temperature
    c. Always auscult the heart because the pulse rate may be lower than the heart rate
    d. Auscult the heart if the patient does not like you to touch its legs

19. The pulse pressure or quality of the pulse:
    a. Is not of clinical significance as it is a subjective measurement
    b. Might be an indicator of possible heart or blood pressure issues
    c. Often feels very strong in older animals
    d. May feel weak if the patient is excited

20. Which of the following endocrine diseases results in weight loss and a ravenous appetite in cats?
    a. Hyperadrenocorticism
    b. Hypoadrenocorticism
    c. Hyperthyroidism
    d. Hypothyroidism

21. When restraining a cat for a blood draw from the medial saphenous vein, the patient is restrained in:
    a. Dorsal recumbency
    b. Lateral recumbency
    c. Medial recumbency
    d. Sternal recumbency

22. Weak, moderate, strong, bounding, or tall are terms often used to describe the patient's:
    a. Attitude
    b. Respiration quality
    c. Pulse quality
    d. Blood pressure

23. The transparent covering of the front of the eye is called the:
    a. Lens
    b. Iris
    c. Pupil
    d. Cornea

24. Which of the following endocrine diseases results in weight gain, bradycardia, exercise intolerance, and lethargy in a dog?
    a. Hyperadrenocorticism
    b. Hypoadrenocorticism
    c. Hyperthyroidism
    d. Hypothyroidism

25. A canine patient is being held in right lateral recumbency for venipuncture. Which of the following veins are most accessible?
    a. Left lateral saphenous
    b. Left medial saphenous
    c. Right jugular
    d. Right lateral saphenous

26. Hypoxemia is defined as:
    a. A decreased circulating blood volume
    b. Low blood oxygen levels
    c. Low tissue oxygen levels
    d. An increase in circulating fluid in the body

27. Which of the following is the most important first step when a dyspneic patient presents to the veterinary hospital?
    a. Obtain thoracic radiographs
    b. Obtain an arterial blood gas
    c. Stabilize the patient before performing any diagnostic testing
    d. Perform a complete physical examination

28. The normal temperature for an equine patient ranges from:
    a. 99° F–101.5° F
    b. 96.8° F–99° F
    c. 101.5° F–102.5° F
    d. 96.8° F–102.5° F

29. Which of the following is an appropriate method for restraining an animal that does not respond well to gentle words and handling?
    a. Force the patient down and proceed with the procedure without full control
    b. Recruit help from the owner for physical restraint
    c. Running the patient around until it is too tired to struggle
    d. Use chemical agents for restraint

30. The normal temperature for a canine patient ranges from:
    a. 99° F–101.5° F
    b. 96.8° F–99F° F
    c. 100.0° F–102.2° F
    d. 96.8° F–102.5° F

31. Which of the following individuals should not participate in the restraining of patients?
    a. Patient owners
    b. Veterinarians
    c. Veterinary technicians
    d. Veterinary assistants

32. The normal temperature for a feline patient ranges from:
    a. 99° F–101.5° F
    b. 96.8° F–99° F
    c. 100° F–102.2° F
    d. 96.8° F–102.5° F

33. Which of the following conditions is a common sign of heart failure?
    a. Tachypnea
    b. Bradypnea
    c. Tachycardia
    d. Bradycardia

34. The most common presenting sign in a patient with undiagnosed severe hypertension is:
    a. Anoxia
    b. Cardiomyopathy
    c. Blindness
    d. Hypothyroidism

35. Which of the following is a precaution that should be undertaken before restraining a cat?
    a. Maximal restraint should be used from the start to prevent any chance of the cat resisting
    b. Make sure all doors, windows, and cabinets are closed
    c. Prepare to use loud sounds as distraction
    d. Take the same restraining approach for every cat

36. The normal heart rate for a feline patient ranges from:
    a. 16–32 bpm
    b. 20–42 bpm
    c. 60–160 bpm
    d. 140–220 bpm

37. Which of the following is the passive expulsion of material from the mouth, pharynx, or esophagus?
    a. Regurgitation
    b. Vomiting
    c. Hematemesis
    d. Hypersalivation

38. During the first few days of life, the normal body temperature of a newborn puppy is:
    a. 94.5° F–97.3° F
    b. 94.7° F–100.1° F
    c. 97.0° F–99.0° F
    d. 99.0° F–101.5° F

39. A nervous dog should be taken out of its cage by:
    a. Throwing a slip lead onto the neck and pulling them out
    b. Luring the animal out with quiet, gentle urging, standing clear of the door
    c. Quickly adjusting your position, reacting to each movement the patient and making sure the dogs knows they cannot escape
    d. Reaching into the cage with your bare hands to restrain the animal

40. The normal heart rate for a canine patient ranges from:
    a. 16–32 bpm
    b. 20–42 bpm
    c. 60–160 bpm
    d. 140–220 bpm

41. An intravenously delivered solution that distributes evenly throughout the interstitial and intravascular space is considered:
    a. Isotonic
    b. Hypotonic
    c. Hypertonic
    d. 0.45% sodium chloride

42. When a female dog is bred, the amount of food (calories) she is fed should be increased:
    a. Immediately after breeding
    b. 1 week after breeding
    c. 2 or 3 weeks after breeding
    d. 5 or 6 weeks after breeding

43. A device used to help make the vein of the limb stand out is:
    a. Capture pole
    b. Elizabethan collar
    c. Muzzle
    d. Tourniquet

44. The normal pulse for an equine patient ranges from:
    a. 16–32 bpm
    b. 28–44 bpm
    c. 60–160 bpm
    d. 140–220 bpm

45. The gastrointestinal tracts of newborn puppies and kittens are uniquely suited to digest and absorb the milk produced by their mothers. The primary sources of energy in this milk is:
    a. Fat and lactose
    b. Fat and protein
    c. Lactose and protein
    d. Protein and starch

46. The loss of body water that has a solute concentration equal to that which remains in the compartment is called:
    a. Isotonic dehydration
    b. Hypovolemia
    c. Hypotonic dehydration
    d. Hypertonic dehydration

47. When two people are lifting a dog that weighs more than 50 lb, the person handling the front of the patient should:
    a. Hold the mouth closed with one hand and lift the patient by the head
    b. Lift the patient with one arm around the chest behind the front legs and the other arm over the back to interlock the fingers of the two hands
    c. Using one hand to restrain each of the thoracic limbs
    d. Wrap one arm around the dog's neck and the other under and around the dog's chest, behind the front leg

48. The normal respiratory rate for an equine patient ranges from:
    a. 6–16 bpm
    b. 28–44 bpm
    c. 60–160 bpm
    d. 140–220 bpm

49. A patient with an increased pack cell volume (PCV) and an elevated total solids (TS) is likely suffering from:
    a. Protein loss
    b. Dehydration
    c. Anemia
    d. Poor perfusion

50. Which of the following is the largest unit of measure?
    a. Microgram
    b. Milligram
    c. Gram
    d. Kilogram

51. Which of the following is the series of joint, segment, and whole-body movements used for locomotion?
    a. Gait
    b. Gallop
    c. Stance
    d. Stride

52. The normal respiratory rate for a feline patient ranges from:
    a. 6–16 bpm
    b. 16–32 bpm
    c. 20–42 bpm
    d. 42–55 bpm

53. Liquid preparations for oral administration may be purchased in several different forms. Which of the following is generally mixed with water and requires shaking well before administration?
    a. Elixir
    b. Emulsion
    c. Suspension
    d. Syrup

54. When preparing to draw up a drug into a syringe from a multidose vial, it is important to:
    a. Wipe the rubber diaphragm of the vial with 70% isopropyl alcohol before inserting the needle into the vial
    b. Wipe the rubber diaphragm of the vial with 70% isopropyl alcohol after inserting the needle into the vial
    c. Inspect the rubber diaphragm for foreign material
    d. Remove the rubber diaphragm

55. Which of the following is the correct progression of wound healing?
    a. Inflammatory phase, proliferative phase, maturation phase
    b. Inflammatory phase, proliferative phase, granulation phase, maturation phase
    c. Proliferative phase, inflammatory phase, maturation phase
    d. Proliferative phase, granulation phase, inflammatory phase, maturation phase

56. The normal respiratory rate for a canine patient ranges from:
    a. 6–16 bpm
    b. 16–32 bpm
    c. 20–42 bpm
    d. 42–55 bpm

57. Which of the following needle sizes has the largest inside diameter?
    a. 16 gauge
    b. 18 gauge
    c. 20 gauge
    d. 22 gauge

58. When filling a prescription or administering medication to a patient, the technician must be familiar with medical abbreviations. Which of the following abbreviations indicates a medication is to be applied to the right ear?
    a. AD
    b. AS
    c. AU
    d. OD

59. Which of the following is the act of manually providing movement of joints without muscle contraction in a repetitive manner?
    a. Active range of motion
    b. Passive range of motion
    c. Proprioception
    d. Stretching

60. The normal systolic blood pressure for a feline patient ranges from:
    a. 120–160 mm Hg
    b. 130–160 mm Hg
    c. 140–180 mm Hg
    d. 160–190 mm Hg

61. When filling a prescription or administering medication to a patient, the technician must be familiar with medical abbreviations. Which of the following abbreviations indicates a medication is to be given once per 24 hours?
    a. s.i.d.
    b. t.i.d.
    c. q.i.d.
    d. q.o.d.

62. When filling a prescription or administering medication to a patient, the technician must be familiar with medical abbreviations. Which of the following abbreviations indicates milliequivalent?
    a. mcg
    b. mEq
    c. mg
    d. mm

63. Which of the following is a nursing intervention to allow a neurologic patient to void urine?
    a. Atonic bladder
    b. Bladder expression
    c. Bladder palpation
    d. Distension urination

64. The normal systolic blood pressure for a canine patient ranges from:
    a. 120–160 mm Hg
    b. 130–160 mm Hg
    c. 140–180 mm Hg
    d. 160–190 mm Hg

65. Understanding common conversions from the metric system, used in veterinary medicine, to the common household systems of measurement can be helpful when instructing clients about dosage. Which of the following is equal to 30 mL?
    a. 1 Tbsp.
    b. 1 tsp.
    c. 1 oz.
    d. 1 cup

66. Which area of the brain is responsible for higher functions such as learning, memory, and interpretation of sensory input (e.g., vision and pain recognition)?
    a. Cerebrum
    b. Thalamus
    c. Hypothalamus
    d. Reticular formation

67. Which of the following statements is true of urinary catheterization?
    a. Disinfecting of the prepuce is not required
    b. The catheter must be disinfected periodically
    c. After the catheter is properly placed, there is no concern for dislodgment
    d. Aseptic technique is not required when handling the collection bag

68. At what age do the permanent canine and premolar teeth in dogs generally erupt?
    a. 3–5 months
    b. 4–6 months
    c. 5–7 months
    d. 6–8 months

69. The work of the respiratory system can be divided into the following four parts. The movement of gases across the alveolar membrane is called:
    a. Diffusion
    b. Distribution
    c. Perfusion
    d. Ventilation

70. Which of the following is a type of pain that can be beneficial in that it can allow the animal to avoid damaging stimuli?
    a. Neuropathic pain
    b. Physiologic pain
    c. Somatic pain
    d. Visceral pain

71. What is the name of the cycle of collecting subjective and objective data, identifying and prioritizing patient problems to be addressed, developing a nursing plan, implementing interventions, and assessing the treatment's effectiveness?
    a. Nursing process
    b. Physical exam
    c. Patient treatment
    d. Diagnosis

72. A bulldog would be described as having what type of head shape?
    a. Brachycephalic
    b. Dolichocephalic
    c. Mesaticephalic/mesocephalic
    d. Prognacephalic

73. Colloid solutions are used for expansion of the patient's plasma volume. Which of these fluid types is a colloid?
    a. Dextrose 5% in water
    b. Hetastarch
    c. Lactated Ringer solution
    d. Normosol R

74. Which of the following is an alkalizing agent that may be added to intravenous fluids to correct metabolic acidosis?
    a. Calcium chloride
    b. Calcium gluconate
    c. Potassium chloride
    d. Sodium bicarbonate

75. Which of the following is defined as an increase in serum creatinine and blood urea nitrogen level?
    a. Anemia
    b. Azotemia
    c. Hypoproteinemia
    d. Isosthenuria

76. The term that best describes a dog with an abnormally short mandible is:
    a. Prognathism
    b. Brachygnathism
    c. Mesaticephalic
    d. Dolichocephalic

77. When performing an electrocardiogram (ECG) with a dog in right lateral recumbency, the green electrode is attached to the:
    a. Right forelimb
    b. Left forelimb
    c. Right hind limb
    d. Left hind limb

78. A common clinical sign of saddle thrombus in the cat is:
    a. Acute onset of front leg pain and paresis
    b. Acute onset of rear leg pain and paresis
    c. Bright red footpads
    d. Bounding pulses in the rear limbs

79. Consumption of colostrum after being born is important to a neonate's health, because:
    a. The neonate immediately requires calories to start growing
    b. Colostrum strengthens the bond between mother and neonate
    c. Passive acquirement of immunoglobulins strengthens the immune system
    d. Colostrum has a palatable taste that encourages neonates to continue suckling

80. Stomatitis is defined as:
    a. Bad breath that is evident when dental work must be completed
    b. Inflammation of the mouth's soft tissue
    c. Resorption of hard dental tissues by odontoclasts
    d. Inflammation and infection of some or all of the tooth's supportive tissues

81. The stomach is located in the left cranial abdomen. When food is ingested, it mixes with gastric juices, and then it propels to which part of the small intestine?
    a. Cecum
    b. Duodenum
    c. Pylorus
    d. Serosa

82. Jaundice might develop as diseases progresses in which of the following organs?
    a. Heart
    b. Intestinal
    c. Kidney
    d. Liver

83. How soon should a kitten receive colostrum to obtain passive immunity?
    a. 8 hours
    b. 16 hours
    c. 24 hours
    d. 48 hours

84. Which of the following is least useful when resuscitating a dog in shock?
    a. D5W
    b. Hetastarch
    c. Hypertonic saline
    d. Plasma-Lyte 48

85. Which of the following is considered a zoonotic disease?
    a. Cholangiohepatitis
    b. Infectious canine hepatitis
    c. Leptospirosis
    d. Toxin-induced liver disease

86. Clients may not want to ask the veterinarian to repeat what he or she has said, especially if the client does not understand a lot of specialized terminology that the vet has used. The veterinary technician should:
    a. Repeat what the veterinarian said using the same terminology to be consistent
    b. Offer a dictionary of medical terms to the client so he or she can look up terms that are not understood
    c. Explain the veterinarian's words using laymen's terms
    d. Suggest the client use the Internet to obtain additional information

87. Which of the following are reasons for cautious drug dosing in neonates?
    a. Neonates have reduced liver function.
    b. The left and right ventricles are of approximately equal size.
    c. Appropriate immunoglobulin production is lacking.
    d. Neonates are susceptible to hypothermia.

88. The first drug of choice for a cat that experiences status epilepticus is:
    a. Diazepam
    b. Pentobarbital
    c. Potassium bromide
    d. Propofol

89. Which of these common radiology terms refers to a negatively charged electrode that produces electrons in the x-ray tube?
    a. Anode
    b. Artifact
    c. Cathode
    d. Collimator

90. Which of these abbreviations commonly used in radiology causes the electrons to move faster, increasing the force of the collision with the target?
    a. kVp
    b. mAs
    c. SID
    d. OID

91. Which of the following is a true feline blood type?
    a. AB
    b. DEA 1
    c. Q
    d. Tr

92. Which of the following is defined as the assessment of the patient through the tactile senses of one's hands and fingers?
    a. Auscultation
    b. Centrifugation
    c. Mentation
    d. Palpation

93. Tension pneumothorax occurs when pressure in the thoracic cavity is:
    a. Less than atmospheric pressure
    b. Equal to atmospheric pressure
    c. Greater than atmospheric pressure
    d. Constant as animal breathes in and out

94. Emesis should not be induced in patients that have ingested:
    a. Anticholinergics
    b. Hydrocarbons
    c. Organophosphates
    d. Salicylates

95. The mucous membranes of a dog in septic shock are:
    a. Cyanotic
    b. Hyperemic
    c. Icteric
    d. Pale

96. Diarrhea is a common clinical sign of a variety of diseases. Which of the following disease is zoonotic?
    a. Canine parvovirus
    b. Campylobacteriosis
    c. Feline infectious enteritis
    d. Inflammatory bowel disease

97. When administering oral liquid medications the patient's neck should be:
    a. Hyperextended
    b. Flexed in a downward angle
    c. Flexed in an upward angle
    d. Held at a neutral angle

98. The most desirable induction agent for an emergency cesarean section in a dog is:
    a. Etomidate
    b. Diazepam
    c. Propofol
    d. Thiopental

99. The underlying disease for most cases of feline aortic thromboembolism is _____ in origin.
    a. Cardiac
    b. Hepatic
    c. Renal
    d. Respiratory

100. Which of the following points are true in gathering patient data during the nursing process?
    a. Past medical history should be ignored because the presenting problem might not be related.
    b. Consulting the veterinarian is unnecessary for a veterinary technician to assess a patient.
    c. The physical exam should be focused on the area of concern for efficiency.
    d. Owner's presenting complaint and description of history should be taken.

101. To reduce intracranial pressure that results from trauma, _____ may be administered every 4 to 8 hours.
    a. Atropine
    b. Dexamethasone
    c. Diazepam
    d. Mannitol

102. Orogastric intubation is sometimes necessary for a variety of reasons. The length of the tube is measured from the nose to which of the following?
    a. Thoracic inlet
    b. 8th rib
    c. 13th rib
    d. Medial canthus

103. Certain medications applied topically to the skin have systemic and local effects. Many drugs commonly administered by the oral route, such as prednisone or methimazole, can be formulated into an ointment for this type of application. Other medications, such as nitroglycerin, are manufactured as a cream to be applied directly to the skin. Which of the following terms indicates this route of medication application?
    a. Diuretic
    b. Emetics
    c. Transdermal
    d. Viscu

104. Four patients present at the same time with emergency conditions. In which order should the patients be triaged?
    a. Dyspnea, dystocia, proptosis, laceration
    b. Proptosis, dyspnea, dystocia, laceration
    c. Laceration, dystocia, dyspnea, proptosis
    d. Dystocia, proptosis, laceration, dyspnea

105. Which of the following conditions will heal best through first intention?
    a. Abscess
    b. Degloving
    c. Simple laceration
    d. Puncture wound

106. A patient is experiencing cardiopulmonary arrest. The most desirable route of drug administration is:
    a. Intratracheal
    b. Intracardiac
    c. Intravenous
    d. Intraosseous

107. Which of the following routes of injectable drug administration is not recommended in dehydrated patients, especially in an emergency situation?
    a. Intramuscular
    b. Intraosseous
    c. Intravenous
    d. Subcutaneous

108. A patient that has been hit by a car and has no palpable pulse or detectable heartbeat requires chest compressions. These compressions should be performed at a rate of:
    a. 60–80 compressions per minute
    b. 80–100 compressions per minute
    c. 100–120 compressions per minute
    d. 120–140 compressions per minute

109. Serum centrifuged in a microhematocrit tube characterized as turbid and white in color is called:
    a. Hemolysis
    b. Hyperproteinemia
    c. Icterus
    d. Lipemia

110. In a patient, what does an elevated total protein measurement accompanied by elevated packed cell volume likely indicate?
    a. Anemia
    b. Dehydration
    c. Hemorrhage
    d. Red blood cell transfusion

111. Where should pressure be applied to minimize hemorrhage to the head of a canine trauma patient?
    a. At the thoracic inlet in both jugular grooves
    b. At the thoracic inlet of the left jugular groove
    c. To the area adjacent and ventral to the mandible
    d. To the lateral points of the temporomandibular joint

112. Which of the following is not included in the veterinary technician practice model?
    a. Technician assessment
    b. Technician evaluation
    c. Technician intervention
    d. Technician prescription

113. A calorie is a very small unit that is not of practical use in the science of animal nutrition. The commonly used unit of measure is the kilocalorie (kcal). One kcal is equal to how many calories?
    a. 10
    b. 100
    c. 1000
    d. 10,000

114. In emergency care cases in which it is not possible to administer large volumes of desired fluids, it may be beneficial to properly administer:
    a. D5W
    b. Hypertonic saline
    c. Hypotonic saline
    d. Isotonic saline

115. What does the presence of petechiae and ecchymoses indicate in a patient?
    a. Anemia
    b. Coagulation disorder
    c. Dehydration
    d. Hypertension

116. During emergency intubation, the cranial nerve _____ may be stimulated, resulting in _____.
    a. I; bradycardia
    b. IV; tachycardia
    c. X; bradycardia
    d. XII; tachycardia

117. Which of the following is an essential amino acid?
    a. Arginine
    b. Alanine
    c. Asparagine
    d. Aspartate

118. Which of the following is a nonessential amino acid?
    a. Histidine
    b. Isoleucine
    c. Methionine
    d. Tyrosine

119. A man phones the veterinary practice to say that he has just hit a dog with his car, and the animal is now lying on the side of the road. It appears to be breathing with minimal distress; however, there is blood coming from both nostrils and there is a small river of dark blood coming from a laceration on the lateral side of its hind leg. The dog can raise its head and is attempting to stand. In advising the man, your recommendation is to do all of the following except:
    a. Be aware for any signs of aggression
    b. Tie the mouth securely closed with your shoelace
    c. Transport the dog on a board lying on its side
    d. Apply direct pressure to the wound

120. What does the presence of peripheral edema indicate?
    a. Coagulation disorder
    b. Hypoproteinemia
    c. Hypotension
    d. Hypoxia

121. A normal central venous pressure (CVP) range is:
    a. 0–5 cm H_2O
    b. 5–10 cm H_2O
    c. 10–15 cm H_2O
    d. 15–20 cm H_2O

122. Which of the following is a water-soluble vitamin?
    a. Vitamin A
    b. Vitamin C
    c. Vitamin E
    d. Vitamin K

123. Rickets is caused by a deficiency of which vitamin?
    a. Vitamin A
    b. Vitamin D
    c. Vitamin E
    d. Vitamin K

124. When monitoring patients on fluids and/or patients that undergo diuresis, urine output is an important consideration. The normal urine production for a healthy dog or cat is approximately:
    a. 0–1 mL/kg/hr
    b. 1–2 mL/kg/hr
    c. 2–3 mL/kg/hr
    d. 3–4 mL/kg/hr

125. On auscultation of the ventral side of the abdomen, which of the following is a normal finding?
    a. Borborygmus
    b. Crackles
    c. No audible sound
    d. Stertor

126. Multiple parameters are measured to determine a category of shock that an animal may be experiencing. In which of the following types of shock is the central venous pressure high?
    a. Cardiogenic
    b. Distributive
    c. Hypovolemic
    d. Septic

127. Most vitamins cannot be synthesized by the body and must be supplied in food. Well-balanced pet foods are formulated to provide the necessary supplementation. What is the one vitamin that can be synthesized from glucose by dogs and cats?
    a. Vitamin A
    b. Vitamin B_6
    c. Vitamin C
    d. Vitamin K

128. Which of the following vitamins is a form of vitamin D?
    a. Cobalamin
    b. Ergocalciferol
    c. Pyridoxine
    d. Thiamin

129. Hypoglycemia is most common in patients that experience:
    a. Anaphylactic shock
    b. Cardiogenic shock
    c. Neurogenic shock
    d. Septic shock

130. For what purpose is an esophageal stethoscope most useful?
    a. Assessing megaesophagus
    b. Detecting ileus
    c. Monitoring anesthetized patients
    d. Routine physical exam

131. Blood levels of total bilirubin are used primarily to evaluate function of the:
    a. Kidneys
    b. Liver
    c. Pancreas
    d. Bile ducts

132. Deficiencies in iron may result in anemia. Which of these minerals may also cause anemia if it is deficient in a dog's or a cat's diet?
    a. Calcium
    b. Phosphorus
    c. Copper
    d. Zinc

133. Macrominerals are minerals that occur in appreciable amounts in the body and account for most of the body's mineral content. Microminerals, often referred to as trace minerals, include a larger number of minerals that are present in the body in very small amounts. Which of these minerals is a trace mineral?
    a. Phosphorus
    b. Magnesium
    c. Sulfur
    d. Zinc

134. A hospital-acquired disease is known as:
    a. Endemic
    b. Nosocomial
    c. Ergasteric
    d. Iatrogenic

135. Taste receptor cells are located at the tip of each taste bud. Taste receptors in dogs and cats are similar, however there are also interesting differences. For which of the following do dogs show a preference that cats do not?
    a. Sweet
    b. Sour
    c. Salty
    d. Bitter

136. A decrease in albumin may occur in cases experiencing:
    a. Chronic liver disease
    b. Carnivorous diet
    c. Gastroenteritis
    d. Vegetarian diet

137. Which of the following describes a canine patient experiencing a fever?
    a. 97.8° F when presenting with pyometra
    b. 100.2° F after being left in a warm car for 30 minutes
    c. 103.9° F when presenting with septic peritonitis
    d. 105.7° F after exercising in heat

138. When palpating pulses, what do bounding pulses indicate?
    a. Adequate cardiovascular function
    b. Elevated diastolic blood pressure
    c. Elevated pulse pressure
    d. Elevated mean arterial pressure

139. With significant dehydration in an otherwise healthy patient, which of the following would likely be seen on a urinalysis and CBC?
    a. Increased urine UG and increased PCV
    b. Increased urine SG and decreased PCV
    c. Decreased urine SG and decreased PCV
    d. Decreased urine SG and increased PCV

140. The majority of water and certain electrolytes, especially sodium, are absorbed in the:
    a. Esophagus
    b. Stomach
    c. Small intestine
    d. Large intestine

141. The domestic cat has a high dietary protein requirement. A diet containing animal tissue is required to meet this need. In addition, this species requires all of the following except:
    a. Ascorbic acid
    b. Arachidonic acid
    c. Preformed vitamin A
    d. Taurine

142. Ketonuria is most commonly associated with what condition?
    a. Liver disease
    b. Urinary tract infection
    c. Renal failure
    d. Diabetes mellitus

143. Which blood pressure measuring device obtains automated readings through sensing pressure oscillations on a cuff?
    a. Doppler ultrasound
    b. Direct blood pressure
    c. Oscillometric device
    d. Stethoscope

144. What does redness, swelling, and purulent discharges from an IV catheter site indicate?
    a. Catheter site infection
    b. Catheter leakage
    c. Catheter occlusion
    d. Normal insertion site

145. Total protein levels are _____ in a dehydrated animal.
    a. Unaffected
    b. Decreased
    c. Increased
    d. Variable

146. Which is *least* likely to be a clinical sign of a patient experiencing allergies?
    a. Face rubbing
    b. Ear problems
    c. Loss of appetite
    d. Skin rashes

147. Current recommendations for feeding critically ill patients are to begin feeding equal to the patient's estimated:
    a. Resting energy requirement (RER)
    b. Resting energy requirement (RER) × 2
    c. Resting energy requirement (RER) × 4
    d. Daily energy requirement (DER) × 4

148. The presence of protein in the urine may indicate:
    a. Acid-base imbalance
    b. Hemolytic anemia
    c. Kidney disease
    d. Diabetes mellitus

149. Arterial blood is most commonly used to analyze:
    a. Hematology
    b. Blood gases
    c. Blood chemistry
    d. Organ function tests

150. Various factors influence a pet's total daily energy expenditure. Which of the following is affected by gender, reproductive status, and age?
    a. Basal metabolic rate
    b. Voluntary muscular activity
    c. Meal-induced thermogenesis
    d. Adaptive thermogenesis

151. Which of the following agencies has no regulatory authority regarding pet food, however is made up of government employees?
    a. AAFCO—Association of American Feed Control Officials
    b. FDA—Food and Drug Administration
    c. FTC—Federal Trade Commission
    d. USDA—United States Department of Agriculture

152. Which clotting disorder is stimulated by hypothyroidism?
    a. Hemophilia A
    b. Von Willebrand disease
    c. Disseminated intravascular coagulation
    d. Coumarin toxicity

153. What is the most appropriate action when a catheter infection is detected?
    a. Disinfect the catheter site and continue use
    b. Measure patient temperature and remove only if there is a fever
    c. Remove the catheter
    d. There is no need for intervention

154. What is the most appropriate action when a catheter is determined to be leaking subcutaneously?
    a. Leave as is, and check the site 3 to 4 hours later
    b. Reduce the fluid rate and continue use
    c. Remove the catheter
    d. There is no need for intervention

155. Hyperkalemia is commonly associated with which endocrine disorder?
    a. Diabetes insipidus
    b. Hyperthyroidism
    c. Hyperparathyroidism
    d. Hypoadrenocorticism

156. The forceful expulsion of stomach contents that requires abdominal contractions is:
    a. Cachexia
    b. Cathartics
    c. Regurgitation
    d. Vomiting

157. If the patient is vomiting fresh or digested blood, this is termed:
    a. Hematemesis
    b. Hematochezia
    c. Hematuria
    d. Hemoabdomen

158. In what endocrine disorder is polyuria and polydipsia not commonly seen?
    a. Hyperadrenocorticism
    b. Diabetes insipidus
    c. Hyperparathyroidism
    d. Diabetes mellitus

159. How do transfusion reactions in the cat differ from transfusion reactions in the dog?
    a. Transfusions are more acute in the cat
    b. Transfusions are more acute in the dog
    c. Cats suffer from severe pruritus
    d. Transfusions are more severe in the dog

160. Which of the following is the least effective method for delivering fluids to a 12% dehydrated patient?
    a. Central intravenous
    b. Intraosseous
    c. Peripheral intravenous
    d. Subcutaneous

161. How does marked dehydration affect an animal's eye?
    a. Lateral nystagmus
    b. Pinpoint pupils
    c. Rotated ventrally
    d. Sunken in the socket

162. An allergic response that is frequently life threatening is the result of:
    a. Agglutination
    b. Hemolysis
    c. DIC
    d. Anaphylaxis

163. The letters "DEA" precede canine blood types. What do these letters stand for?
    a. Detectable erythrocyte antibody
    b. Detectable erythrocyte antigen
    c. Dog erythrocyte antibody
    d. Dog erythrocyte antigen

164. Which of the following describes a patient suffering from dystocia?
    a. Hard, painful nipple, and galactostasis
    b. Hypocalcemia, muscle spasms, fever, tachycardia, and seizures
    c. In hard labor for 30 to 60 minutes with no new young produced
    d. Vaginal discharge, vomiting, diarrhea, dehydration, anorexia, polyuria, and polydipsia

165. Which of the following is a technique to keep from joints becoming stiff?
    a. Cold compress
    b. Coupage
    c. Passive range of motion
    d. Warm compress

166. Coagulation tests are useful for diagnosing:
    a. Rodenticide poisoning
    b. Thyroid function
    c. Adrenal function
    d. Ethylene glycol poisoning

167. When a medical history of a patient with diarrhea is obtained, it is important to question the owner regarding the duration, severity, frequency, amount, and quality. This information can assist in localizing diarrhea as involving the small or large bowel. Which of these is a common indication of small bowel diarrhea?
    a. Decreased volume of feces
    b. Mucus in feces
    c. Normal frequency of bowel movements
    d. Tenesmus

168. Painful straining at urination or defecation is:
    a. Hematochezia
    b. Hematuria
    c. Melena
    d. Tenesmus

169. What is the underlying cause of icterus?
    a. Anemia
    b. Hyperbilirubinemia
    c. Ketonuria
    d. Hyperhemoglobinemia

170. Fresh frozen plasma can be stored up to _____ and still contain clotting factors.
    a. 1 month
    b. 12 months
    c. 36 months
    d. 60 months

171. Pancreatitis occurs in both dogs and cats. Which of the following statements is false?
    a. Acute pancreatitis is seen more commonly in dogs
    b. Chronic pancreatitis is more common in cats
    c. Chronic pancreatitis is often caused by dietary indiscretion
    d. Acute pancreatitis is often caused by dietary indiscretion

172. Treatment of acute pancreatitis includes administration of intravenous fluid therapy, analgesics, antiemetics, mucosal protectants, and antibiotics to prevent secondary sepsis. Treatment also includes which of the following?
    a. Feeding a low-protein, high-fat diet
    b. Feeding a bland, low-fat diet
    c. Feeding a low-carbohydrate, high-fat diet
    d. Feeding a diet high in fat and calories

173. Frozen fresh plasma (FFP) must be separated and frozen within _____ hours to maintain all coagulation factors in normal concentrations.
    a. 2
    b. 8
    c. 12
    d. 6

174. Which of the following choices characterizes the skin turgor in a dehydrated dog or cat?
    a. Prolonged
    b. Normal
    c. Shortened
    d. Skin turgor is not a reliable indicator of hydration status

175. What type of anemia is associated with icterus?
    a. Responsive
    b. Nonresponsive
    c. Hemolytic
    d. Megaloblastic

176. With the exception of cats, most animals have a total blood volume equivalent to ____ of their body weight.
    a. 7%
    b. 15%
    c. 25%
    d. 40%

177. Which of the following choices characterizes the pulse rate and quality in a moderately dehydrated dog?
    a. Pulse rate increased
    b. Pulse rate decreased
    c. Pulse rate inconsistent
    d. Pulses not palpable

178. Which of the following choices characterizes the mucous membrane color and capillary refill time in a patient in hypovolemic shock?
    a. Pale, prolonged
    b. Pink, normal
    c. Red, rapid
    d. Yellow, normal

179. Myasthenia gravis is commonly associated with:
    a. Megaesophagus
    b. Exercise intolerance
    c. Aspiration pneumonia
    d. All of the above

180. Goals for the medical management of chronic kidney disease include all of the following *except:*
    a. Slowing progression of the disease
    b. Treating concurrent disease
    c. Correcting electrolyte imbalances
    d. Restoring loss of kidney function

181. Which of the following is a postpartum complication caused by hypocalcemia?
    a. Eclampsia
    b. Galactostasis
    c. Mastitis
    d. Metritis

182. Vaccines may be given by any of the following routes, *except:*
    a. Subcutaneously
    b. Intramuscularly
    c. Intranasally
    d. Intraperitoneal

183. Pemphigus is a group of autoimmune disorders that affects the:
    a. Blood and lymph systems
    b. Skin and oral mucosa
    c. Eyes
    d. Hooves and claws

184. Signs of immune-mediated thrombocytopenia (ITP) include all of the following conditions, *except:*
    a. Petechiae
    b. Ecchymoses
    c. Thrombocytosis
    d. Anemia

185. When the medical history of a patient with diarrhea is obtained, it is important to question the owner regarding the duration, severity, frequency, amount, and quality. This information can assist in localizing diarrhea as involving the small or large bowel. Which of these is a common indication of large bowel diarrhea?
    a. Increased volume of feces
    b. Mucus in feces
    c. Normal frequency of bowel movements
    d. Weight loss

186. Nasoesophageal (NE) feeding tubes may be used to provide short-term enteral nutrition to dogs and cats. Which of the following statements regarding NE feeding tubes is false?
    a. Can be used for the continuous delivery of liquid food and/or water
    b. Can be used for boluses of liquid food and/or water
    c. Can often be placed without sedation
    d. Can be used in unconscious patients

187. Which of the following is defined as the assessment of the patient through listening to sounds through a stethoscope?
    a. Auscultation
    b. Centrifugation
    c. Mentation
    d. Palpation

188. When setting up an IV fluid line to be used without an infusion pump, the drip chamber should be:
    a. Filled completely to the top
    b. Filled to the halfway line on the chamber
    c. Left empty
    d. Allowed to fill by gravity

189. Many hospitalized veterinary patients receive fluid therapy. The veterinary technician is responsible for many aspects of fluid therapy. Which of the following is the responsibility of the veterinarian and not the technician?
    a. Calculating fluid rate
    b. Ordering the fluid type
    c. Initiating fluid therapy
    d. Monitoring the infusion

190. Cats exposed to feline leukemia virus typically respond in any of the following ways, *except:*
    a. Not becoming infected at all
    b. Becoming temporarily infected, developing immunity, and overcoming the infection
    c. Becoming infected and continuing to shed the virus indefinitely without becoming ill
    d. Becoming infected, becoming ill within 3 days, and dying within a week

191. Which of the following types of fluids is used primarily to replace intravascular volume?
    a. Hypertonic crystalloid
    b. Isotonic crystalloid
    c. Synthetic colloid
    d. Whole blood

192. What is the predominant method for transmission of feline immunodeficiency virus in cats?
    a. Grooming
    b. Bite wounds
    c. Urine
    a. Feces

193. Pinkeye or contagious conjunctivitis in cattle is caused by:
    a. *Haemophilus aegypti*
    b. *Moraxella bovis*
    c. *Streptococcus pyogenes*
    d. *Staphylococcus aureus*

194. How many drops per minute is equivalent to 20 mL/hr using a 60 drops/mL drip set?
    a. 10
    b. 20
    c. 60
    d. 120

195. Which of the following allows for oxygen supplementation with minimal stress and handling of the patient?
    a. Mask oxygen
    b. Nasal cannula
    c. Oxygen cage
    d. Transtracheal catheter

196. Inflammation, infection, sepsis, neoplasia, and reaction to transfusion of blood products are common causes of:
    a. Hyperthermia
    b. Hypothermia
    c. Pyrexia
    d. Pyridoxine

197. Which of the following is a common cause of bradycardia?
    a. Hypovolemia
    b. Hypoxia
    c. Hypokalemia
    d. Hyperkalemia

198. Polyuria is:
    a. A lack of urine production
    b. The production of excessive amounts of urine
    c. A lack of water intake
    d. Excessive protein in the urine

199. A urolith is a pathologic stone formed from mineral salts found in the urinary tract. Which of the following is not a factor in the formation of uroliths?
    a. Urine pH
    b. Urine concentration
    c. Urine saturation
    d. Urine protein

200. Lower urinary tract infections (UTIs) can be caused by a variety of bacteria; the most common pathogen in small animals is *Escherichia coli*. Which of the following statements is true?
    a. Bacterial infections of the bladder are common in the dog and are rare in the healthy cat
    b. Bacterial infections of the bladder are common in the cat and are rare in the healthy dog
    c. Male dogs are more prone to infection than female dogs
    d. Treatment for bacterial infections consists of appropriate antimicrobial therapy for 2 to 4 days

201. Oliguria is:
    a. Excessive eating
    b. Green urine
    c. Excessive bilirubin in the urine
    d. Decreased urine output

202. Urinary tract infection is a common secondary complication in cats and dogs with:
    a. Congestive heart failure
    b. Diabetes mellitus
    c. Hepatic lipidosis
    d. Hyperthyroidism

203. Common signs of bacterial infections of the urinary tract include hematuria, pollakiuria, urinating in inappropriate places, and which of the following?
    a. Azotemia
    b. Dehydration
    c. Dysuria
    d. Elevated BUN

204. Anuria is:
    a. Decreased urine output
    b. Decreased drinking
    c. Complete lack of urine production
    d. Excessive drinking

205. Painful urination is recorded as:
    a. Dysuria
    b. Hematuria
    c. Pyuria
    d. Proteinuria

206. Which of the following is *false* regarding nonpharmacologic interventions to provide pain relief?
a. Stress from boredom, thirst, anxiety, and the need to urinate and defecate can mimic pain.
b. The need for physical comfort of the patient is alleviated when adequate pain medication is administered.
c. The patient may need to be placed in a position to reduce pain, to allow for easier breathing, and to promote sleep.
d. Each patient has unique emotional needs.

207. How might anesthesia affect an animal's eye?
a. Lateral nystagmus
b. Pinpoint pupils
c. Rotated ventrally
d. Sunken in the socket

208. Hemolytic anemia is characterized by the destruction of:
a. Erythrocytes
b. Leukocytes
c. Lymphocytes
d. Monocytes

209. Which of the following laboratory tests would not be used to diagnose immune-mediated hemolytic anemia (IMHA)?
a. Autoagglutination test
b. CBC
c. Coombs test
d. Fructosamine

210. The veterinary technician can play an important role in pain management by:
a. Monitoring urine and fecal output
b. Changing the medication when it is ineffective
c. Communicating directly with the clinician about particular concerns
d. Directing the veterinary assistant to provide medications

211. Which of the following signs would a regurgitating patient show?
a. Forceful contraction of the abdomen and diaphragm
b. Restlessness
c. Salivation
d. Undigested food in the expelled substance

212. What does the presence of green fluid in the vomitus indicate?
a. Gastric or esophageal disorder
b. Gastrointestinal ulceration
c. Involvement of bile in the duodenum
d. Pyloric outflow obstruction

213. Which of the following characteristics do cats exhibit when they experience pain?
a. Sleeping continuously, overeating, and attention-seeking behaviors
b. Resentment of being handled, aggression, and abnormal posture
c. Hyperactivity, pupillary enlargement, and tail swishing
d. Hypotension, hypocapnia, hypopnea, bradycardia

214. During hospitalization, how often should pain assessment be performed?
a. Every 4–6 hours
b. Every 30 minutes to 1 hour
c. Every 12–24 hours
d. Every 8 hours

215. Which of the following drugs is a commonly used antiemetic?
a. Apomorphine
b. Chlorpromazine
c. Hydrogen peroxide
d. Xylazine

216. Patients with myasthenia gravis may also suffer from megaesophagus and regurgitation. These patients are at increased risk for:
a. Acephalus
b. Aspiration
c. Asteatosis
d. Astrocytoma

217. Which of the following choices characterizes the mucous membrane color and capillary refill time in a patient with liver disease?
a. Pale, prolonged
b. Pink, normal
c. Red, rapid
d. Yellow, normal

218. What do black "coffee grounds" in the vomitus indicate?
a. Gastric or esophageal disorder
b. Gastrointestinal ulceration
c. Involvement of bile in the duodenum
d. Pyloric outflow obstruction

219. When a veterinary technician is trying to distinguish pain from dysphoria, which of the following would the technician do?
a. Place the patient on comfortable blankets
b. Speak in low tones and interact with the animal, which makes the patient feel better, but behaviors resume when the interactions stop
c. Move the animal to a different ward
d. Reverse the analgesic medication

220. Which of the following is a zoonotic disease that is spread by fleas?
    a. *Borrelia burgdorferi*
    b. *Rickettsia rickettsii*
    c. *Ehrlichia*
    d. *Yersinia pestis*

221. Which of the following types of cancer commonly arises from cartilage or bone?
    a. Adenocarcinoma
    b. Sarcoma
    c. Lymphoma
    d. Carcinoma

222. Massage is an example of which type of rehabilitation technique?
    a. Manual therapy
    b. Effleurage techniques
    c. Physical modalities
    d. Therapeutic exercise

223. What does high-frequency diarrhea with straining and mucus indicate?
    a. Involvement of the stomach
    b. Involvement of the jejunum or ileum
    c. Involvement of the large intestine
    d. Colitis

224. Which of the following describes a patient suffering from pyometra?
    a. Hard, painful nipple, and galactostasis
    b. Hypocalcemia, muscle spasms, fever, tachycardia, and seizures
    c. In hard labor for 30 to 60 minutes with no new young produced
    d. Vaginal discharge, vomiting, diarrhea, dehydration, anorexia, polyuria, and polydipsia

225. Visceral pain is common among companion animals. Which of the following is *not* an example of visceral pain?
    a. Pancreatitis
    b. Gastroenteritis
    c. Bowel ischemia
    d. Osteosarcoma

226. Which of the following might a dysphoric or delirious animal experience because of opioid overdose?
    a. Thrashing and yowling continuously
    b. Claustrophobia
    c. Only rare response to soothing interaction
    d. Chewing on cage doors

227. Technicians administering IV chemotherapy drugs via an IV catheter must be vigilant. If you suspect some of the drug may have leaked out of the vessel into the surrounding tissue, you should:
    a. Immediately remove the IV catheter
    b. Leave the IV catheter in place
    c. Continue to administer the drug
    d. No action is required

228. A blood sampling from neonatal puppies and kittens is generally most easily obtained using the:
    a. Cephalic vein
    b. Jugular vein
    c. Lateral saphenous vein
    d. Medial saphenous vein

229. Which of the following is the shortest portion of the small intestine?
    a. Cecum
    b. Duodenum
    c. Ileum
    d. Jejunum

230. Which of the following behaviors is commonly associated with clinical signs of pain in dogs?
    a. Vocalization and increased appetite
    b. Playful actions and excessive licking of the owners
    c. Panting, anorexia, and depression
    d. Increased attention to the environment

231. Which device for measuring blood pressure is used to obtain manual blood pressure measurements, turning blood flow into an audible signal?
    a. Doppler ultrasound
    b. Direct blood pressure
    c. Oscillometric device
    d. Stethoscope

232. What does frank blood in the diarrhea indicate?
    a. Involvement of the stomach
    b. Involvement of the jejunum or ileum
    c. Involvement of the large intestine
    d. Colitis

233. The large intestine begins at the:
    a. Ascending colon
    b. Ileocecocolic valve
    c. Cecum
    d. Transverse colon

234. The energy required for a normal animal in a fasting state in a thermoneutral environment, awake but resting, is the:
    a. Basal energy requirement
    b. Resting energy requirement
    c. Maintenance energy requirement
    d. Daily energy requirement

235. It is sometimes difficult to distinguish normal from pain-associated behaviors in cats and dogs. Which of the following behaviors are most likely to be normal, nonpainful behaviors?
    a. Decreased appetite
    b. Unusual aggression
    c. Stretching all four legs when the abdomen is touched
    d. Decreased social interaction

236. Which of the following is most beneficial in preventing gastrointestinal ulceration?
    a. Antibiotic administration
    b. Enteral feeding
    c. Famotidine
    d. Withholding food (NPO)

237. Which of the following is true of artificial warming devices?
    a. Warm water blankets are the most effective in preventing hypothermia
    b. Commercial warming devices do not require insulation because they are tested to be safe
    c. Can solely provide sufficient heat support to prevent hypothermia
    d. Should be directed at warming the core as opposed to the periphery

238. Treatment for joint mobility includes:
    a. ROM
    b. Stretching exercises
    c. a and b
    d. None of the above

239. The U.S. Food and Drug Administration regulates pet food labels, and labels are required to contain the name of the product. Using chicken as an example, a label that includes "Chicken Dinner" in the product name must contain:
    a. At least 70% chicken
    b. At least 10% chicken
    c. At least 3% chicken
    d. Less than 3% chicken

240. The principal display panel (PDP) is required to contain all of the following *except:*
    a. Manufacturer's name
    b. Brand name
    c. Net weight
    d. Nutritional claim

241. The most common types of pain experienced by horses are:
    a. Ocular and head pain
    b. Spine and pelvic pain
    c. Orthopedic and abdominal/colic pain
    d. Foot and dental pain

242. Which of the following is optional (not required) on the information panel of all pet foods?
    a. Feeding guidelines
    b. Freshness date
    c. Manufacturer or distributor
    d. Nutritional adequacy statement

243. The guaranteed analysis panel on a cat food label is required to include all of the following *except:*
    a. Minimum percentage of crude protein
    b. Minimum percentage of crude fat
    c. Maximum percentage of moisture
    d. Minimum percentage of taurine

244. Which of the following are effects of hypothermia?
    a. Increased metabolic rate
    b. Decreased clotting time
    c. Cardiac dysfunction
    d. Increased peripheral blood flow

245. Which of the following clinical signs might a cow in pain exhibit?
    a. Dullness and depression
    b. Inappetence and grinding teeth
    c. A stance with one foot behind the other
    d. All of the above

246. What is the definition of obesity?
    a. 10% heavier than the optimal weight for the breed in question
    b. 20% heavier than the optimal weight for the breed in question
    c. An increase in fat tissue mass sufficient to contribute to disease
    d. None of the above

247. Which of the following drugs is a commonly used emetic?
    a. Acepromazine
    b. Apomorphine
    c. Chlorpromazine
    d. Prochlorperazine

248. Which of these drugs is a laxative used most commonly in small animals with chronic constipation?
    a. Diphenoxylate
    b. Lactulose
    c. Loperamide
    d. Paregoric

249. A traumatic cause of OA in dogs indicates obesity as a risk factor. What is the most common traumatic cause of OA in dogs?
    a. Ruptured cruciate ligaments
    b. Torn Achilles group
    c. Hip dysplasia
    d. Phalangeal fracture

250. Which of the following is detrimental to a patient with limited mobility?
    a. Passive range of motion exercises
    b. Sling walking
    c. Adjusting position as little as possible to prevent pain
    d. Neck and head being slightly elevated

251. What is "porphyrin staining" in rodents?
    a. Hair standing on end
    b. Color of cage litter from urine
    c. Red tears which may encircle the eye
    d. None of the above

252. How is pain typically characterized in rabbits?
    a. Reduction in food and water intake
    b. Bruxism
    c. Closed eyes
    d. Lateral recumbency

253. Which of these is an antiulcer drug used to treat ulcers of the stomach and upper small intestine?
    a. Cimetidine
    b. Famotidine
    c. Ranitidine
    d. Sucralfate

254. When attaching an ECG, which leg should have the red lead attached to it?
    a. Right foreleg
    b. Left foreleg
    c. Right hind leg
    d. Left hind leg

255. Which of the following is a sign of insulin overdose in treated diabetic patients?
    a. Muscle wasting
    b. Polyuria
    c. Severe lethargy and seizures
    d. Vomiting and halitosis

256. Which statement regarding first-intention wound healing is false?
    a. It occurs without infection
    b. It occurs when the skin edges are held together in apposition
    c. It usually has some degree of suppuration
    d. It occurs with minimal scar formation

257. Which of the following agencies is responsible for approving new pet food ingredients?
    a. AAFCO—Association of American Feed Control Officials
    b. FDA—Food and Drug Administration
    c. FTC—Federal Trade Commission
    d. USDA—United States Department of Agriculture

258. Which of the following is a common cause of tachycardia:
    a. Hypoxia
    b. Hyperkalemia
    c. Hypocalcemia
    d. Toxin ingestion

259. If an animal goes home with a bandage, the client should observe the bandage daily and remove it if any of the following are observed, *except:*
    a. If skin irritation appears at the edge of the bandage
    b. All bandages should be removed 24 hours after application
    c. If the bandage is wet
    d. If the position of the bandage has shifted

260. Which of the following describes a patient suffering from eclampsia?
    a. Hard, painful nipple, and galactostasis
    b. Hypocalcemia, muscle spasms, fever, tachycardia, and seizures
    c. In hard labor for 30 to 60 minutes with no new young produced
    d. Vaginal discharge, vomiting, diarrhea, dehydration, anorexia, polyuria, and polydipsia

261. When feeding the patient through a gastrostomy tube, the technician should:
    a. Rapidly inject the fluids and food
    b. Flush the tube with water
    c. Flush the tube with air
    d. Feed a full days' caloric requirement immediately after placement

262. Which of these drugs is an antacid used to reduce acidity of the stomach?
    a. Amphojel
    b. Misoprostol
    c. Omeprazole
    d. Sucralfate

263. A semipermanent feeding tube may be placed in all of the following ways, *except:*
    a. Through the nose
    b. Through a pharyngostomy site
    c. Through a gastrostomy site
    d. Through the mouth

264. Which of the following are small bones that support part of the lateral walls of the throat?
    a. Palatine bones
    b. Pterygoid bones
    c. Turbinates
    d. Vomer bone

265. It is important that the nursing care provided to paralyzed patients focuses on patient comfort. The prevention of decubital ulcers can be accomplished by all of the following procedures, *except:*
    a. Frequent turning or repositioning the patient
    b. Adequate padding in the cage or bed
    c. Appropriate analgesic therapy
    d. Massage

266. Which of the following is a technique used to increase blood flow to improve drainage and healing to an area?
    a. Cold compress
    b. Coupage
    c. Passive range of motion
    d. Warm compress

267. A proptosed globe:
    a. Can be caused by overzealous restraint of the animal
    b. Is not considered an emergency
    c. Can most easily occur in dolichocephalic breeds, such as collies
    d. Is commonly a consequence of conjunctivitis

268. The metabolic alterations that occur after nutritional support is started in a severely malnourished, underweight, and/or starved patient is known as:
    a. Refeeding syndrome
    b. Starvation
    c. Simple starvation
    d. None of the above

269. Proper splint and bandage care includes all of the following, *except:*
    a. Washing the splint or bandage daily
    b. Preventing the bandage or splint from becoming wet
    c. Inspecting the bandage or splint daily for any change, such as swelling above or below the splint or bandage
    d. Inspecting the bandage or splint for any shifting or change in position on the limb

270. Serum centrifuged in a microhematocrit tube characterized as transparent and yellow or orange in color is called:
    a. Hemolysis
    b. Hyperproteinemia
    c. Icterus
    d. Lipemia

271. A chest tube is placed when an animal has:
    a. Subcutaneous emphysema
    b. Pulmonary edema
    c. Ascites
    d. Pneumothorax

272. Refeeding syndrome occurs in disease conditions such as:
    a. Starvation from feline hepatic lipidosis
    b. Overall malnutrition
    c. Prolonged diuresis
    d. All of the above

273. Which of the following are the bones in the tail of a dog?
    a. The cervical vertebrae
    b. The coccygeal vertebrae
    c. The lumbar vertebrae
    d. The sacral vertebrae

274. Which of the following agents has been associated with causing neurologic disorders in cats?
    a. Chlorhexidine
    b. Povidone iodine
    c. Quaternary ammonium compounds
    d. Hexachlorophene

275. Which blood pressure measuring technique requires an arterial catheter?
    a. Doppler ultrasound
    b. Direct blood pressure
    c. Oscillometric device
    d. Stethoscope

276. Anterior drawer movement detects a problem with the:
    a. Elbow
    b. Stifle
    c. Hip
    d. Hock

277. Nutrients given in excess of the patient's needs _____ in a critically ill patient, as they would in a healthy patient.
    a. Will be used
    b. Will not be used
    c. Occasionally will be used
    d. Will be stored as fat for later use

278. What does the presence of subcutaneous fluid around an IV catheter site indicate?
    a. Catheter site infection
    b. Catheter leakage
    c. Catheter occlusion
    d. Normal insertion site

279. Clear fluid removed from thoracic cavity is known as:
    a. Pleural effusion
    b. Pulmonary edema
    c. Ascites
    d. Pyothorax

280. Which of the following choices characterizes skin turgor in an overhydrated dog or cat?
    a. Prolonged
    b. Normal
    c. Shortened
    d. Skin turgor is not a reliable indicator of hydration status

281. Abscesses are generally allowed to heal open to provide continuous drainage. This type of wound healing is considered:
    a. Primary intention
    b. Second intention
    c. Third intention
    d. Fourth intention

282. Chronic mitral valvular disease (endocardiosis) affects more than one third of patients older than:
    a. 2 years
    b. 5 years
    c. 8 years
    d. 10 years

283. The prevalence of dilated (congestive) cardiomyopathy in cats has decreased markedly since 1987, following the discovery that _____ deficiency was the principal cause.
    a. Glutamine
    b. Taurine
    c. Arginine
    d. Copper

284. What is the most appropriate wound-flushing solution?
    a. Hydrogen peroxide
    b. Isotonic saline
    c. Povidone-iodine solution
    d. Tap water

285. How might a neurologic issue affect an animal's eye?
    a. Lateral nystagmus
    b. Pinpoint pupils
    c. Rotated ventrally
    d. Sunken in the socket

286. Which of the following choices characterizes the mucous membrane color and capillary refill time in a patient with systemic inflammation?
    a. Pale, prolonged
    b. Pink, normal
    c. Red, rapid
    d. Yellow, normal

287. Most of the clinical signs seen in an animal in shock from excessive blood loss are attributable to:
    a. Acidosis
    b. Alkalosis
    c. Cell death
    d. Redistribution of blood flow

288. Within a few _____ of ingesting high levels of sodium, normal dogs and cats easily excrete the excess in their urine.
    a. Hours
    b. Days
    c. Months
    d. Weeks

289. Abnormalities in potassium or magnesium homeostasis may cause all of the following *except*:
    a. Cardiac dysrhythmias
    b. An increase in myocardial contractility
    c. Profound muscle weakness
    d. A potentiation of the effects of drugs

290. Which fatty acids have been shown to have a significant effect on survival times when used in dogs diagnosed with dilated cardiomyopathy (DCM) or chronic valvular disease (CVD)?
    a. Omega-3
    b. Omega-6
    c. Omega-9
    d. None of the above

291. All of the following are clinical signs a horse may show when experiencing respiratory disease, *except*:
    a. Stertor
    b. Bilateral nasal discharge
    c. Bradycardia
    d. Cough

292. Which of the following are abnormal lung sounds heard in an equine patient on auscultation of the lower respiratory system?
    a. Stridor
    b. Wheezes
    c. Stertor
    d. Increased airflow

293. Projectile vomiting is most associated with:
    a. Gastric or esophageal disorder
    b. Gastrointestinal ulceration
    c. Involvement of bile in the duodenum
    d. Pyloric outflow obstruction

294. Which tests may be recommended for an equine patient that is experiencing upper airway complications?
    a. BAL
    b. TTW
    c. MRI
    d. Pulmonary function testing

295. All of these are typical clinical signs of advanced arthritis in dogs *except:*
    a. Reduced appetite
    b. Stiffness
    c. Lameness
    d. Difficulty in rising

296. A respiratory disease that produces swelling of abscesses of the submandibular and retropharyngeal lymph nodes is known as:
    a. Strangles
    b. Equine influenza
    c. Herpes
    d. Viral arteritis

297. Which part of the gastrointestinal system is associated with melena?
    a. Involvement of the stomach
    b. Involvement of the jejunum or ileum
    c. Involvement of the large intestine
    d. Colitis

298. A causative agent of rhinopneumonitis is:
    a. *Streptococcus equi*
    b. Equine herpes virus
    c. *Aspergillus spp*
    d. None of the above

299. All of the following are risk factors for developing osteoarthritis in dogs, *except:*
    a. Trauma
    b. Obesity
    c. Large/giant breeds
    d. Spaying or neutering

300. Which of the following is commonly seen in cats older than 10 years but is very rare in dogs?
    a. Hyperadrenocorticalism
    b. Hypoadrenocorticism
    c. Hypothyroidism
    d. Hyperthyroidism

301. Which of the following is not generally a symptom of osteoarthritis in cats?
    a. Changes in mobility
    b. Changes in activity level
    c. Changes in grooming
    d. Changes in eating habits

302. Which of the following is described as seizures involving loss of consciousness with tonic-clonic whole body movements, possibly with salivation, urination, and defecation?
    a. Absence seizures
    b. Focal seizures
    c. Generalized seizures
    d. Myoclonus

303. Which equine respiratory can cause abortion?
    a. Strangles
    b. Equine influenza
    c. Herpes
    d. Equine infectious anemia

304. Nutritional deficiencies and excesses in avian patients might result in:
    a. Immune dysfunction
    b. Increased susceptibility to infectious diseases
    c. Metabolic and biochemical derangements
    d. All of the above

305. Which of the following is described as seizures involving specific parts of the body, many times without a loss of consciousness?
    a. Absence seizures
    b. Focal seizures
    c. Generalized seizures
    d. Myoclonus

306. Which of the following is described as a transient alteration in consciousness, with or without external signs?
    a. Absence seizures
    b. Focal seizures
    c. Generalized seizures
    d. Myoclonus

307. Which of the following conditions is an allergic airway disease experienced by equine patients?
    a. Heaves
    b. Viral arteritis
    c. Inflammatory airway disease
    d. Exercise-induced pulmonary hemorrhage

308. Which of the following conditions matches a patient exhibiting a head tilt, facial paresis, nystagmus, positional strabismus, and ataxia?
    a. Brachycephalic syndrome
    b. Horner syndrome
    c. Wobbler syndrome
    d. Vestibular syndrome

309. Ferrets are which of the following?
    a. Carnivores
    b. Herbivores
    c. Omnivores
    d. Granivores

310. Pleuropneumonia in horses occurs when:
    a. Viral infections spread from lung tissue to the pleural space
    b. Viral infections spread from the plural space to lung tissue
    c. Bacterial infections spread from the plural space to lung tissue
    d. Bacterial infections spread from lung tissue to the pleural space

311. Which of the following is characterized as droopy eyelids, protruding nictitans, and miosis?
    a. Brachycephalic syndrome
    b. Horner syndrome
    c. Wobbler syndrome
    d. Vestibular syndrome

312. A contagious viral disease that produces limb swelling in horses is:
    a. Equine infectious anemia
    b. Equine viral arteritis
    c. Heaves
    d. Herpes

313. Lagomorphs have a rapid gut transit time resulting in starch and simple sugars not being completely digested in the:
    a. Large intestine
    b. Stomach
    c. Small intestine
    d. Colon

314. It is difficult to determine truly how much food is being ingested by the following small mammal(s), which hoard food items:
    a. Hamsters
    b. Rabbits
    c. Guinea pigs
    d. Ferrets

315. Which of the following is described as ataxia and paresis resulting from spondylosis of the vertebrae?
    a. Brachycephalic syndrome
    b. Horner syndrome
    c. Wobbler syndrome
    d. Vestibular syndrome

316. Equine anaplasmosis exhibits all of the following clinical signs, *except:*
    a. Anemia
    b. Icterus
    c. Excitement
    d. Stiffness

317. Clinical signs of gastric ulcers include:
    a. Bruxism
    b. Pyrexia
    c. Hyposalivation
    d. All of the above

318. Because Guinea pigs lack the enzyme involved in synthesizing glucose to ascorbic acid, they require a dietary source of which of the following?
    a. Vitamin K
    b. Vitamin B
    c. Vitamin C
    d. All of these

319. Nutritional protein for ferrets should come from:
    a. Carbohydrates
    b. Animal-based ingredients
    c. Plant-based ingredients
    d. Fiber

320. Which of the following is the recommended method to prevent further exposure to chemicals spilled on an animal's fur (not caustic on touch)?
    a. Applying chemical solvents
    b. Bathed with mild dishwashing detergent
    c. Induce emesis
    d. Wipe it off with a dry towel

321. Phenylbutazone toxicosis in horses can produce:
    a. Liver insufficiency
    b. Oral, gastric, and colonic ulcerations
    c. Icterus
    d. Limb edema

322. A prescription for a controlled substance must be signed and dated when issued. The prescription must include the patient's (owner's) full name and address, the practitioner's full name and address, and the practitioner's DEA number. Which of the following is not required on the prescription?
    a. Drug name and strength
    b. Quantity prescribed and number of refills authorized
    c. Directions for use
    d. Drug manufacturer's name and address

323. All of the following can result from colitis in horses, *except:*
    a. Endotoxemia
    b. Electrolyte loss
    c. Hypervolemia
    d. Hypovolemia

324. Which of the following is typically the largest vein to collect blood from a bird?
    a. Cutaneous ulnar vein
    b. Left jugular vein
    c. Medial metatarsal vein
    d. Right jugular vein

325. You must give a dog 250 mg of a medication that comes in tablets labeled 100 mg each. How many tablets will you give?
    a. 1½
    b. 2
    c. 2¼
    d. 2½

326. Complications of colitis in an equine patient could include:
    a. Founder
    b. Stertor
    c. Stridor
    d. Bruxism

327. What is the most common neoplasia seen in horses?
    a. Lymphosarcoma
    b. Osteosarcoma
    c. Lymphoma
    d. All of the neoplasms listed occur equally among the equine species

328. It is safe to draw ≤1% of a bird's body weight of blood. For a 450 g bird, how much blood can be taken safely?
    a. 0.45 mL
    b. 4.5 mL
    c. 45 mL
    d. 450 mL

329. All of the following are examples of viral equine encephalitis, *except:*
    a. Eastern
    b. Western
    c. Pacific
    d. West Nile

330. A dog weighs 88 lb. What is this dog's weight in kilograms?
    a. 20 kg
    b. 24 kg
    c. 40 kg
    d. 44 kg

331. Clinical signs of West Nile encephalitis include:
    a. Hypoesthesia
    b. Bilateral nasal discharge
    c. Ataxia
    d. Mandibular lymph node swelling

332. When hemorrhaging from a broken blood feather occurs, what is the appropriate course of action?
    a. Apply pressure to the broken edge
    b. Apply styptic powder to the feather
    c. Cut the feather at the base
    d. Pull the feather out along the follicle

333. When should horses receive vaccines for encephalomyelitis viruses?
    a. Autumn, before the first freeze
    b. Before breeding
    c. Spring, before mosquito season
    d. At 3 months of age

334. A cat requires 60 mg of a liquid medication of strength 120 mg/mL. What quantity of the medication should be administered?
    a. 2.0 mL
    b. 0.5 mL
    c. 0. 2 mL
    d. 5.0 mL

335. _____ is a highly fatal neurologic disease in horses, characterized by a stiff, stilted gait, hyperexcitability, seizure, and coma.
    a. West Nile
    b. Tetanus
    c. Equine degenerative myelopathy
    d. Herpes

336. Which of the following is a common venipuncture site for a reptile?
    a. Basilic vein
    b. Caudal tail vein
    c. Cephalic vein
    d. Jugular vein

337. A symptom of botulism is:
    a. Dysphagia
    b. Bruxism
    c. Pyrexia
    d. Tachycardia

338. A dog on intravenous fluids has initially received 25% of the 1000 mL in the IV bag. How many mL has it received?
    a. 100 mL
    b. 250 mL
    c. 350 mL
    d. 500 mL

339. If a dog that weighs 25 kg has received 250 mL of IV fluids, how many mL/kg of body weight has it received?
    a. 5
    b. 10
    c. 15
    d. 25

340. Acute renal failure in horses is most often a result of:
    a. Colic
    b. Toxicity
    c. Age
    d. Hereditary factors

341. Which of the following is defined as an irreversible, progressive loss of functioning renal tissue?
    a. Acute kidney injury
    b. Chronic kidney disease
    c. Acute liver failure
    d. Chronic liver disease

342. Which of the following is the appropriate treatment when a patient experiences severe heartworm infestation and caval syndrome?
    a. Adulticide therapy
    b. Microfilaricide therapy
    c. Surgical removal
    d. No treatment is needed, as it is transient

343. What is an average amount of water intake per day for a full-sized horse?
    a. 20–30 mL/day
    b. 5–15 L/day
    c. 20–30 L/day
    d. 20–30 gal/day

344. A cat is to receive 90 kcal of a canned food at each meal. The food has a caloric density of 360 kcal per can. How much of this food should the cat be fed at each meal?
    a. 0.25 can
    b. 0.20 can
    c. 0.50 can
    d. 1 can

345. The cell is the basic unit of the body. Cells contain all of the following, *except:*
    a. Cell membrane
    b. Cytoplasm
    c. Neuron
    d. Nucleus

346. What is an average amount of urine output per day, for a full-sized horse?
    a. 20–30 mL/day
    b. 1–3 L/day
    c. 5–15 L/day
    d. 5–15 gal/day

347. Which of the following is a sign of common complications to heartworm adulticide therapy?
    a. Ecchymoses, anemia
    b. Hemoptysis, dyspnea
    c. Hematuria, stranguria
    d. Melena, lethargy

348. Which of the following is the most common clinical sign of severe hypertension?
    a. Acute blindness
    b. Syncope
    c. Tachycardia
    d. Weakness

349. Which of the following is a common contributor to pancreatitis specific to dogs?
    a. Blunt force trauma
    b. Dietary indiscretion
    c. Pancreatic hypoperfusion
    d. Pancreotoxic drugs

350. Which of the following is another term for red blood cells?
    a. Epithelial cells
    b. Glandular cells
    c. Osteoblasts
    d. Erythrocytes

351. The highly convoluted _____ extends from the glomerular capsule to the connection with the collecting duct.
    a. Nephron
    b. Renal tubule
    c. Ureter
    d. Urethra

352. The veterinary technician can use both subjective and objective observations to determine the patient's state. All of the following are examples of objective observations, *except:*
    a. Body temperature
    b. Capillary refill time
    c. Demeanor
    d. Heart rate

353. All of the following may contribute to PU/PD in a horse, *except:*
    a. Lactation
    b. Psychogenic water drinking
    c. Glucocorticoid administration
    d. Acute renal failure

354. Which of the following is a technique used to used to help loosen purulent material within the pulmonary parenchyma?
    a. Cold compress
    b. Coupage
    c. Passive range of motion
    d. Warm compress

355. When monitoring a condition, the SOAP method may be used to ensure completeness. SOAP stands for:
    a. Subjective, objective, assessment, and planning
    b. Study, objective, assessment, and planning
    c. See, objective, assessment, and planning
    d. Subjective, objective, appraisal, and planning

356. Dermatophilosis in horses is also known as:
    a. Ringworm
    b. Rain rot
    c. Culicoides hypersensitivity
    d. Arcoid

357. Which of the following is an endocrine disease most commonly seen in cats?
    a. Chronic kidney disease
    b. Diabetes mellitus
    c. Hyperthyroidism
    d. Hypothyroidism

358. Production of fresh, bright red blood in the feces, indicating blood loss in the lower gastrointestinal tract, is:
    a. Dyschezia
    b. Hematochezia
    c. Melena
    d. Tenesmus

359. Moon blindness in horses is also known as:
    a. Ringworm
    b. Rain rot
    c. Corneal ulceration
    d. Equine recurrent uveitis

360. Which of the following endocrine diseases results in weight gain, muscle weakness, polyuria, polydipsia, skin and hair coat abnormalities, and a pot-bellied appearance in a dog?
    a. Hyperadrenocorticism
    b. Hypoadrenocorticism
    c. Hyperthyroidism
    d. Hypothyroidism

361. Which of the following is an appropriate element for an isolation ward?
    a. Sharing all equipment available to nonisolated patients
    b. Positive-pressure air-ventilation system
    c. Double-door entryway with an anteroom
    d. Two walls of cage banks facing each other

362. Passage of large volumes of pale, fatty feces, usually associated with exocrine pancreatic insufficiency, is referred to as:
    a. Anuria
    b. Coprophagia
    c. Steatorrhea
    d. Oliguria

363. When passing urine is painful and uncomfortable, it is known as which of the following?
    a. Dysuria
    b. Poikuria
    c. Polyuria
    d. Stranguria

364. Equine recurrent uveitis results from:
    a. An immune mediated condition
    b. Ocular trauma
    c. Antibiotic toxicity
    d. Corticosteroid therapy

365. Which of the following is not a part of a standard set of personal protective gear in an isolation ward?
    a. Filtered respirator mask
    b. Gloves
    c. Gown
    d. Shoe cover

366. Nauseous patients often:
    a. Are unable to urinate
    b. Vomit every time they eat
    c. Appear unusually depressed and may intermittently lick their lips
    d. All of the above

367. Conditions that may induce a coughing reflex include all of the following, *except:*
    a. Bronchitis
    b. Infectious rhinotracheitis
    c. Intestinal foreign body
    d. Left-sided congestive heart failure

368. To perform coupage, cupped hands should be used to tap firmly on the chest wall, starting:
    a. Caudally and working forward
    b. Cranially and working upward
    c. Caudally and working backward
    d. Cranially and working backward

369. *Pica* is a term used to describe:
    a. A partial reduction in appetite
    b. Ingestion of an animal's own feces
    c. Cravings for eating unusual food or objects
    d. Loss of desire to eat

370. All of the following are common locations for decubital ulcers in recumbent horses, *except:*
    a. Pelvis
    b. Elbow
    c. Head
    d. Hock

371. Why do tortoises require ultraviolet light in their habitat?
    a. To prevent vitamin A deficiency
    b. To promote cholecalciferol synthesis
    c. To reduce vitamin D level
    d. To regulate body temperature

372. Which of the following is not used to determine a patient's dehydration status?
    a. Capillary refill time (CRT)
    b. Eye position
    c. Discharge in the pinna
    d. Packed cell volume (PCV)

373. Which of the following methods of delivering fluids should not be used in severely dehydrated patients?
    a. Intraosseous fluid administration
    b. Intravenous fluid administration
    c. Subcutaneous fluid administration
    d. Intraperitoneal fluid administration

374. Recumbent equine patients should be rotated every:
    a. 2–3 hours
    b. 4–6 hours
    c. 8–10 hours
    d. 12–14 hours

375. Which of the following animals are strict carnivores?
    a. Dogs
    b. Ferrets
    c. Prairie dogs
    d. Rabbits

376. Which of the following are dorsal to the abdominal region?
    a. The cervical vertebrae
    b. The thoracic vertebrae
    c. The lumbar vertebrae
    d. The sacral vertebrae

377. Clinical signs associated with endotoxemia include:
    a. Fever
    b. Bradycardia
    c. Cyanotic mucous membranes
    d. Leukocytosis

378. Which of the following is seen as chalky-white or cream-colored urine in rabbits?
    a. Coprophagy
    b. Dysbiosis
    c. Dystrophic calcification
    d. Vitamin A deficiency

379. Which of the following complications associated with intravenous catheters is the term used to describe the formation of a blood clot resulting from an impeded blood flow?
    a. Thrombophlebitis
    b. Thrombus
    c. Air embolism
    d. Septicemia

380. After the medical resolution of colic, horses should be fed:
    a. Twice daily
    b. Three times daily
    c. Frequent, small meals
    d. A calorically dense food

381. Which of the following is true of hamsters?
    a. Male hamsters often attack newly introduced female hamsters
    b. Hamsters live 4–5 years
    c. Female hamsters may hide their young in their cheek pouches, leading to death
    d. The best method of restraint is to pick them up by the tail

382. Inappetent horses should be fed:
    a. Twice daily
    b. A calorically dense food
    c. Fresh grass
    d. High-fat food

383. Hypostatic pneumonia in hospitalized patients may be prevented by:
    a. Starting a course of antibiotics when the patient is admitted to the hospital
    b. Turning the patient every 4 hours
    c. Ensuring that the patient is fully awake and able to protect its own airway in advance of extubation
    d. All of these

384. Which of the following might be useful in the prevention of muscle atrophy?
    a. Passive limb movement
    b. Hydrotherapy
    c. Massage
    d. All of the above

385. Physical therapy for companion animals presents multiple therapeutic benefits, improves the quality of life, and speeds functional recovery. Which of the following may be helped by physical therapy?
    a. Pain management
    b. Combating acute and chronic inflammatory processes
    c. Reducing edema
    d. All of the above

386. Septic thrombophlebitis is more likely to occur in which of the following equine patients?
    a. Patients experiencing endotoxemia
    b. Patients receiving enteral nutrition
    c. Patients that are recumbent
    d. Septic thrombophlebitis does not occur in horses

387. Which of the following describes a patient suffering from mastitis?
    a. Hard, painful nipple, and galactostasis
    b. Hypocalcemia, muscle spasms, fever, tachycardia, and seizures
    c. In hard labor for 30 to 60 minutes with no new young produced
    d. Vaginal discharge, vomiting, diarrhea, dehydration, anorexia, polyuria, and polydipsia

388. Which of the following increases the supply of oxygen and nutrients to the tissues, while encouraging muscle relaxation? It is used to encourage the breakdown and mobilization of adhesions in damaged tissues, soften fascia, and prevent injury.
    a. Effleurage
    b. Petrissage
    c. Percussion
    d. Vibration

389. Life-threatening anaphylactic reactions are reported in equine patients that receive IV doses of:
    a. Aminoglycosides
    b. Procaine penicillin
    c. Trimethoprim-sulfa
    d. Metronidazole

390. Which of the following is one of the most important components of the successful rearing of lambs?
    a. The establishment of a strong ram–lamb bond
    b. The establishment of a strong ewe–lamb bond
    c. The establishment of a strong lamb–lamb bond
    d. The establishment of a strong ram–ewe bond

391. Which type of visit is not considered an outpatient service?
    a. Examination
    b. Vaccination
    c. Lab work
    d. Surgery

392. Which of the following qualifies an individual as a credentialed veterinary technologist?
    a. A 4-year Bachelor of Science degree in veterinary technology accredited by the AVMA
    b. A diploma from an accredited high school
    c. A 4-year Bachelor of Science degree in Animal Science
    d. An Associate of Science degree in veterinary technology

393. Which of the following team members is considered the face of the veterinary practice?
    a. Veterinary assistants
    b. Veterinarians
    c. Receptionists
    d. Veterinary technicians

394. What is the purpose of a safety program?
    a. To reduce or eliminate the possibility of injury or illness for everyone on the premises
    b. To reduce or eliminate the possibility of injury or illness for employees only
    c. To make OSHA happy
    d. To reduce or eliminate the possibility of injury or illness for clients only

395. Which potent chemical is used for "cold sterilization" of hard instruments?
    a. Ethylene oxide
    b. Formalin
    c. Glutaraldehyde
    d. Formaldehyde

396. Which of the following can result from long-term work in an indoor kennel with barking dogs?
    a. Ear ablation
    b. Hearing loss
    c. Ear infections
    d. Hyphema

397. How high can noise levels in veterinary dog wards reach?
    a. 220 dB
    b. 440 dB
    c. 110 dB
    d. 880 dB

398. Which of the following describes the transmission path of a zoonotic disease?
    a. From animals to humans
    b. From animals to animals
    c. From humans to humans
    d. From humans to zoos

399. Which of the following routes may expose veterinary technicians to organisms that cause disease?
    a. Inhalation
    b. Ingestion
    c. Needle sticks
    d. All of the above

400. All of the following are adverse side effects with the use of corticosteroids in horses, *except:*
    a. Laminitis
    b. Anuria
    c. Progression of joint disease
    d. Poor wound healing

401. Coupage is contraindicated in patients that have:
    a. Proptosed eye
    b. Fractured ribs
    c. Pulmonary disease
    d. Fractured femur

402. Orally administered drugs travel through the gastrointestinal tract, and most are absorbed in the small intestine. After absorption across the intestinal wall, orally administered drugs:
    a. Enter the stomach where the remainder of the drug is absorbed
    b. Enter the hepatic portal circulation and are routed directly to the liver
    c. Enter the kidney and are eliminated in the urine
    d. Enter the colon and are eliminated in the feces

403. Colostrum ingestion terminates _____ post birth.
    a. 8 hours
    b. 12 hours
    c. 24 hours
    d. 48 hours

404. Calf scours is common among young dairy and beef calves, and it is characterized by:
    a. Muscle weakness
    b. Diarrhea
    c. Hyperglycemia
    d. Hyperthermia

405. The movement of drug from the systemic circulation into the body tissues is known as which of the following?
    a. Therapeutic effect
    b. Protein binding
    c. Distribution
    d. Redistribution

406. A disease that is not caused by microorganisms but is usually a result of a disturbance in the normal metabolism of the animal is:
    a. A contagious disease
    b. An infectious disease
    c. A noninfectious disease
    d. A vector

407. Glomerulonephritis and pyelonephritis are two causes of:
    a. Cardiac disease
    b. Hepatic disease
    c. Renal disease
    d. Thyroid disease

408. Which of the following types of uroliths are found in alkaline urine?
    a. Struvite uroliths
    b. Ammonium urate uroliths
    c. Calcium oxalate uroliths
    d. Cystine uroliths

409. Nutritional myodegeneration is also known as:
    a. Scours
    b. Bacterial enteritis
    c. Bovine viral diarrhea
    d. White muscle disease

410. White muscle disease can be treated with:
    a. Selenium
    b. Vitamin E
    c. First cut of alfalfa with higher levels of protein
    d. Both a and b

411. Which of the following may be caused by right-sided heart failure?
    a. Aortic stenosis
    b. Mitral valve dysplasia
    c. Dysrhythmias
    d. Tricuspid dysplasia

412. Addison's disease is also known as which of the following:
    a. Hyperadrenocorticalism
    b. Hypoadrenocorticism
    c. Hypothyroidism
    d. Hyperthyroidism

413. Small ruminants are considered highly susceptible to enterotoxemia and should be vaccinated every _____ months.
    a. 3
    b. 6
    c. 10
    d. 12

414. Rumen fluid with a pH less than _____ suggests grain overload.
    a. 3.5
    b. 5.5
    c. 7.5
    d. 9.0

415. A vascular abnormality in which the hepatic portal vein empties directly into the caudal vena cava is:
    a. Hepatic lipidosis
    b. Portosystemic shunt
    c. Cardiomyopathy
    d. Aortic stenosis

416. Which of the following terms is used to describe a high-pitched, discontinuous inspiratory sound associated with the reopening of airways that closed during expiration?
    a. Crackle
    b. Stertor
    c. Stridor
    d. Wheeze

417. Rumen indigestion may result from:
    a. Undercooked feeds
    b. Vaccination
    c. Slow transition within the rumen environment
    d. Rapid feed change

418. Mucous membranes that appear deep brick red in color and appear injected are:
    a. Pale
    b. Icteric
    c. Hyperemic
    d. Cyanotic

419. Sites for intraosseous catheter placement include:
    a. The cranial aspect of the greater tubercle of the humerus
    b. The trochanteric fossa of the proximal femur
    c. The flat medial aspect of the proximal tibia
    d. All of these

420. Clinical signs of rumen indigestion include all of the following *except:*
    a. Anorexia
    b. Malodorous diarrhea
    c. Reduced rumen motility
    d. Increased rumen motility

421. Which of the following terms is used to describe passing larger volumes of urine than normal?
    a. Fomite
    b. Poikuria
    c. Polyuria
    d. Vector

422. Which of the following terms refers to excessive salivation?
    a. Borborygmus
    b. Dyschezia
    c. Polyphagia
    d. Ptyalism

423. The medical treatment for lactic acidosis in ruminants is:
    a. Rapid removal of rumen contents
    b. Intravenous administration of calcium
    c. Intramuscular injection of sodium bicarbonate
    d. Lactic acidosis can not be treated

424. Which of the following terms refers to the passive, retrograde movement of ingested material to a level above the upper esophageal sphincter?
    a. Expectoration
    b. Hematemesis
    c. Regurgitation
    d. Vomiting

425. Which plane across the body divides it into cranial (head-end) and caudal (tail-end) parts that are not necessarily equal?
    a. Sagittal plane
    b. Transverse plane
    c. Median plane
    d. Dorsal plane

426. Rumen tympany is also referred to as:
    a. Lactic acidosis
    b. Tetany
    c. Bloat
    d. Rumenitis

427. Which is a special term used only to describe positions or directions on the head?
    a. Cranial
    b. Caudal
    c. Rostral
    d. Ventral

428. Which surface of an animal's leg is the one closest to its body?
    a. Medial
    b. Lateral
    c. Proximal
    d. Distal

429. The technician who is involved in performing a professional dental cleaning should be capable of:
    a. Performing assessment
    b. Periodontal debridement
    c. Polishing
    d. All of the above

430. The American Veterinary Dental College (AVDC) position statement indicates it is appropriate for veterinary technicians to perform:
    a. Dental cleanings
    b. Root canals
    c. Surgical extractions
    d. All of the above

431. Dogs have all of the following types of teeth *except:*
    a. Canines
    b. Elodont teeth
    c. Molars
    d. Premolars

432. Which of the following terms is used to describe the tooth surface facing the lips?
    a. Rostral
    b. Caudal
    c. Lingual
    d. Vestibular

433. Which of the following may be caused by left-sided heart failure?
    a. Mitral valve dysplasia
    b. Pulmonic stenosis
    c. Neoplasia
    d. Myocarditis

434. Which of the following terms refers to a structure with a location that is closer to the crown of the tooth in relation to another structure?
    a. Palatal
    b. Mesial
    c. Coronal
    d. Apical

435. Treatment of free gas bloat in ruminant patients includes all of the following *except:*
    a. Passing an orogastric tube
    b. Administration of calcium
    c. Exercise restriction
    d. Rumen trocarization

436. Treatment of frothy gas bloat in ruminant patients includes the administration of all of the following products, *except:*
    a. Dioctyl sodium sulfosuccinate (DSS)
    b. Poloxalene
    c. Household detergent
    d. Calcium

437. Most mammals have a first set of teeth, which are replaced with permanent or adult teeth. This first set of teeth is called:
    a. Malocclusions
    b. Occlusion
    c. Deciduous
    d. Cingulum

438. How many adult teeth does the normal cat have?
    a. 30
    b. 32
    c. 40
    d. 42

439. The heart is an organ that is commonly affected by age. Chronic valvular disease (CVD) results from thickening of the heart valves, and it affects many:
    a. Young dogs
    b. Older dogs, especially smaller dogs
    c. Large breed dogs
    d. Cats

440. Hardware disease in ruminants is also known as:
    a. Grain overload
    b. Rumen tympany
    c. Traumatic reticuloperitonitis
    d. Polioencephalomalacia

441. Bovine viral diarrhea can manifest with all of the following clinical symptoms, *except:*
    a. Oral ulcers
    b. Pyrexia
    c. Bloat
    d. Lethargy

442. Chronic renal disease is one of the diseases seen most commonly in geriatric patients, especially cats. In addition to causing increased polyuria and polydipsia, renal disease may also cause:
    a. Anemia
    b. Anorexia
    c. Gastric upset
    d. All of the above

443. Which of the following treatments used to treat heartworm disease in dogs is a common microfilaricide treatment?
    a. Thiacetarsamide
    b. Melarsomine dihydrochloride
    c. Ivermectin
    d. All of the above

444. Increased intraocular pressure (IOP), caused by more aqueous fluid being produced than leaving the eye, might result in:
    a. Pannus
    b. Keratoconjunctivitis sicca
    c. Glaucoma
    d. Chronic superficial keratitis

445. The cornea is composed of four layers. Which of the following is not one of the four layers of the cornea?
    a. Epithelium
    b. Stroma
    c. Endothelium
    d. Sclera

446. Treatment for bovine viral diarrhea is:
    a. IV fluid administration
    b. Anti-inflammatory administration
    c. Anthelmintic therapy
    d. There is no treatment for BVD

447. Overproduction of tears is always the result of:
    a. Ocular pain or irritation
    b. Sad or frightened patients
    c. Ingesting too much protein in the patient's diet
    d. All of the above

448. The term used to describe a group of hereditary eye diseases seen in many breeds of dogs, which causes loss of night vision or low-light vision, is:
    a. Pannus
    b. Keratoconjunctivitis sicca
    c. Progressive retina atrophy
    d. Chronic superficial keratitis

449. Pyrexic cows experiencing bovine respiratory disease syndrome commonly have a temperature of:
    a. 99° F–101.5° F
    b. 96.8° F–99° F
    c. 100° F–102.2° F
    d. 104° F–107° F

450. The mass treatment of animal populations before the onset of disease is termed:
    a. Metaphylaxis
    b. Preconditioning
    c. Megascript
    d. All of the above

451. External parasites are responsible for many skin problems seen in small-animal medicine. All of the following may be treated with shampoos and dips, *except:*
    a. Fleas
    b. Ticks
    c. Ear mites
    d. Mange mites

452. The current recommended location for administering a rabies vaccine to a cat is:
    a. Between the shoulder blades
    b. The right shoulder
    c. The right rear leg
    d. The left rear leg

453. In the veterinary hospital, barrier nursing should be practiced:
    a. To keep the staff's uniforms free of pet hair
    b. To prevent the staining of staff uniforms
    c. To avoid transmitting infection among patients
    d. All of the above

454. Which of these endocrine disorders can result from the failure of the pituitary gland to produce antidiuretic hormone (ADH)?
    a. Diabetes insipidus
    b. Cushing's disease
    c. Hypothyroidism
    d. Insulinoma

455. BRDS, which affects primarily feedlot calves and dairy calves younger than 6 months of age, is caused by:
    a. Respiratory viruses
    b. Bacteria
    c. Stress
    d. All of the above

456. Ovine progressive pneumonia (OPP) causes all of the following, *except:*
    a. Mastitis
    b. Arthritis
    c. Neurologic signs
    d. Pyometra

457. Which of the following types of cells makes up bone?
    a. Osteoblasts
    b. Osteocytes
    c. Osteoclasts
    d. All of the above

458. The bones of the head and trunk are referred to as the:
    a. Axial skeleton
    b. Appendicular skeleton
    c. Visceral skeleton
    d. Metacarpal bones

459. *Coccidioides* is commonly referred to as:
    a. Erhlichia
    b. Anaplasmosis
    c. Valley Fever
    d. Aspergillosis

460. Which of the following are the two small bones that form part of the orbit of the eye?
    a. Ossicles
    b. Malleus
    c. Incus
    d. Lacrimal

461. Retained placentas in dairy cattle may result from all of the following, *except:*
    a. Delivery of twins
    b. Abortion
    c. Vitamin D deficiency
    d. Dystocia

462. Postpartum uterine infections are known as:
    a. Fetal membranes
    b. Metritis
    c. Pseudopregnancy
    d. Milk fever

463. The two zygomatic bones are also known as the:
    a. Malar bones
    b. Maxillary bones
    c. Lacrimal bones
    d. Nasal bones

464. Which of the following are four thin, scroll-like bones that fill most of the space in the nasal cavity and are also called the nasal conchae?
    a. Palatine bones
    b. Pterygoid bones
    c. Turbinates
    d. Vomer bone

465. A condition that is characterized by the accumulation of fluid in the uterus and one or more corpus lutea in the ovaries is known as:
    a. Fetal membranes
    b. Metritis
    c. Pseudopregnancy
    d. Milk fever

466. Which of the following types of vertebrae are unique in that they form a single solid structure?
    a. The cervical vertebrae
    b. The thoracic vertebrae
    c. The lumbar vertebrae
    d. The sacral vertebrae

467. How many grams per week of growth is normal for a kitten that is less than 6 months of age?
    a. 20 g
    b. 50 g
    c. 100 g
    d. 200 g

468. A metabolic disorder in which there is a severe decline in the serum calcium, usually occurring within 48 hours of calving, is known as:
    a. Fetal membranes
    b. Metritis
    c. Pseudopregnancy
    d. Milk fever

469. The most caudal sternebra is called the:
    a. Sternebra
    b. Manubrium
    c. Xiphoid
    d. Anticlinal

470. The most proximal bone of the thoracic limb is the:
    a. Humerus
    b. Scapula
    c. Tubercle
    d. Greater tubercle

471. The antebrachium is made up of which two bones?
    a. Humerus and radius
    b. Humerus and scapula
    c. Ulna and radius
    d. Radius and scapula

472. The anatomical term *synarthroses* refers to:
    a. Fibrous joints
    b. Palatine bones
    c. Vomer bone
    d. Pterygoid bones

473. Uterine infections in ruminants are associated with all of the following *except:*
    a. Unbalanced prepartum diets
    b. Viruses
    c. Delivery of twins
    d. Bacterium

474. Clinical symptoms of milk fever include:
    a. Staggering gate
    b. Bilateral nasal discharge
    c. Polyuria
    d. Lacrimation

475. The effect of the omega-3 fatty acids on cardiac patients may be attributed to:
    a. Anti-inflammatory effects
    b. Improved appetite
    c. Antiarrhythmic effects
    d. All of the above

476. The American Veterinary Dental College (AVDC) supports veterinary technicians with advanced training who are performing which of the following procedures?
    a. Charting dental lesions
    b. Taking dental radiographs
    c. Performing nonsurgical subgingival root planing
    d. All of the above

477. Milk fever can be prevented by:
    a. Feeding a high-calcium diet during the dry period
    b. Feeding a low-calcium diet during the dry period
    c. The slow administration of calcium intravenously
    d. The oral administration of 50% dextrose

478. Spheroidal joints are also called:
    a. Trochoid joints
    b. Pivot joints
    c. Gliding joints
    d. Ball-and-socket joints

479. Which of the following is commonly seen in dogs but is rare in cats?
    a. Hyperadrenocorticalism
    b. Hypoadrenocorticism
    c. Hypothyroidism
    d. Hyperthyroidism

480. Ketosis in dairy cows may result from all of the following *except:*
    a. Deficient energy intake
    b. Abomasal displacement
    c. Metritis
    d. Milk fever

481. Caseous lymphadenitis is:
    a. The most common cause of lymph node abscess in small ruminants
    b. A major cause of carcass condemnation in sheep
    c. Endemic
    d. All of the above

482. Which of the following is not a common risk factor for obesity in dogs?
    a. Age
    b. Feeding semimoist food
    c. Feeding homemade diets
    d. Feeding dry dog food

483. Which of the following allows the body to withdraw calcium from the bone when blood calcium levels are low?
    a. Osteoblasts
    b. Osteocytes
    c. Osteoclasts
    d. Hematopoiesis

484. Copper toxicity results from the accumulation of copper in the:
    a. Liver
    b. Kidneys
    c. Gallbladder
    d. Lymph nodes

485. Keratoconjunctivitis in sheep or goats can be treated with:
    a. Penicillin
    b. Tetracycline
    c. Aminoglycoside
    d. Phenylbutazone

486. Which of the following bones are usually clearly visible in young animals but may become indistinguishable in older animals?
    a. Interparietal bones
    b. Occipital bone
    c. Parietal bones
    d. Temporal bones

487. In general, how many days should be allowed for diet changes in dogs and cats?
    a. 5 to 7 days
    b. 1 to 3 days
    c. 48 to 72 hours
    d. 28 days

488. As a dog or cat transitions from immature to mature, the recommended diet change is for the:
    a. Increase in calories
    b. Decrease in fat and increase in fiber
    c. Addition of table scraps
    d. Decrease in fiber

489. Which of the following is/are antioxidants?
    a. Vitamin A, vitamin E, vitamin C
    b. L-Carnitine
    c. Vitamin
    d. Krebs cycles

490. Which of the following has the least influence on the acceptability of food to dogs and cats?
    a. Salt content
    b. Size
    c. Shape
    d. Color

491. Interdigital necrobacillosis is also known as:
    a. Polioencephalomalacia
    b. Foot rot
    c. Hardware disease
    d. Hairy heel wart

492. Laminitis in cattle is a diffuse, aseptic inflammation of the:
    a. Coronary band
    b. Wall
    c. Coffin bone
    d. Corium

493. Horses are which of the following?
    a. Ruminants
    b. Omnivores
    c. Hindgut fermenters
    d. Carnivores

494. Puppies, kittens, and nursing mothers require:
    a. Higher levels of protein in their diet than adult maintenance requirements
    b. Vitamin supplementation
    c. Higher levels of fiber than are required in adult maintenance diets
    d. Fewer calories than adult maintenance requirements

495. Which of the following is/are examples of preservatives?
    a. Omega-3 oils
    b. Sucrose, dextrose
    c. Lactated Ringer
    d. Vitamin E

496. Which of the following organisms is responsible for ringworm in cattle?
    a. *Trichophyton verrucosum*
    b. *Microsporum gypseum*
    c. *Epidermophyton floccosum*
    d. *Microsporum canis*

497. Contagious ecthyma is a common viral disease of small ruminants that is zoonotic. What is this disease also known as?
    a. Orf
    b. Sore mouth
    c. Sorf
    d. Both a and b

498. Corticosteroids are used for which of the following?
    a. Decreasing appetite
    b. Stimulating tear production
    c. Increasing appetite
    d. Improving hair coat

499. Chondroitin sulfates are an example of:
    a. Flavor enhancement
    b. Nutraceuticals
    c. Dentifrices
    d. Parenteral medications

500. All of the following processes should be completed for piglets raised in confinement, *except:*
    a. Iron injections at 3 days of age
    b. Clipping needle teeth
    c. Tail docking
    d. Removing dewclaws

501. The typical gestation period for pigs is:
    a. 42 days
    b. 63 days
    c. 114 days
    d. 147 days

502. Another term for exertional rhabdomyolysis is:
    a. Polydipsia
    b. Azoturia
    c. Anorexia
    d. Pyrexia

503. Which of the following vitamins is/are water soluble?
    a. Vitamins A and D
    b. Vitamins E and K
    c. Vitamins B$_{12}$ and C
    d. Vitamins A and E

504. Patients with pancreatitis or hyperlipidemia should avoid foods that are:
    a. High in protein
    b. Low in protein
    c. High in fats
    d. Low in fats

505. Taurine and L-carnitine have been found to aid in:
    a. Inappetence
    b. Dysphagia
    c. Cardiac muscle function
    d. Temperament

506. Potassium deficiency results in:
    a. Neurologic disease
    b. Weight gain
    c. Increased palatability
    d. Improved growth

507. The typical gestation period for dogs is:
    a. 42 days
    b. 63 days
    c. 114 days
    d. 147 days

508. In the equine large intestine, the optimum pH for microbial activity that promotes volatile fatty acid (VFA) absorption is:
    a. 6.5
    b. 6.7
    c. 7.1
    d. 6.1

509. AAFCO feeding trials are used to evaluate pet foods in all of the following life stages, *except:*
    a. Senior
    b. Gestation and lactation
    c. Adult maintenance
    d. Growth

510. Porcine stress syndrome is also known as:
    a. Malignant hypothermia
    b. Malignant hyperthermia
    c. Sodium ion toxicosis
    d. Porcine parvovirus

511. According to AAFCO rules, a pet food indicating "beef" on the label must have how much beef in the food?
    a. 70%
    b. 50%
    c. 40%
    d. 25%

512. If the client wants to feed a preservative-free food to a pet, which food should you recommend?
    a. Canned food
    b. Dry food
    c. Semimoist food
    d. A combination of dry and semimoist foods

513. Porcine stress syndrome results in all of the following, *except:*
    a. Muscle tremors
    b. Death
    c. Hypothermia
    d. Dyspnea

514. Which of the following statements about cats is true?
    a. Cats need more protein in their diets than dogs
    b. It is important to provide plenty of variety by buying different brands of foods
    c. Hairballs are a sign of illness in a cat
    d. Giving liver as a treat can result in vitamin A deficiency

515. Which of the following diets is intended to be dispensed under the supervision of veterinarians in the context of a valid veterinarian-client-patient relationship (VCPR)?
    a. Veterinary therapeutic
    b. Holistic
    c. Raw
    d. Over-the-counter

516. Swine wallow in mud to:
    a. Forage for food
    b. Thermoregulate
    c. Remove parasites
    d. Prevent sunburn

517. Kittens are generally fed a growth formula food until they are approximately how old?
    a. 10–12 months
    b. 18 months
    c. 2 years
    d. 6 months

518. Most clients offer treats to their pets. How many treats can safely be given each day?
    a. Not more than 20% of the pet's diet in treats
    b. As long as the pet isn't overweight, there's no limit on the number of treats that may be offered
    c. If the treats are low in calories, it should not matter
    d. Not more than 10% of the pet's diet in treats

519. What is the average weight of an adult pot bellied pig?
    a. 50 lb
    b. 120 lb
    c. 220 lb
    d. 450 lb

520. Which amino acid must be present in cat food but not in dog food?
    a. L-Carnitine
    b. Glutamine
    c. Taurine
    d. Lysine

521. The list of ingredients appear on a pet food label in order of:
    a. Dietary importance
    b. Nutrient bioavailability
    c. Caloric percentage
    d. Weight

522. What is the most common nutritional disease of pot bellied pigs?
    a. Calcium deficiency
    b. Vitamin E deficiency
    c. Obesity
    d. Malnourishment

523. Which government agency is responsible for inspecting the ingredients used in pet foods?
    a. USDA
    b. FDA
    c. AAFCO
    d. FTC

524. A bitch's food caloric needs are highest:
    a. During the first trimester
    b. During the fourth week of lactation
    c. During the third trimester
    d. Just before weaning

525. An atypical heart sound associated with a functional or structural valve abnormality is known as:
    a. Arrhythmia
    b. Fibrillation
    c. Murmur
    d. Infarct

526. Semimoist food is not recommended for an animal that is:
    a. Diabetic
    b. Geriatric
    c. Growing
    d. Lactating

527. If "fish flavor" is stated on the pet food label, how much fish must be in the food?
    a. 5%
    b. 8%
    c. 15%
    d. An amount that is detectable by the pet

528. Which of the following is an example of a product designator from a pet-food label?
    a. Beef entrée
    b. Cat food
    c. Nine Lives
    d. Complete and balanced for adult dogs

529. An equine that is about to turn 1 year old is referred to as a:
    a. Yearling
    b. Foaling
    c. Weanling
    d. Filly

530. What does the guaranteed analysis on the pet-food label mean?
    a. It states the exact measurements of the nutrients and moisture levels in the food
    b. It is a combination of maximum and minimum nutrient and moisture levels in the food
    c. It states the maximum levels of each nutrient in the food
    d. It states the minimum levels of each nutrient in the food

531. The difference between the amount of a nutrient consumed and the amount absorbed by the body is described as:
    a. Dry-matter basis
    b. Energy density
    c. Digestibility
    d. Hydrolyzation

532. Which of the following is an acceptable method of making food more palatable to the pet?
    a. Warming the food
    b. Adding onion salt to the food
    c. Heating the food above body temperature
    d. Adding warm milk to the food

533. Fats are composed of triglycerides, which include:
    a. Two fatty acids to a glycerol chain
    b. Three fatty acids attached to three glycerol chains
    c. Three fatty acids attached to a glycerol chain
    d. One fatty acid attached to one glycerol chain

534. A male donkey that has not been castrated and is capable of breeding is referred to as a:
    a. Jenny
    b. Dam
    c. Jack
    d. Sire

535. The process of giving birth to pigs is referred to as:
    a. Stag
    b. Freshening
    c. Farrowing
    d. Kidding

536. Most veterinary therapeutic diets fall into this category, which should be prescribed and monitored by animal health professionals:
    a. All purpose
    b. Premium
    c. Specific purpose
    d. Value

537. Pet foods that use food ingredients that have not been exposed to insecticides, pesticides, or medications such as antibiotics or growth promotants, are known as:
    a. Organic
    b. Raw
    c. Natural
    d. Holistic

538. Pet food recipes found in books and on the Internet are almost always:
    a. Perfectly balanced for dogs and cats
    b. Complete and healthy
    c. Highly palatable
    d. Incomplete and unbalanced

539. The number of animals within a population that becomes sick can be defined as:
    a. Morbidity
    b. Mortality
    c. Chronic
    d. Acute

540. A collection of blood in the cranial portion of the ventral cavity is known as:
    a. Pneumothorax
    b. Pneumonia
    c. Hematothorax
    d. Hemostasis

541. The most common error in feeding growing puppies is providing:
    a. Too much food
    b. Too little food
    c. The right amount of food
    d. Too much milk

542. Cats that act hungry and tend to overeat should be:
    a. Free fed
    b. Meal fed twice a day
    c. Fed once a day
    d. Fed once a week

543. The most common form of malnutrition in hospitalized animals is _____ because of the reluctance or inability to eat voluntarily.
    a. Lack of energy and protein intake
    b. Lack of sugar
    c. Lack of carbohydrates
    d. Lack of minerals

544. Which type of feeding is the most physiologic and often the safest route?
    a. Intravenous
    b. Intraosseous
    c. Oral
    d. Subcutaneous

545. Which of the following is not true of nasoesophageal (NE) or nasogastric (NG) tubes?
    a. Inexpensive
    b. Easy to place
    c. Useful for short-term feeding support
    d. Costly and inefficient

546. An overgrowth of scar tissue at the site of injury is known as:
    a. Papule
    b. Petechia
    c. Laceration
    d. Keloid

547. Osteomalacia is known as the:
    a. Hardening of bones
    b. Softening of bones
    c. Collection of abnormal cells that accumulate within the bones
    d. Thickened skin

548. Inadequate intake of protein and energy may result in:
    a. A dry, dull hair coat and excessive pigmentation
    b. Pyoderma
    c. Skin depigmentation and crusting around the eyes
    d. Hair loss and dry, dull hair coat

549. Which factor influences the success of a dietary elimination trial?
    a. Type of protein contained in the elimination diet
    b. Use of a homemade diet
    c. Concurrent allergic skin disease
    d. All of the above

550. Foods effective in the management of an adverse food reaction include:
    a. Novel protein diets
    b. Foods that contain high levels of proteins
    c. Foods that contain a single carbohydrate source
    d. Foods that use only natural preservatives

551. What is the name of the third party that evaluates veterinary dental foods and approves an oral care seal on its veterinary products?
    a. Veterinary Oral Health Council
    b. American Veterinary Dental Association
    c. Academy of Veterinary Oral Health
    d. Veterinary Dental Society

552. What structure connects muscles to bones?
    a. Ligaments
    b. Tendons
    c. Foramen
    d. Process

553. Acute diarrhea is usually caused by:
    a. Malignancy
    b. Diet or dietary indiscretion
    c. Histoplasmosis
    d. Pythiosis

554. Which of the following is not a typical sign of inflammatory bowel disease (IBD) in cats?
    a. Vomiting
    b. Diarrhea
    c. Weight gain
    d. Weight loss

555. Increased frequency of defecation and loose and watery stools are common when the _____ is involved.
    a. Small intestine
    b. Large intestine
    c. Colon
    d. Stomach

556. A comprehensive nutritional history for patients presenting with acute diarrhea should include:
    a. Ingestion of trash or any unusual foods
    b. The diet fed
    c. The household member responsible for feeding the pet
    d. All of the above

557. Inflammation of all bones or inflammation of every part of one bone is known as:
    a. Panosteitis
    b. Polypathia
    c. Pandemic
    d. Osteoporosis

558. The term *amyoplasia* refers to the:
    a. Lack of muscle formation or development
    b. Paralysis of muscles
    c. Muscular weakness or partial paralysis restricted to one side of the body
    d. Any disease of a muscle

559. Patients suffering with short-bowel syndrome (SBS) should be fed the following type of diet in the long term:
    a. High-protein, high-fat diets
    b. Low-fat, highly digestible diets
    c. High-fat, highly digestible diets
    d. High-protein, moderately digestible diets

560. Dehydration is frequently encountered in patients suffering from GI disorders. Which of the following factors causes this?
    a. Reduced oral water consumption
    b. Vomiting
    c. Diarrhea
    d. All of the above

561. If vomiting patients lose hydrogen and chloride ions in excess of sodium and bicarbonate, which of the following should be expected?
    a. Acidemia
    b. Neutrality
    c. Alkalemia
    d. None of the above

562. Hydremia refers to which of the following?
    a. Inadequate supply of blood to a part of the body
    b. Disorder in which there is excess fluid in the blood
    c. Low red blood cell count
    d. The narrow, pointed bottom of the heart

563. The accumulation of fluid in the abdominal cavity is defined as:
    a. Auscultate
    b. Infarct
    c. Ascites
    d. Edema

564. Enteral feeding tubes of all types should be flushed:
    a. Before and after use
    b. After use only
    c. Before use only
    d. Never

565. Which type of nutrition is defined as providing nutrients intravenously?
a. Parenteral
b. Enteral
c. Oral
d. Emergency

566. Feeding dog food to a cat is _____ advised.
a. Never
b. Sometimes
c. Seldom
d. Frequently

567. An abnormally low white blood cell count is referred to as:
a. Normocytic
b. Leukocytosis
c. Leukopenia
d. Anemia

568. A lack of digestion is referred to as which of the following?
a. Bradypeptic
b. Apepsia
c. Monogastric
d. Anastomosis

569. All but one of the following make up the five vital assessments:
a. Temperature
b. Pain
c. Weight
d. Nutrition

570. Which nutrient is the most important for patients with acute or chronic vomiting?
a. Protein
b. Vitamins
c. Minerals
d. Water

571. Acute diarrhea is typically the result of which of the following?
a. Diet
b. Parasites
c. Infectious disease
d. All of the above

572. The goals of the nutritional management of hepatic disease include:
a. Providing substrates to support hepatocellular repair and regeneration
b. Maintaining normal metabolic processes
c. Avoiding toxic byproduct accumulation
d. All of the above

573. Melena refers to which of the following?
a. Passing of dark, tarry feces containing blood that has been acted on by bacteria in the intestines
b. A semifluid mass of partially digested food that enters the small intestine from the stomach
c. A protein produced by living cells that initiates a chemical reaction but is not affected by the reaction
d. To fall back into a disease state after an apparent recovery

574. Which of the following is a technique used to decrease blood flow and minimize inflammation?
a. Cold compress
b. Coupage
c. Passive range of motion
d. Warm compress

575. What percentage in excess of the optimal weight for their breed classifies dogs and cats as obese?
a. ≥20%
b. 10%–19%
c. 35%
d. 50%

576. When reintroducing exercise into the pet's and owner's daily regimen to promote weight loss, the following recommendation should be made:
a. Start with a moderate exercise plan
b. Exercise should include running
c. Exercise as much as possible on the first day
d. Exercise is not necessary

577. Sebaceous glands that deposit cat scent are located in all of the following areas, *except:*
a. Around the lips and chin
b. Between the toes
c. The tip of the tail
d. The perianal area

578. What amino acid does a cat require in its diet to avoid dilated cardiomyopathy?
a. Cysteine
b. Taurine
c. Guanine
d. Isoleucine

579. The most accurate formula to determine the pet's resting energy requirement is:
a. RER kcal/day = 50 (ideal body weight in kg) 0.75
b. RER kcal/day = 70 (ideal body weight in kg) 0.50
c. RER kcal/day = 70 (ideal body weight in kg) 0.75
d. RER kcal/day = 75 (ideal body weight in kg) 0.75

580. Specific recommendations that support a successful weight-loss program include:
    a. Using an 8 oz measuring cup to measure food
    b. Appropriate exercise for the pet
    c. Emphasizing feeding consistency including feeding the pet from its designated dish only
    d. All of the above

581. The most common cause of FLUTD in cats less than 10 years of age is:
    a. Struvite uroliths
    b. Feline idiopathic cystitis (FIC)
    c. Calcium oxalate crystals
    d. Urethral plugs

582. Which of the following is a clinical symptom of thromboemboli in cats?
    a. Chronic onset or rear leg pain
    b. Acute onset of rear leg pain
    c. Palpable pulses in rear limbs
    d. Warm foot pads

583. Causes of congenital heart disease include all of the following, *except:*
    a. Genetics
    b. Viruses
    c. Nutrients
    d. Drugs

584. Litter box management for cats with FLUTD includes:
    a. Using only covered litter boxes
    b. Using highly-scented litter so the unappealing urine odor is masked
    c. Having one litter box per cat—plus one additional
    d. Always using scoopable litter

585. Diagnostic evaluation of felines with recurrent or persistent lower urinary tract signs should include:
    a. Urinalysis
    b. Diagnostic imaging
    c. Thyroid testing
    d. Both a and b

586. To evaluate urine for crystalluria:
    a. Urinalysis should be performed within 30 minutes of sample collection
    b. Evaluation is best performed after urine has been refrigerated for 12 hours
    c. Sample should always be sent out for evaluation
    d. Ultrasound is the most reliable means of evaluation

587. Which of the following are clinical symptoms seen in a cat with heartworm disease?
    a. Diarrhea
    b. Left-sided chronic heart failure
    c. Weight gain
    d. Vomiting

588. The FDA's Center for Veterinary Medicine (CVM) regulates pet foods in cooperation with the individual states. Which of the following is not a responsibility of the FDA?
    a. Establishing certain animal food-labeling regulations
    b. Specifying certain permitted ingredients such as drugs and additives
    c. Enforcing regulations about chemical and microbiologic contamination
    d. Enforcing manufacturing procedures

589. Adverse reaction to food is an abnormal response to which of the following?
    a. Ingested toxin
    b. Ingested food
    c. Inhaled food
    d. Inhaled toxin

590. Protein malnutrition in patients with hepatic disease manifests clinically as:
    a. Hypoalbuminemia weight gain, and muscle atrophy
    b. Weight loss, muscle atrophy, and hypoalbuminemia
    c. Muscle atrophy, hyperalbuminemia zinc accumulation
    d. Vitamin K accumulation, weight loss, and muscle atrophy

591. Small frequent meals help the patient with hepatic disease by:
    a. Optimizing blood flow through the liver
    b. Managing fasting glucose
    c. Minimizing hepatic encephalopathy
    d. All of these

592. In cats, hepatic lipidosis often occurs as a result of which of the following?
    a. Thyroid disease
    b. Anorexia and weight loss
    c. Lower urinary tract disease
    d. Cardiac disease

593. Chronic hepatitis may be a result of:
    a. Copper accumulation, infectious diseases, drugs
    b. Breed-associated hepatitis, autoimmune disease, copper deficiency
    c. Infectious diseases, unknown etiology, zinc accumulation
    d. Autoimmune disease, vitamin K deficiency, drugs

594. When administrating oral medications to cats, which of the following techniques should be practiced?
    a. Placing medication inside a piece of cheese
    b. Flushing water with a syringe into the mouth after the tablet has been given
    c. Placing the tablet or capsule on the back of the tongue and holding the mouth shut
    d. Cats cannot take oral medications

595. Clinical signs of acute gastritis may include:
    a. Anorexia
    b. Polyuria
    c. Polydipsia
    d. Anuria

596. The accumulation of inflammatory cells within the lining of the small intestine, stomach, or large bowel is known as:
    a. Acute gastritis
    b. Chronic gastritis
    c. Inflammatory bowel disease
    d. Colitis

597. Hematuria can be determined to exist:
    a. When there is any positive reading for blood on the dipstick
    b. If intact erythrocytes are present in the microscopic examination of the urine sediment
    c. Only if there is a red tint to the urine sample
    d. Whenever there is a case of feline idiopathic cystitis

598. Methods for increasing water intake in cats include:
    a. Placing ice cubes in water
    b. Adding broth to foods
    c. Providing water fountains
    d. All of the above

599. A key nutritional component to managing the inflammation seen in FIC is:
    a. Adding salt to the cat's food
    b. Adding omega-3 fatty acids to the diet
    c. Feeding only once daily
    d. Feeding various types of food

600. Currently the recommended treatment(s) for cats with FIC include:
    a. Nutritional management
    b. Environmental enrichment
    c. Stress reduction
    d. All of the above

601. The most common sign in dogs and cats with allergic disease is:
    a. Reluctance to eat
    b. Lethargy
    c. Pruritus
    d. Hyperpigmentation

602. All of the following information should be provided to clients when their pet has been diagnosed with inflammatory bowel disease, *except:*
    a. A definitive diagnosis requires a biopsy
    b. Therapy will only be required until the clinical signs resolve
    c. A special diet will be required for the remainder of the animal's life
    d. Pets cannot eat table food

603. Which of the following medications is most commonly implicated in cases of gastric ulcers in horses, dogs, and cats?
    a. NSAIDs
    b. Antibiotics
    c. Parasiticides
    d. Immunotherapy

604. All of the following are among the most commonly diagnosed skin disorders in cats *except:*
    a. Miliary dermatitis
    b. Eosinophilic granuloma complex
    c. Adverse reaction to food
    d. Hyperthyroidism

605. Colostrum is rich in all of the following nutrients, except:
    a. Protein
    b. Growth Factors
    c. Energy
    d. Hormones

606. Feline eosinophilic granuloma complex involves which three conditions?
    a. Indolent ulcers, eosinophilic plaques, and linear granulomas
    b. Indolent ulcers, eosinophilic granulomas, and linear plaques
    c. Linear ulcers, eosinophilic plaques, and linear granulomas
    d. Eosinophilic ulcers, indolent granulomas, and linear plaques

607. Intestinal lymphangiectasia is defined as:
    a. A protein-losing stomach disease
    b. A fat-losing stomach disease
    c. A fat-losing intestinal disease
    d. A protein-losing intestinal disease

608. Which of the following factors is most important in the nutritional management of inflammatory skin disorders?
    a. Assessment of current foods being fed and identification of an appropriate feeding plan
    b. Assessment of the feeding method and elimination of corn from the diet
    c. Determination of an appropriate feeding plan including the elimination of gluten from the diet
    d. Assessment of the feeding plan and elimination of carbohydrates from the diet

609. Which of the following factors influences the success of a dietary elimination trial for pets suffering from adverse food reactions?
    a. Type of protein contained in the elimination diet
    b. Complete elimination of all other foods and treats
    c. Concurrent allergic skin disease
    d. All of the above

610. Feline obstipation is also known as:
    a. IBD
    b. Megacolon
    c. Constipation
    d. All of the above

611. Acute onset of hepatic disease may result from all of the following drugs, *except:*
    a. Acetaminophen
    b. Phenobarbital
    c. Antifungals
    d. Vitamin K

612. Dogs and cats with diabetes mellitus (DM) typically present to the veterinary hospital with which of the following signs?
    a. Polydipsia and lethargy
    b. Weight gain and lethargy
    c. Lethargy and chronic kidney disease (CKD)
    d. All of the above

613. What is a relatively new option to manage hyperthyroidism in cats?
    a. Thyroidectomy
    b. Nutritional management
    c. Anti-thyroid medications
    d. Radioactive iodine

614. What percent of hyperthyroid cats remained euthyroid when fed ≤0.32 ppm iodine DMB as the sole source of nutrition?
    a. 60%
    b. 80%
    c. 90%
    d. 75%

615. Clinical signs associated with liver disease could include:
    a. Melena
    b. Anuria
    c. Weight gain
    d. Hyposalivation

616. Which of the following hormones is produced by the thyroid gland?
    a. Triiodothyronine
    b. Tetraiodothyronine
    c. Calcitonin
    d. All of the above

617. If a patient is 12–15% dehydrated, which characteristics would you expect to see?
    a. Death
    b. Slightly dry mucous membranes
    c. Prolonged capillary refill time
    d. Eyes are sunken in orbits

618. Which of the following is intended to provide long-term solutions for feline hyperthyroidism?
    a. Surgery and oral anti-thyroid drugs
    b. Radioactive iodine therapy and oral anti-thyroid drugs
    c. Surgery and radioactive iodine therapy
    d. Radioactive iodine therapy *only*

619. Feline hyperthyroidism is a result of:
    a. Malnutrition
    b. Excessive production of thyroid hormone
    c. Excessive production of the pituitary glands
    d. Diets containing excessive protein

620. Poorly controlled diabetic patients may experience muscle wasting because of:
    a. Fat being catabolized to meet energy needs
    b. Protein being catabolized to meet energy needs
    c. Carbohydrates being catabolized to meet energy needs
    d. All of the above

621. All of the following are symptoms of hyperthyroid disease, *except:*
    a. Weight gain
    b. Polyphagia
    c. Vomiting
    d. Increased appetite

622. Which of the following hormones does the pancreas produce?
    a. Oxytocin
    b. Glucagon
    c. Glycogen
    d. Calcitonin

623. Key nutritional factors in the management of skin disorders include:
    a. Carbohydrates, essential fatty acids, and calcium
    b. Proteins, essential fatty acids, and calcium
    c. Proteins, essential fatty acids, copper, and zinc
    d. Proteins, carbohydrates, essential fatty acids, copper, and zinc

624. A paraneoplastic syndrome manifested by weight loss and a decrease in body condition, despite adequate nutritional intake, is known as:
    a. Cancer anorexia
    b. Cancer cachexia
    c. Inappetence
    d. None of the above

625. Key nutritional factors in animals with cancer include which of the following?
    a. Soluble carbohydrate, protein, and omega-3 fatty acids
    b. Soluble carbohydrate, polyphenols, and cysteine
    c. Insoluble carbohydrate, polyphenols, and arginine
    d. Insoluble carbohydrate, protein, and calcium

626. Which of the following types of diabetes are more common in dogs?
    a. Insulin dependent diabetes
    b. Type 1 diabetes
    c. Non–insulin-dependent diabetes
    d. Both a and b

627. Copper storage disease is an inherited autosomal recessive trait that is prevalent in:
    a. Afghan hounds
    b. Bedlington terriers
    c. Pekinese dogs
    d. Cats

628. The liver's main responsibility is:
    a. Maintaining homeostasis
    b. Removing waste products from the body
    c. Both a and b
    d. None of the above

629. The most common electrolyte disturbance in vomiting cats and dogs is:
    a. Hypokalemia
    b. Hypochloremia
    c. Hypernatremia
    d. All of the above

630. In clinical trials of dogs with spontaneous cancer, high levels of omega-3 fatty acids and arginine in food were shown to benefit dogs with:
    a. Lymphoma
    b. Nasal carcinomas
    c. Hemangiosarcomas
    d. All of the above

631. Which of the following types of diabetes are more common in cats?
    a. Non–insulin-dependent diabetes
    b. Type 2 diabetes
    c. Insulin-dependent diabetes
    d. All of the above

632. Which statement(s) regarding vitamin supplementation in dogs is/are true?
    a. The vitamin E level should be appropriate to the levels of polyunsaturated fatty acids in the food
    b. Vitamin E can reverse cancer cachexia
    c. Mega doses of vitamins are recommended for dogs receiving commercial dry food diets
    d. All of the above

633. Which of the following is considered to be the most commonly detected electrolyte disturbance when providing nutritional support to a patient suffering from refeeding syndrome?
    a. Hyponatremia
    b. Hypochloremia
    c. Hypokalemia
    d. Hypomagnesemia

634. Common symptoms of diabetes in both dogs and cats include:
    a. Bradypnea/bradycardic
    b. Polyuria/polydipsia
    c. Weight gain/pitting edema
    d. All of the above

635. Which of the following conditions can be life threatening?
    a. Hyperglycemia
    b. Hypoglycemia
    c. Polyuria
    d. Polyphagia

636. Which disease involves the adrenal glands?
    a. Diabetes
    b. Addison's
    c. IBD
    d. Eclampsia

637. Clinical signs that a patient may present with that would indicate small intestine diarrhea include:
    a. Mucus
    b. Hematochezia
    c. Increased stool volume
    d. Dyschezia

638. Clinical signs that a patient may present with that would indicate large intestinal diarrhea include:
    a. Halitosis
    b. Borborygmus
    c. Tenesmus
    d. Steatorrhea

639. Which of the following toxic plants would have an effect on the cardiovascular system?
    a. Oleander
    b. Marijuana
    c. Morning glory
    d. Tobacco

640. Which of the following toxic plants would have an effect on the kidneys of cats?
    a. Apricot seeds
    b. Easter lily
    c. Onion
    d. Mistletoe

641. Which heart condition is most common in Pomeranians?
    a. Patent ductus arteriosus
    b. Aortic stenosis
    c. Atrial septal defect
    d. Ventricular septal defect

642. If a patient is 5–6% dehydrated, which characteristics would you expect to see?
    a. 5–6% is not clinically detectable
    b. Subtle loss of skin elasticity
    c. Prolonged capillary refill time
    d. Eyes are sunken in orbits

643. Which of the following symptoms would be common in dogs experiencing anemia?
    a. Anorexia
    b. Weakness
    c. Tachypnea
    d. All of the above

644. Which of the following diseases would cause a patient to become anemic?
    a. Iron deficiency
    b. Lethargy
    c. Alopecia
    d. Viral infection of the upper respiratory tract

645. Opaque pupillary opening and progressive vision loss may be seen in patients with:
    a. Calcivirus
    b. Parvovirus
    c. Cataracts
    d. Distemper

646. Which of the following may contribute to ringworm in companion animals?
    a. *Microsporum canis*
    b. *M. gypseum*
    c. *Trichophyton mentagrophytes*
    d. All of the above

647. What is a cause of flea allergy dermatitis?
    a. Environmental allergens, including trees, grasses and pollens
    b. *Ctenocephalides* infestation
    c. *Blastomyces* infestation
    d. Mite infestation

648. Which of the following would contribute to geriatric vestibular syndrome?
    a. Increased intraocular fluid production
    b. Otitis media
    c. *Coccidioides immitis*
    d. *Histoplasum capsulatum*

649. The accumulation of triglycerides in the liver would be known as:
    a. Renal lipidosis
    b. Hepatic lipidosis
    c. Hyperthyroidism
    d. Hypothyroidism

650. Which of the following diseases exhibit coughing, fever, and mucopurulent discharge?
    a. Kennel cough
    b. Canine parvovirus
    c. Canine distemper
    d. Infectious canine tracheobronchitis

651. Which of the following contribute to Lyme disease?
    a. *Rickettsia rickettsii*
    b. *Scabies scabei*
    c. *Staphylococcus*
    d. *Borrelia burgdorferi*

652. Viral rhinotracheitis is caused by:
    a. Canine distemper
    b. Canine parvovirus
    c. Heresvirus
    d. von Willebrand's

653. Which of the following may be a viral enteritis?
    a. Parvovirus
    b. Coronavirus
    c. Rotavirus feline
    d. All of the above
    e. None of the above

654. Petechial hemorrhage, ecchymosis, epistaxis, and lethargy might be seen with:
    a. Thrombocytopenia
    b. Urolithiasis
    c. Renal failure
    d. Pyometra

655. The overingestion of fats may contribute to:
    a. Patella luxation
    b. Cushing's disease
    c. Pancreatitis
    d. Panosteitis

656. All of the following diseases are of orthopedic descent, *except:*
    a. Osteochondrosis dessicans
    b. von Willebrand's disease
    c. Panosteitis
    d. Arthritis

657. All of the following would be considered a core vaccine, *except:*
    a. Distemper
    b. Rabies
    c. Canine adenovirus
    d. Leptospira

658. All of the following would be considered a core vaccine, *except:*
    a. Modified live panleukopenia
    b. Herpes-calicivirus
    c. Leukemia
    d. Rabies

659. What is the known duration of immunity for *Bordetella bronchiseptica?*
    a. 6 months
    b. 1 year
    c. 3 years
    d. 5 years

660. When charting a medical record, in what portion of the record is the TPR logged?
    a. Subjective
    b. Objective
    c. Assessment
    d. Plan

661. If a patient presents with a heart murmur that can be heard with the stethoscope bell slightly off of the thoracic wall, which grade would the heart murmur receive?
    a. $\frac{1}{6}$
    b. $\frac{4}{6}$
    c. $\frac{6}{6}$
    d. Murmurs are not graded

662. When choosing a specific restraint mechanism for a patient, which of the following should be taken into consideration before restraining?
    a. Available equipment
    b. The individual patient's behavior
    c. Whether the client is watching
    d. There are no considerations in advance of restraint

663. Which of the following devices are used to immobilize a patient with chemical restraint?
    a. Muzzle
    b. Towel
    c. Drugs
    d. Sandbags

664. Which of the following knots are used to secure the ends of two ropes together or to form a nonslipping noose?
    a. Square knot
    b. Nonslip knot
    c. Surgeon's knot
    d. Reefer's knot

665. Which of the following is a false statement?
    a. Use minimal restraint with a cat to start the procedure
    b. Treat all cats the same when it comes to handling
    c. Use distraction techniques when retraining cats
    d. Use towels to restrain cats, versus muzzles

666. All of the following procedures can be completed with a feline patient in sternal recumbency *except:*
    a. Administration of ophthalmic medications
    b. SQ injections
    c. Cystocentesis
    d. Cleaning ears

667. All of the following are signs of anxiety in a dog, *except:*
    a. Ears stand tall
    b. An averted gaze
    c. Raised hair along the back
    d. Tail straight out

668. _____ feet is known as the "kill zone" in cattle, when considering restraint.
    a. 2–4 feet
    b. 4–6 feet
    c. 6–8 feet
    d. 8–10 feet

669. What device is used to restrain cattle?
    a. Nose ring
    b. Nose lead
    c. Chute
    d. Halter

670. The "blind spot" for horses is:
    a. Between their eyes
    b. Below their noses
    c. To the left of their heads
    d. To the right of their heads

671. In which direction can a horse kick?
    a. Directly behind itself
    b. To the front of itself
    c. To its side
    d. All of the above

672. A horse's tail can indicate his/her attitude. What does a horse do with the tail when he/she has fear?
    a. Wringing or circling
    b. Held straight down
    c. Tightly clamped
    d. Held with an arch

673. What are the main tools of equine restraint?
    a. Halter
    b. Lead rope
    c. Nose twitch
    d. Only a and b

674. All of the following are distraction techniques for an equine patient, *except:*
    a. Rocking an ear
    b. Skin roll
    c. Hand twitch
    d. Tail jacking

675. A hurdle is used to capture:
    a. Sheep
    b. Cows
    c. Pigs
    d. Horses

ⓔ *Answers and rationales available on Evolve*
http://evolve.elsevier.com/Prendergast/QAvettech/

Diagnostic Imaging

Brooke Lockridge, RDMS

QUESTIONS

1. Which one of the following imaging modalities produces images without the use of radiation?
   a. X-ray
   b. Ultrasound
   c. Fluoroscopy
   d. CT

2. To obtain a radiographic image of both temporomandibular joints of a small animal, which of the following is the best position?
   a. Dorsal recumbency
   b. Ventral recumbency
   c. Right lateral recumbency
   d. Sternal recumbency

3. When obtaining a lateral projection of the skull of small animals, where should the centering of the image occur?
   a. Midway between the tip of the nose to just caudal to the occipital protuberance at the base
   b. Lateral canthus of the eye socket
   c. Between the eyes
   d. Above the base of the tongue and just below the palate, approximately at the commissure of the mouth

4. Which grade level on the ossification index for newborn foals does a closed metacarpal and metatarsal physes describe?
   a. Grade 1
   b. Grade 2
   c. Grade 3
   d. Grade 4

5. What element is found within the transducer of an ultrasound machine?
   a. Bucky
   b. Piezoelectric ceramics
   c. Magnets
   d. All of the above

6. To obtain a dorsoventral view of the abdomen of a rabbit, where should the center of the beam be focused?
   a. Center over the heart
   b. Center over the liver
   c. Center of the body cranial to caudal
   d. Center over the thoracolumbar area

7. What happens to crystals within the ultrasound transducer when strong, short electrical pulses strike them?
   a. They harden
   b. They melt
   c. They vibrate
   d. They break apart

8. What is the speed of sound through fat tissue?
   a. 330 m/s
   b. 600 m/s
   c. 1460 m/s
   d. 1480 m/s

9. At what age in foals does the closure of the proximal growth plate of P2 occur?
   a. 4–22 weeks
   b. 18–30 weeks
   c. 22–38 weeks
   d. 18–38 weeks

10. A deformity, in which the interior angle of the joint, viewed frontally, is <180 degrees, is known as what?
    a. Axial rotation
    b. Windswept
    c. Valgus deformity
    d. Varus deformity

11. Where should the cassette be held when obtaining a dorsomedial-palmarolateral oblique view of the carpus of a horse?
    a. Against the palmarolateral aspect of the leg
    b. Against the medial aspect of the leg
    c. Against the palmaromedial aspect of the leg
    d. Against the palmar aspect of the carpus

12. What is the speed of sound through bone?
    a. 330 m/s
    b. 600 m/s
    c. 1600 m/s
    d. 4080 m/s

13. Which of the following radiographic terms describes the caudal surface of the hind limb distal to the carpus?
    a. Plantar
    b. Dorsopalmar
    c. Palmar
    d. Caudocranial

14. Approximately how many shades of gray are incorporated into the display of an image obtained through ultrasound?
    a. 50 shades of gray
    b. 100 shades of gray
    c. 226 shades of gray
    d. 256 shades of gray

15. What is the correct definition of the abbreviation *B-mode* in ultrasound?
    a. Brightness
    b. Bits
    c. Binary
    d. Power mode

16. Which of the following best describes the use for Doppler ultrasound?
    a. Doppler uses a motion mode that simultaneously creates a B-mode image while displaying the motion of the tissues over a two-dimensional scale
    b. Doppler is used to image the flow of blood and other liquids as well as to measure their velocity
    c. Doppler units display the different shades of gray
    d. None of the above

17. When using color-flow Doppler in ultrasound, what do the displayed red and blue colors mean?
    a. Blue colors are veins, and red colors are arteries
    b. Blue colors are arteries, and red colors are veins
    c. The colors show blood flow; blue indicates flow away, and red indicates flow toward
    d. The colors show different velocities of blood

18. Which radiographic view provides the best accuracy for evaluating major fracture dislocation and conformational abnormalities in horses?
    a. Lateral view
    b. Medial oblique view
    c. The flexed lateral view
    d. Dorsopalmar view

19. What is the difference between color Doppler and power Doppler ultrasound?
    a. Color Doppler indicates velocity and power Doppler indicates direction of flow
    b. Power Doppler is sensitive to slow flow and color Doppler indicates direction of flow
    c. Power Doppler indicates direction of flow and color Doppler indicates slow flow
    d. Color Doppler indicates arteries and power Doppler indicates veins

20. Pulse wave imaging can detect velocities up to a maximum of _____ m/s.
    a. 0.5
    b. 1.0
    c. 1.4
    d. 2.2

21. Which of the following best describes the Nyquist point in ultrasound?
    a. The point at which the maximum blood velocity is reached
    b. The point of deepest penetration
    c. The point at which a drop-out signal is reached and an image is no longer produced
    d. The Nyquist point is not an ultrasound concern

22. Dental film should be placed in the mouth with the dimple facing:
    a. Up and pointing rostrally
    b. Up and pointing caudally
    c. Down and pointing rostrally
    d. Down and pointing caudally

23. Which of the following allows for measurements of very high blood flow velocities in ultrasound?
    a. Color Doppler
    b. PW Doppler
    c. CW Doppler
    d. Harmonics

24. What does the gain control knob adjust on the ultrasound machine?
    a. The power output
    b. The brightness of the image
    c. The PRF scale used in PW Doppler
    d. The depth of the image

25. What does the TGC or time gain compensation allow on the ultrasound machine?
    a. It allows the amount of time it takes sound to travel through a medium to be changed
    b. It provides a faster time frame for clearer images with motion
    c. It allows adjustment of the gain at various depths
    d. None of the above

26. Which of the following is the best view for judging a major fracture dislocation and conformational abnormalities?
    a. Lateral view
    b. Flexed lateral view
    c. Medial oblique
    d. Dorsopalmar view

27. What is the maximum number of focal points that are recommended for use in ultrasound?
    a. 2
    b. 3
    c. 4
    d. 5

28. Which of the following frequencies will allow for the deepest level of penetration in ultrasound?
    a. 4 MHz
    b. 5 MHz
    c. 9 MHz
    d. 12 MHz

29. The ability to distinguish between two objects that are adjacent to each other, yet perpendicular to the sound wave in ultrasound, is described as:
    a. Axial resolution
    b. Lateral resolution
    c. Longitudinal resolution
    d. Azimuthal resolution

30. To obtain a lateromedial view of the femorotibial joint of the horse, the cassette should be placed against which surface?
    a. Cranial aspect
    b. Caudal aspect
    c. Lateral aspect
    d. Medial aspect

31. Which of the following is the proper way to disinfect an ultrasound probe?
    a. Autoclave
    b. Gas sterilization
    c. Wipe with a glutaraldehyde-based disinfectant
    d. Immerse in an alcohol-based cleaner

32. Which of the following ultrasound artifacts will likely be produced when the sound wave strikes a metal object or a pocket of air?
    a. Edge shadowing
    b. Comet tail
    c. Mirror image
    d. Acoustic enhancement

33. Which of the following is the correct abbreviation to perform a *caudalocranial* radiograph?
    a. CdCr
    b. Dpa
    c. CrCd
    d. Cr

34. Which of the following is the correct definition for the ultrasound term *hypoechoic*?
    a. Bright gray
    b. Dark gray
    c. White
    d. Black

35. Which of the following can the piezoelectric crystal within an ultrasound probe do?
    a. Convert electrical energy into mechanical energy
    b. Convert mechanical energy into electrical energy
    c. Change shape in the presence of an electrical current
    d. All of the above

36. For a dorsolateral-palmaromedial oblique of the metacarpus of a horse, on which surface should the cassette be placed?
    a. The medial aspect
    b. The palmar aspect
    c. The palmaromedial aspect
    d. The palmarolateral aspect

37. Which of the following radiographic terms describes the view when the primary x-ray beam enters the dorsal surface and exits the ventral surface of the patient?
    a. Dorsoventral
    b. Ventrodorsal
    c. Craniocaudal
    d. Caudocranial

38. To obtain a craniocaudal view of the tibia of a small animal, that patient should be in which of the following positions?
    a. Sternal recumbency
    b. Dorsal recumbency
    c. Right lateral recumbency
    d. Left lateral recumbency

39. To perform an ultrasound in the intercostal region, which transducer would be ideal?
    a. Linear probe
    b. Microconvex probe
    c. Phase array probe
    d. All of the above produce the same images

40. When scanning in the sagittal plane, where is the cranial aspect of the patient's body displayed on the ultrasound monitor?
    a. Left side of the monitor
    b. Right side of the monitor
    c. Top of the monitor
    d. Bottom of the monitor

41. In the equation $Z = pV$ used in ultrasound, what does the letter Z represent?
    a. Density
    b. Acoustic velocity
    c. Acoustic impedance
    d. None of the above

42. What is the speed of sound through air?
    a. 330 m/s
    b. 600 m/s
    c. 1540 m/s
    d. 4080 m/s

43. When using a dental x-ray unit, the end of the cone should be positioned at _____ inches from the patient's anatomy.
    a. 2
    b. 4
    c. 6
    d. 10

44. Which of the following image receptors is used in dental imaging?
    a. Film
    b. Phosphor plates
    c. Neither
    d. Both

45. A biarticular fracture is also known as a:
    a. Corner fracture
    b. Slab fracture
    c. Chip fracture
    d. Biarticular fractures do not exist

46. What size of power outlet is required to run a digital dental unit?
    a. 70 kV
    b. 110 V
    c. 110 kV
    d. 8 mA

47. What is the purpose of the foil backing found on dental x-ray film?
    a. To absorb exiting remnant radiation
    b. To be able to mold to the shape of the tooth
    c. To create a waterproof barrier around the film
    d. None of the above

48. Which of the following is the correct order to process dental film?
    a. Passed through the developer, then the fixer, then the wash
    b. Passed through the fixer, wash, developer, then the wash again
    c. Passed through the developer, wash, fixer, then the wash again
    d. Passed through the wash, developer, fixer, and wash again

49. Which of the following radiographic terms describes the radiographic views distal to the carpus obtained by passing the primary x-ray beam from the dorsal direction to the palmar surface of the forelimb?
    a. Plantar
    b. Dorsopalmar
    c. Palmar
    d. Caudocranial

50. What is the typical kilovoltage preset on a dental unit?
    a. 110 kV
    b. 25 kV
    c. 50 kV
    d. 70 kV

51. Which of the following correctly describes a CT image?
    a. A two-dimensional image
    b. A matrix of pixel or picture elements
    c. A three-dimensional image
    d. A matrix of voxels
    e. Both c and d
    f. Both a and b

52. A computer tomography x-ray tube can rotate how many degrees?
    a. 270 degrees
    b. 180 degrees
    c. 360 degrees
    d. None, it does not rotate

53. When using computed tomography, what Hounsfield unit does blood have?
    a. −50 HU
    b. 160 HU
    c. 80 HU
    d. None of these

54. The number of detectors that are covered by the x-ray beam in CT scanning is known as which type of field of view?
    a. Display field of view
    b. Scan field of view
    c. Raw data
    d. Image data

55. Anything below what Hounsfield unit is displayed as black on CT imaging?
    a. −750 HU
    b. 0 HU
    c. 250 HU
    d. None; black is not displayed on CT

56. Which of the following Hounsfield units on CT imaging appears as white?
    a. −755 HU
    b. 120 HU
    c. 1200 HU
    d. 1260 HU

57. Modern CT scanners use multislice technology and are able to acquire image slices thinner than which of the following sizes?
    a. 10 mm
    b. 1 cm
    c. 10 cm
    d. 1 mm

58. What does the term *pitch* refer to in CT imaging?
    a. The calculation of an unknown value based on two known values on either side
    b. A ratio between the table movement in mm and the CT slice thickness
    c. A type of helical scanning
    d. None of the above

59. IV contrast used with CT imaging will help to view all of the following, *except:*
    a. Veins
    b. Arteries
    c. Bone marrow
    d. Infection of the extremities

60. When using the shaded-surface display process with CT, which Hounsfield units should be selected to view bone?
    a. −750 HU
    b. 160 HU
    c. −200 HU
    d. −800 HU

61. Which of the following best describes the term *fulcrum*?
    a. The point of interest
    b. The distortion of the resolution of anatomy above and below the region of interest
    c. A series of boxes or individual shades of information
    d. None of the above

62. Which of the following best describes the word *tomography*?
    a. Cut or section
    b. Whole
    c. Point of interest
    d. A series of boxes or individual shades of information

63. Which of the following imaging modalities can cause radiation burns if the unit is too close to the skin and remains in exposure mode for too long?
    a. CT
    b. MRI
    c. Fluoroscopy
    d. Ultrasound

64. What does the acronym ALARA stand for?
    a. As low as reasonably achievable
    b. Animal limited anatomical radiation assessment
    c. As large as radiation accepts
    d. None of the above

65. Atoms that emit particles and energy to become stable are known as:
    a. Photons
    b. Radionuclides
    c. Radioactive decay
    d. Isotopes

66. What is an isotope termed when it is radioactive?
    a. Photon
    b. Radionuclide
    c. Radioisotope
    d. None of the above; isotopes do not become radioactive

67. Which particles have high linear energy transfer (LET) with low penetrability?
    a. Alpha particles
    b. Beta particles
    c. Gamma particles
    d. Both a and b

68. Which of the following types of tissue absorb the most radiation?
    a. Bone
    b. Soft tissue
    c. Fat
    d. Bone, fat, and soft tissue absorb the same amount of radiation

69. For a mediolateral view of the tarsal joint of a horse, the cassette should be placed in which position?
    a. On the lateral surface
    b. On the medial surface
    c. On the plantar surface
    d. On the plantaromedial surface

70. Which of the following kV will produce more scatter and secondary radiation?
    a. 40 kV
    b. 60 kV
    c. 70 kV
    d. 110 kV

71. Which of the following is considered to be a cardinal rule for radiation protection?
    a. Distance
    b. Time
    c. Shielding
    d. All of the above

72. When obtaining a dorsopalmar view of the carpus of a horse, where should the cassette be held?
    a. Against the palmarolateral aspect of the leg
    b. Against the medial aspect of the leg
    c. Against the palmaromedial aspect of the leg
    d. Against the palmar aspect of the carpus

73. Which time frame is the most critical for limiting radiation exposure to an unborn fetus of an employee?
    a. 2nd trimester
    b. 3rd trimester
    c. Between 2 and 10 weeks gestation
    d. After 35 weeks

74. Which radiographic view provides the best option for detecting slab fractures in horses?
    a. Lateral view
    b. Medial oblique view
    c. Flexed lateral view
    d. Dorsopalmar view

75. *Meters to measure the rate of exposure* is also known as:
    a. Dosimeter
    b. Fluoroscopy
    c. Collimation
    d. Shielding

76. Which of the following is the best method for storing lead x-ray gowns?
    a. Folded and kept in a drawer to prevent overexposure
    b. Hung up by the shoulders when not in use
    c. Draped across the table with the tail end hanging off the side
    d. None of the above

77. Which of the following locations is best for storing a dosimeter badge?
    a. In the x-ray room
    b. At home with the employee
    c. In a box on a window sill to receive natural light
    d. In a dry, cool place away from the x-ray room

78. How often should x-ray equipment in a veterinarian's office be tested?
    a. Every 6 months
    b. Every year
    c. Every 2 years
    d. Only once when the equipment is installed

79. To what level of kV radiation are most lead aprons effective?
    a. 50 kV
    b. 70 kV
    c. 90 kV
    d. 125 kV

80. All of the following people are allowed to view individual dosimetry reports, *except:*
    a. OSHA inspector
    b. Owner of the practice
    c. Only the employee exposed
    d. All team members

81. Which of the following can occur if DNA is affected by radiation?
    a. Cell death
    b. Cell damage may be obvious, with portions of the DNA compromised
    c. Cell may display no immediate effects, but damage may have occurred internally that will affect the individual later, when mitosis occurs
    d. All of the above

82. Which imaging modality is superior for demonstrating the brain and spinal cord?
    a. Ultrasound
    b. MRI
    c. X-ray
    d. Fluoroscopy

83. What is a major safety concern with MRI machines?
    a. The amount of radiation emitted
    b. The intensity of the magnet on the patient
    c. The potential projectile effect with metallic objects within the vicinity of the machine
    d. MRI machines are extremely safe and contain no safety concerns

84. What is the term used to describe a medical magnet's field strength?
    a. Gauss
    b. Tesla
    c. Polarity
    d. Precession

85. Which type of magnet consists of two slabs of magnetic material facing each other?
    a. Permanent magnets
    b. Electromagnets
    c. Resistive magnets
    d. Superconducting magnets

86. Which of the following is the most common medical magnet?
    a. Resistive magnets
    b. Superconducting magnets
    c. Permanent magnets
    d. Electromagnets

87. Which of the following correctly defines the term *shims* in reference to MRI?
    a. Pieces or plates of metal used to correct the magnetic field within the magnet
    b. Coils or assemblies within the magnetic bore that enable the machine to create images in any plane
    c. Devices that receive radio-wave signals from a body part that is covered or contained by them
    d. None of the above

88. Which repetition time shows the T1 decay response of the tissues using MRI?
    a. 899 ms
    b. 1500 ms
    c. 546 ms
    d. 1680 ms

89. What does the MRI unit use to manipulate hydrogen atoms in and out of an excited energy state?
    a. Helium
    b. Water
    c. Radio waves
    d. Oxygen

90. In MRI what are the various shades of gray referred to as?
    a. Densities
    b. Signal intensities
    c. Hypoechoic
    d. Hyperechoic

91. How does cerebrospinal fluid appear on a true T1-weighted image of MRI?
    a. White
    b. Black
    c. Different shades of gray
    d. None of the above

92. What does MRI require to highlight injections, tumors, or vascular disease?
    a. Gadolinium
    b. Iodine contrast
    c. Barium
    d. None of the above

93. How is gadolinium that is used in MRI excreted from the body?
    a. Liver
    b. Kidneys
    c. Lungs
    d. GI tract

94. Which of the following radiographic terms describes the radiographic projection obtained by passing the primary x-ray beam from the caudal surface to the cranial surface of a structure?
    a. Plantar
    b. Dorsopalmar
    c. Palmar
    d. Caudocranial

95. MRI machines produce noise in which of the following ranges?
    a. 20–30 dB
    b. 40–50 dB
    c. 60–90 dB
    d. 100–110 dB

96. Which of the following factors should all personnel understand about MRI machines?
    a. No loose metallic objects can be near the machine
    b. It consists of a strong magnetic field
    c. The magnet is always on
    d. Every patient/employee should be screened for safety purposes
    e. All of the above

97. For a dorsopalmar view of the metacarpus of a horse, which surface should the cassette be on?
    a. The medial aspect
    b. The palmar aspect
    c. The palmaromedial aspect
    d. The palmarolateral aspect

98. In which imaging modality is Technetium 99m used?
    a. MRI
    b. Ultrasound
    c. Nuclear medicine
    d. Fluoroscopy

99. Which of the following is the best view for detecting distal corner fractures?
    a. Lateral view
    b. Flexed lateral view
    c. Medial oblique
    d. Dorsopalmar view

100. The amount of radioisotope used for each examination in a nuclear medicine study is measured in which of the following units?
    a. kV
    b. mAS
    c. mCi
    d. MHz

101. What is the term used to describe an area that indicates higher radiation has been emitted in nuclear medicine?
    a. Cold spot
    b. Hot spot
    c. Gamma photon burst
    d. None of the above

102. In dental radiographs, periapical disease appears as a:
    a. Radiopaque area around the apex of the tooth
    b. Radiolucent area around the apex of the tooth
    c. Radiopaque area inside the tooth pulp
    d. Radiolucent area inside the tooth pulp

103. When does the soft tissue phase occur in nuclear medicine?
    a. 5–10 minutes after injection
    b. Immediately during injection
    c. 2–3 hours after injection
    d. 48 hours after injection

104. What does the color blue indicate on a nuclear medicine study?
    a. High activity
    b. Low activity
    c. No activity
    d. Normal anatomy

105. Which of the following is the correct abbreviation to perform a *dorsopalmar* radiograph?
    a. CdCr
    b. Dpa
    c. CrCd
    d. Cr

106. What is the half-life of the radioisotope Technetium Tc 99m used in nuclear medicine studies?
    a. 1 hour
    b. 6 hours
    c. 24 hours
    d. 48 hours

107. Which parts of a patient's body are considered radioactive after they have received the radioisotope?
    a. Skin
    b. Hair
    c. Waste products
    d. All of the above

108. Which of the following PPE must the handler wear when a patient is considered radioactive?
    a. Lab coat only
    b. Lab coat and gloves
    c. Lab coat, gloves, and disposable boots
    d. Lab coat, gloves, disposable boots, and a dosimeter badge

109. Radiographic projections are named according to which of the following?
    a. The direction in which the central beam anatomically enters the body parts, followed by the area of exit of the x-ray beam
    b. The direction in which the central beam anatomically leaves the body parts, followed by the area of entrance of the x-ray beam
    c. The side of the patient to which the film is closest, followed by the exposed side
    d. Radiation that bounces off objects

110. The term *ventral recumbency* refers to the patient lying on the _____.
    a. Back
    b. Abdomen
    c. Right side
    d. Left side

111. The abbreviation *Cd* in x-ray positioning refers to which of the following?
    a. Cranial
    b. Caudal
    c. Ventral
    d. Palmar

112. The term *proximal* refers to which of the following abbreviations?
    a. Pa
    b. Pr
    c. Pl
    d. Di

113. The abbreviation *CrCd* refers to which of the following?
   a. Craniocaudal
   b. Mediolateral
   c. Dorsopalmar
   d. Dorsoplantar

114. Which of the following radiographic terms describes the view when the primary x-ray beam enters the cranial surface and exits the caudal surface of the patient?
   a. Dorsoventral
   b. Ventrodorsal
   c. Craniocaudal
   d. Caudocranial

115. The term *oblique* is generally used in reference to which of the following?
   a. Abdomen
   b. Spine
   c. Limbs
   d. Head

116. The term *rostral* refers to toward the _____.
   a. Head
   b. Nose
   c. Tail
   d. Middle

117. The median plane divides the body into which of the following?
   a. Left/right portions
   b. Anterior/posterior portions
   c. Cranial/caudal portions
   d. None of the above

118. When a patient is receiving an x-ray and is in the right lateral recumbent position, what marker should be used to denote the correct side?
   a. Left
   b. Right
   c. Front
   d. Hind

119. When viewing a lateral radiograph, the cranial part of the animal is in which direction in relation to the illuminator?
   a. To the left
   b. To the right
   c. To the top
   d. To the bottom

120. The area of interest when obtaining an x-ray should be closest to what?
   a. The end of the table
   b. The back of the table
   c. The image receptor
   d. The restrainer

121. For a lateromedial view of the metacarpus of a horse, which surface should the cassette be on?
   a. The medial aspect
   b. The palmar aspect
   c. The palmaromedial aspect
   d. The palmarolateral aspect

122. What does it mean to collimate the x-ray beam?
   a. To use the highest kV possible
   b. To limit the beam exposure just to the area of interest within the film
   c. To allow for full exposure of the entire film
   d. None of the above

123. Which of the following will help prevent motion artifacts?
   a. Low milliamperage
   b. High milliamperage
   c. Higher kVp
   d. Lower kVp

124. For a dorsoplantar view of the tarsal joint of a horse, the cassette should be placed in which position?
   a. On the lateral surface
   b. On the medial surface
   c. On the plantar surface
   d. On the plantaromedial surface

125. When obtaining an x-ray of a vomiting patient, which position is ideal?
   a. Right lateral recumbency
   b. Left lateral recumbency
   c. Dorsal/ventral
   d. Ventral/dorsal

126. Which of the following are ways to determine if the animal is properly positioned in the lateral view?
   a. Coxofemoral joints are superimposed
   b. Intervertebral foramina are different sizes
   c. Rib heads are perpendicular
   d. Transverse processes are perpendicular at the origin from the vertebral bodies

127. Which of the following are ways to determine whether the animal is properly positioned in the ventrodorsal view?
    a. Rib and abdominal symmetry
    b. Wings of the ilium are symmetrical
    c. Coxofemoral joints are superimposed
    d. Rib heads are superimposed
    e. Both a and b
    f. Both c and d

128. When obtaining a foramen magnum projection of the skulls of small animals, where should the centering of the image occur?
    a. Midway between the tip of the nose to just caudal to the occipital protuberance at the base
    b. Lateral canthus of the eye socket
    c. Between the eyes
    d. Above the base of the tongue and just below the palate, approximately at the commissure of the mouth

129. All of the following organs are normally seen on a radiograph, *except:*
    a. Liver
    b. Kidney
    c. Pancreas
    d. Bladder

130. All of the following organs are seen on ultrasound, *except:*
    a. Lungs
    b. Adrenal glands
    c. Pancreas
    d. Gallbladder

131. In a dorsoventral view on a small animal x-ray, which organ appears in the shape of a question mark?
    a. Colon
    b. Spleen
    c. Right kidney
    d. Diaphragm

132. When viewing a radiograph, which organ lies in the cranial abdomen between the diaphragm and stomach in small animals?
    a. Adrenal glands
    b. Pancreas
    c. Liver
    d. Spleen

133. When do fetal skeletons of small animals become visible on x-ray?
    a. 20–25 days
    b. 42–45 days
    c. 55–60 days
    d. 65–70 days

134. If pneumonia is suspected in small animals, which of the following radiographic views should be performed?
    a. Both lateral views
    b. Dorsoventral view
    c. Both lateral views and ventrodorsal view
    d. Right lateral and dorsoventral views

135. Which of the following could cause a false diagnosis of a pneumothorax on a radiograph?
    a. Underexposure of film
    b. Overexposure of film
    c. Panting
    d. Motion artifacts

136. Which radiographic view is best suggested for imaging the lungs?
    a. Right lateral
    b. Left lateral
    c. VD
    d. DV

137. What is the maximum permissible dose of radiation a person can receive per year?
    a. 1000 millirems/yr
    b. 2000 millirems/yr
    c. 2500 millirems/yr
    d. 5000 millirems/yr

138. How long should veterinary facilities maintain dosimetry reports?
    a. 5 years
    b. 20 years
    c. 30 years
    d. 1 year following separation of an employee

139. What is the best exposure time for a thoracic radiograph?
    a. At any point during the respiratory cycle
    b. At maximum inspiration
    c. At maximum expiration
    d. While the patient is panting

140. Before taking a radiograph of a patient, what is the proper way to obtain a measurement of the area of interest?
    a. With the patient standing
    b. When the patient is in the position in which it is to be x-rayed
    c. When the thinnest part is targeted
    d. With the patient lying in the dorsal recumbent position

141. When obtaining a caudocranial view of the scapula of a small animal, where should the central ray be located?
    a. Center of the scapula
    b. Center of the humerus
    c. At the level of the eighth rib
    d. At the first thoracic vertebral body

142. The only dental radiographic view that can be made with a true parallel technique is:
    a. Rostral maxillary
    b. Parallel mandibular view
    c. Rostral mandibular view
    d. Parallel oblique view

143. When obtaining a caudocranial view of the humerus of a small animal, in which position should the animal be?
    a. Ventral recumbency
    b. Left lateral recumbency
    c. Dorsal recumbency
    d. Right lateral recumbency

144. If the mA or exposure time is doubled, what happens to the film density?
    a. It is halved
    b. It is doubled
    c. It stays the same
    d. It is unrelated to the mA or exposure time

145. What does the milliamperage control on the x-ray machine affect?
    a. The amount of radiation that is produced
    b. The amount of incoming voltage
    c. The current to the cathode
    d. Both a and c

146. The degree of blackness on a radiograph is described as:
    a. Radiographic density
    b. Radiographic contrast
    c. Focal-film distance
    d. Radiographic fogging

147. What occurs when the object is not parallel to the recording surface of an x-ray?
    a. Distortion
    b. Penumbra
    c. Foreshortening
    d. Fogging

148. When an x-ray photon strikes an object, which of the following can occur?
    a. The object rejects the photon
    b. The photon penetrates the object
    c. The photon reduces scatter radiation
    d. X-ray photons do not leave the housing unit

149. Scatter radiation has a _____ wavelength than the primary beam used in an x-ray.
    a. Shorter
    b. Longer
    c. Wider
    d. Thinner

150. What is the typical wavelength of a medical x-ray?
    a. 0.05–0.01 mm
    b. 0.05–0.01 m
    c. 0.05–0.01 nm
    d. 0.05–0.01 dm

151. Lead shutters installed in the tube head of the x-ray machine are referred to as:
    a. Filters
    b. Diaphragms
    c. Cones
    d. Collimators

152. When obtaining a view of the tympanic bullae of small animals, where should the centering of the image occur?
    a. Midway between the tip of the nose to just caudal to the occipital protuberance at the base
    b. Lateral canthus of the eye socket
    c. Between the eyes
    d. Above the base of the tongue and just below the palate, approximately at the commissure of the mouth

153. For what are grids used on an x-ray machine?
    a. To decrease scatter radiation and to increase the contrast on the radiograph
    b. To absorb the less penetrating x-rays as they leave the tube head
    c. To restrict the primary beam to the size of the cone used
    d. The limit the size of the primary beam to the size of the diaphragm used

154. When obtaining a dorsolateral-palmaromedial oblique view of the carpus of a horse, where should the cassette be held?
    a. Against the palmarolateral aspect of the leg
    b. Against the medial aspect of the leg
    c. Against the palmaromedial aspect of the leg
    d. Against the palmar aspect of the carpus

155. A grid is a series of thin, linear strips made of alternating radiodense and radiolucent material. Of what are the radiodense strips made?
    a. Aluminum
    b. Fiber
    c. Lead
    d. Plastic

156. Where is the grid located in reference to an x-ray machine?
    a. Below the cassette
    b. Between the patient and the cassette
    c. On top of the patient
    d. Within the housing unit

157. Which of the following causes a black irregular border on one end of the film?
    a. Rough handling of the film before exposure
    b. Expired film
    c. Light exposure while still in the box in advance of exposure
    d. Exposure to radiation while still in storage

158. Which of the following will cause a fogged film?
    a. Chemical spills on the screen
    b. Exposure resulting from static electricity
    c. Exposure to excessive scatter radiation
    d. Foreign materials between the film and the screen

159. What causes grid lines on the entire film?
    a. Patient motion
    b. Poor film-screen contact
    c. Grid not being centered with the primary beam
    d. Focal-film distance not being in the range of the grid's focus

160. What is the correct temperature for an automatic processor tank that is used to develop x-ray film?
    a. 35° C
    b. 95° F
    c. 68° F
    d. Both a and b
    e. Both a and c

161. Decreased radiographic density with poor contrast results from which of the following?
    a. The film was overdeveloped
    b. The film was overexposed
    c. The film was underexposed
    d. The film was developed in chemicals that were too hot

162. To obtain a whole body view of the abdomen of a rabbit, where should the center of the beam be focused?
    a. Center over the heart
    b. Center over the liver
    c. Center of the body cranial to caudal
    d. Center over the thoracolumbar area

163. To obtain a mediolateral view of the brachioantebrachial joint of a horse, how should the leg be positioned?
    a. Adducted
    b. Abducted
    c. Extended cranially
    d. Extended caudally

164. To obtain a lateral view of the tibia of a small animal, the patient should be in which of the following positions?
    a. Sternal recumbency
    b. Right lateral recumbency
    c. Left lateral recumbency
    d. Both b and c

165. Which of the following is the best view of the carpal joint for detecting slab fractures?
    a. Lateral view
    b. Flexed lateral view
    c. Medial oblique
    d. Dorsopalmar view

166. Which of the following conditions results from uneven development of film?
    a. Uneven chemical levels
    b. Low-grade light leak in the darkroom
    c. Film developed in chemicals that are too cold
    d. Underexposed film

167. Which of the following causes the entire film to be clear?
    a. Final wash was conducted improperly
    b. There was no exposure
    c. The film was placed in the fixer before the developer
    d. Both b and c

168. When obtaining a lateral view of the cervical vertebrae of a small animal, which of the following techniques should *not* be performed?
    a. Overextend the limbs caudally
    b. Place a pad beneath the mandible to superimpose the wings of the atlas
    c. Place a pad under the neck to prevent sagging of the spine
    d. Place the wings of the atlas and center of the spine of the scapula in the longitudinal center of the primary beam

169. What is the topographic radiographic landmark for the caudal cervical vertebrae?
    a. Base of the skull
    b. Center of the spine of the scapula
    c. At the C4 level
    d. At the T4 level

170. What is the cranial landmark for an x-ray of the thoracic vertebrae in the lateral position?
    a. The base of the skull
    b. Halfway between the xiphoid process and the last rib
    c. Spine of the scapula
    d. Wings of the ilium

171. When obtaining a radiograph of the thoracic vertebrae, what level should be measured for the kVp setting?
    a. The cranial end of the thoracic vertebrae
    b. The caudal end of the thoracic vertebrae
    c. The lowest point of the thorax
    d. The highest point of the thorax

172. Which of the following is the correct abbreviation to perform a *cranial* radiograph?
    a. CdCr
    b. Dpa
    c. CrCd
    d. Cr

173. When imaging the lumbosacral vertebrae in the lateral position, which of the following should be done to ensure proper exposure?
    a. Decrease the kVp
    b. Increase the kVp
    c. Increase the mAs
    d. Decrease the mAs

174. To obtain a dorsopalmar x-ray of the metacarpus and digits, in which position should the patient be?
    a. Right lateral recumbency
    b. Left lateral recumbency
    c. Sternal recumbency
    d. Dorsal recumbency

175. When obtaining a ventrodorsal x-ray of the thorax, what is the cranial landmark?
    a. The base of the skull
    b. The manubrium
    c. Halfway between the xiphoid and the last rib
    d. The ilium wings

176. What is the caudal landmark for obtaining an abdominal x-ray in the lateral position?
    a. Three rib spaces cranial to the xiphoid
    b. Greater trochanter of the femur
    c. The ilium wings
    d. The manubrium

177. Which of the following is the best technique to consider for an abdominal x-ray?
    a. Peak inspiration
    b. Peak expiration
    c. Panting
    d. Consideration of breathing techniques is not necessary for abdominal x-rays

178. What caudal landmark is used when obtaining a lateral x-ray of the pelvis?
    a. Border of the ischium
    b. Wings of the ilium
    c. The xiphoid process
    d. The greater trochanter of the femur

179. Which of the following radiographic terms describes the view when the primary x-ray beam enters the caudal surface and exits the cranial surface of the patient?
    a. Dorsoventral
    b. Ventrodorsal
    c. Craniocaudal
    d. Caudocranial

180. When obtaining a caudocranial x-ray of the stifle joint, what should be palpated to determine the amount of rotation necessary for an exact caudocranial projection?
    a. The greater trochanter of the femur
    b. The tibial tuberosity
    c. The patella
    d. The manubrium

181. Which of the following terms is used to describe the white appearance on an x-ray?
    a. Radiolucent
    b. Radiopaque
    c. Hyperechoic
    d. Hypoechoic

182. You are looking at your dental radiograph and notice that the tooth is elongated. This happened because the beam was perpendicular to the:
    a. Film
    b. Tooth
    c. Bisecting angle
    d. Wrong tooth

183. Which contrast is commonly used for GI studies when perforation is *not* suspected?
    a. Barium sulfate
    b. Meglumine diatrizoate
    c. Sodium diatrizoate
    d. Betadine

184. How long does it take for barium sulfate to travel from the stomach to the colon?
    a. 30 minutes
    b. 1 hour
    c. 2 hours
    d. 3 hours

185. Which of the following is not a form of barium sulfate that can be administered to patients?
    a. Powder
    b. Colloid suspension
    c. Pastes
    d. Injectable

186. Which of the following could be considered as negative-contrast agents used in radiography?
    a. Oxygen
    b. Air
    c. Carbon dioxide
    d. All of the above
    e. b and c only

187. In which of the following circumstances should water-soluble organic iodides be avoided?
    a. Suspected bowel perforation
    b. Dehydrated patients
    c. Overhydrated patients
    d. Kidney failure

188. Exposing a reptile to cool conditions, such as a cool metal surface, will cause what?
    a. Temporary lethargy and immobility
    b. Temporary excitement
    c. Rapid breathing
    d. Aggressiveness

189. For a dorsolateral-plantaromedial oblique view of the tarsal joint of a horse, the cassette should be placed in which position?
    a. On the lateral surface
    b. On the medial surface
    c. On the plantar surface
    d. On the plantaromedial surface

190. When positioning a lizard in right lateral recumbency before taking an x-ray, the left limbs are always _____ to the right limbs.
    a. Cranial
    b. Caudal
    c. Lateral
    d. Medial

191. During an x-ray, a tabletop technique is most commonly used for exotic companion animals, except when the species' girth exceeds which diameter?
    a. 2–5 cm
    b. 5–10 cm
    c. 10–12 cm
    d. 12–15 cm

192. When using a Plexiglas tube to obtain an x-ray, which of the following should be adjusted?
    a. The mAs should be increased
    b. The mAs should be decreased
    c. The kVp should be increased
    d. The kVp should be decreased

193. Which of the following is *not* considered a physical restraint?
    a. Tape
    b. Radiolucent Plexiglas
    c. Gloved hands
    d. Foam pads

194. Which of the following contains a filament consisting of a tightly coiled tungsten wire and is the site of electron generation in the x-ray tube?
    a. Anode
    b. Cathode
    c. B-mode
    d. Transducer

195. What is the amount used to express the dose equivalent that results from exposure to ionizing radiation known as?
    a. REM
    b. ALARA
    c. MPD
    d. Sv

196. The protective lead equipment required for wear during x-ray exposure can decrease the primary beam exposure by how much?
    a. 15%
    b. 25%
    c. 50%
    d. 100%

197. Film badges, TLDs, and OSL badges contain 3–4 elements for filtration. Which element monitors the highest level of exposure to radiation?
    a. Open window
    b. Plastic
    c. Aluminum
    d. Copper

198. Which type of monitoring badge is the most common method of monitoring ionizing radiation?
    a. Thermoluminescent dosimeters
    b. Film badges
    c. Optically stimulated luminescence badges
    d. Ion chambers

199. Digital radiography, CT, MRI, and ultrasound are stored using a universally accepted format known as?
    a. CCD
    b. DICOM
    c. MOD
    d. PACS

200. When obtaining a lateromedial view of the carpus of a horse, where should the cassette be held?
    a. Against the palmarolateral aspect of the leg
    b. Against the medial aspect of the leg
    c. Against the palmaromedial aspect of the leg
    d. Against the palmar aspect of the carpus

201. To obtain a flexed lateromedial view of the carpus of a horse, the limb should be flexed approximately how many degrees?
    a. 15 degrees
    b. 30 degrees
    c. 60 degrees
    d. 90 degrees

202. For standard radiographs of the tarsus of a horse, which of the following is the correct weight distribution?
    a. The affected limb should be suspended with no weight on it for the duration of the x-ray
    b. There should be 25% weight bearing on the affected limb
    c. There should be 50% weight bearing on the affected limb
    d. The weight should be evenly distributed on all four legs

203. For a lateromedial view of the tarsal joint of a horse, the cassette should be placed in which position?
    a. On the lateral surface
    b. On the medial surface
    c. On the plantar surface
    d. On the plantaromedial surface

204. To obtain a flexed dorsoplantar radiographic view of the tarsal joint of a horse, at what angle should the primary beam direction be?
    a. 15 degrees
    b. 45 degrees
    c. 60 degrees
    d. 90 degrees

205. For a standard radiograph of the metacarpus of a horse, the limb of interest should be in which position compared to the ground?
    a. Parallel
    b. Perpendicular
    c. At 45 degrees
    d. At 60 degrees

206. All of the following statements are true, *except:*
    a. Only personnel necessary to complete the procedure should be in the x-ray room at the time of exposure
    b. Persons younger than 18 years and pregnant women must not be in the x-ray room during the examination
    c. Personnel who assist with radiographic examinations should have a rotating duty roster to minimize exposure to any one person
    d. Sandbags, sponges, tape, or other restraining devices should not be used for positioning the patient rather than manual restraint

207. To obtain a dorsopalmar view of the fetlock joint of a horse, the primary beam needs to be angled _____ degrees proximal to distal.
    a. 10
    b. 20
    c. 45
    d. 60

208. To obtain a dorsopalmar view of the interphalangeal joint, what should the primary beam angle be proximal to distal?
    a. 15–20 degrees
    b. 30–45 degrees
    c. 45–60 degrees
    d. 90 degrees

209. Before imaging the coffin bone in horses, which of the following tasks should be performed in preparation?
    a. Hoof should be trimmed to the new sole level
    b. The horseshoes need to be removed
    c. The sulcus should be packed with radiolucent material
    d. All of the above

210. To obtain a caudocranial view of the femorotibial joint of the horse, the cassette should be placed against which surface?
    a. Cranial aspect
    b. Caudal aspect
    c. Lateral aspect
    d. Medial aspect

211. To obtain a craniocaudal view of the brachioantebrachial joint of a horse, how should the leg be positioned?
    a. Adducted
    b. Abducted
    c. Extended cranially
    d. Extended caudally

212. To obtain a caudocranial view of the tibia of a small animal, the patient should be in which of the following positions?
    a. Sternal recumbency
    b. Dorsal recumbency
    c. Right lateral recumbency
    d. Left lateral recumbency

213. To obtain a dorsoventral view of the thorax of a rabbit, where should the center of the beam be focused?
    a. Centered over the heart
    b. Centered over the liver
    c. Center of the body cranial to caudal
    d. Centered over the thoracolumbar area

214. Which of the following is the best restraint to use in avian radiography?
    a. Manual restraint
    b. Physical restraint
    c. Chemical restraint
    d. None; birds should not be restrained for x-rays

215. Which should be avoided when manually restraining a bird?
    a. Grasping the patient around the neck
    b. Grasped by the mandibular articulation
    c. Grasping the feet and gently stretching the bird
    d. All of the above should be avoided

216. For a lateral avian view, where would the left wings and limbs be positioned?
    a. Cranially to the right wings and limbs
    b. Caudally to the right wings and limbs
    c. Lateral to the right wings and limbs
    d. Superimposed to the right wings and limbs

217. For a ventrodorsal avian radiographic view, the keel should be in which position related to the spine?
    a. Superimposed
    b. Lateral
    c. Caudal
    d. Cranial

218. For larger species of birds, which technique can be used to obtain a craniocaudal appendicular skeletal radiograph?
    a. Tape the limb to a Plexiglas plate
    b. Tape the limb directly on the cassette
    c. Use a gloved hand placed behind the hock to restrain the limb for exposure
    d. Both a and c

219. When restraining a sedated bird for a lateral x-ray, where should the wings be properly taped?
    a. On the most distal end
    b. Across the humerus
    c. Across the radius-ulna
    d. The wings should not be taped

220. For an avian lateral view, where should the dependent limb be placed compared to the contralateral limb?
    a. Lateral
    b. Medial
    c. Superimposed
    d. Cranial

221. For smaller-sized patients, which radiographic technique is preferred?
    a. Grid technique
    b. Lower mA
    c. Tabletop technique
    d. Higher kVp

222. When obtaining a dorsoventral view of the whole body of a rodent, how should the front legs be positioned?
    a. Extended caudally
    b. Extended cranially
    c. Superimposed
    d. Abducted from the body

223. What is an essential factor when using a nonscreen film to x-ray a snake?
    a. The snake needs to move continuously across the film
    b. Movement needs to be minimal
    c. The snake needs to be short and thin
    d. Nonscreen films should never be used to x-ray a snake

224. For digital radiography, what does the postprocessing step of image manipulation allow?
    a. Magnification
    b. Rotation
    c. Contrast adjustment
    d. All of the above
    e. a and b only

225. Which of the following is *not* an advantage of digital x-ray versus analog x-ray?
    a. Elimination of the darkroom
    b. Image postprocessing
    c. Elimination of damaging radiation
    d. Exposure latitude and contrast optimization

226. A feature of digital radiography that is related to the bit depth of each pixel and the software that accompanies the digital-imaging system is referred to as which of the following?
    a. Spatial resolution
    b. Contrast optimization
    c. Dynamic range
    d. Exposure latitude

227. What is a concern of *exposure creep* with the use of digital x-rays?
    a. Underexposed x-ray
    b. Unnecessary patient and personnel exposure because of ionizing radiation
    c. Excessive film blackening
    d. Exposure creep is only an issue in analog x-rays

228. Horses have approximately how many carpal bones?
    a. 4
    b. 5
    c. 6
    d. 7

229. Which radiographic view of the carpal joint of a horse provides the best view to judge the width of the cartilage spaces?
    a. Lateral
    b. Dorsopalmar
    c. Medial oblique
    d. Flexed lateral

230. Which of the following is the best view for assessing the distal radial growth plate for closure in horses?
    a. Lateral view
    b. Flexed lateral view
    c. Medial oblique
    d. Dorsopalmar view

231. How does the adjacent bone density appear in fresh carpal chips in horses?
    a. Decreased
    b. Increased
    c. Normal

232. Which of the following does *not* describe an old carpal chip seen on x-ray in horses?
    a. Sharp fragment margination
    b. Decreased adjacent bone density
    c. Presence of osteoarthritis
    d. Normal or cool surrounding tissue

233. Which of the following is the most serious of all carpal fractures seen in horses?
    a. Corner fracture
    b. Slab fracture
    c. Chip fracture
    d. All chip fractures are equal in severity

234. Which radiographic view provides the best accuracy for detecting carpal fractures in horses?
    a. Lateral view
    b. Medial oblique view
    c. Flexed lateral view
    d. Dorsopalmar view

235. Which of the following is *not* a radiographic characteristic of the bones of a newborn foal?
    a. Smooth
    b. Fused
    c. Round
    d. Wider joint spaces

236. At what age does the first radiographic appearance of the crena seen in foals occur?
    a. 18–38 weeks
    b. 22–38 weeks
    c. 4–22 weeks
    d. 0–4 weeks

237. Which of the following is *not* considered a key radiographic feature of carpal or tarsal bone immaturity?
    a. Increased calcification
    b. Increased number of visible vascular canals causing increased porosity
    c. Abnormally tapered profile
    d. One or more fringed margins

238. A deformity in which the interior angle of the joint, viewed frontally, is greater than 180 degrees is known as what?
    a. Axial rotation
    b. Windswept
    c. Valgus deformity
    d. Varus deformity

239. An unossified carpal or tarsal bone describes which grade level on the ossification index for newborn foals?
    a. Grade 1
    b. Grade 2
    c. Grade 3
    d. Grade 4

240. Which of the following is the correct abbreviation indicating performance of a *craniocaudal* radiograph?
    a. CdCr
    b. Dpa
    c. CrCd
    d. Cr

241. Which of the following radiographic terms describes the caudal surface of the forelimb distal to the carpus?
    a. Plantar
    b. Dorsopalmar
    c. Palmar
    d. Caudocranial

242. Which of the following radiographic terms describes the view when the primary x-ray beam enters the ventral surface and exits the dorsal surface of the patient?
    a. Dorsoventral
    b. Ventrodorsal
    c. Craniocaudal
    d. Caudocranial

243. Radiographs of long bones must include which of the following?
    a. The joint proximal to the long bone
    b. The joint distal to the long bone
    c. Both the joint proximal and the joint distal to the long bone
    d. The long bone only, excluding joints proximal and distal

244. Radiographs of joints must include which of the following?
    a. The bones proximal to the joint
    b. The bones distal to the joint
    c. Only the joint needs to be imaged, excluding any surrounding bones
    d. ⅓ of the bones proximal and distal to the joint

245. Films that are properly collimated will have which of the following appearances?
    a. Black, fully exposed edges of the film of a finished radiograph
    b. Clear, unexposed areas on all four edges of the film of a finished radiograph
    c. Clear, unexposed areas of the 2 long edges of a finished radiograph
    d. Clear, unexposed areas of the 2 short edges of a finished radiograph

246. When using a V-trough to aid in obtaining a radiograph, what needs to be measured before taking the x-ray?
    a. The thinnest portion of the body to be radiographed
    b. The thickest portion of the body to be radiographed
    c. The V-trough only
    d. The V-trough and the thickest portion of the body to be measured

247. When obtaining a radiograph, the thickest part of the area of interest is placed toward what?
    a. The anode end of the x-ray tube
    b. The cathode end of the x-ray tube
    c. The center of the x-ray beam
    d. Closest to the radiographer

248. To decrease magnification of an x-ray, which of the following would help?
    a. Patients are positioned as close to the x-ray cassette as possible
    b. Patients are positioned are far away from the x-ray cassette as possible
    c. There should be as much collimation as possible
    d. There should be as little collimation as possible

249. When capturing analog radiographs, which of the following descriptions refers to "splitting the plate"?
    a. Creating a smaller x-ray cassette to use for small patients
    b. Using a lead shield on half of the film to prevent exposure and to allow for 2 views to be obtained on the same film.
    c. Collimating the beam to accommodate for small patients on a large cassette
    d. Combining two small cassettes to accommodate a larger patient

250. What view is required for the evaluation of the nasal passages of small animals?
    a. Dorsoventral view
    b. Lateral view
    c. Rostrocaudal view
    d. Open-mouth view
    e. All of the above
    f. a and b only

251. What is the correct place of measurement for radiographs of the nasal passages of small animals?
    a. The most rostral end of the cranium
    b. The most caudal end of the cranium
    c. Slightly rostral to the widest area of the cranium
    d. At the widest portion of the cranium

252. When obtaining a VD projection of the skull of small animals, where should the centering of the image occur?
    a. Midway between the tip of the nose and just caudal to the occipital protuberance at the base
    b. Lateral canthus of the eye socket
    c. Between the eyes
    d. Above the base of the tongue and just below the palate, approximately at the commissure of the mouth

253. To obtain a radiographic image of the right temporomandibular joint of a small animal, which of the following is the best position?
    a. Dorsal recumbency
    b. Ventral recumbency
    c. Right lateral recumbency
    d. Left lateral recumbency

254. To obtain a radiograph of the VD extended hip projection, where is the center of the beam focused?
    a. Greater trochanter of femur
    b. Midline between the left and right ischial tuberosity
    c. At the level of the 7th vertebrae
    d. At the midfemur

255. To obtain a lateral projection of the pelvis, which area should be used for measurement?
    a. At the highest level of the trochanter
    b. The thickest part of the pelvis
    c. The thinnest part of the pelvis
    d. The level of the 7th vertebrae

256. To obtain a radiograph of the CdCr projection of the scapula of a small animal, which of the following is the correct position for the patient?
    a. Sternal recumbency
    b. Lateral recumbency
    c. Dorsal recumbency
    d. Standing

257. To obtain a CdCr projection of the humerus of small animals, where should the measurement be taken?
    a. Measure from the table to the midshaft humerus
    b. Measure the thickest part of the humerus
    c. Measure on the dorsal side from the table to the height of the scapula
    d. Measure the midshaft humerus

258. To obtain a flexed lateral projection of the carpus of small animals, where should the measurement be taken?
    a. Caudal to the carpal joint
    b. The thickest part of the flexed joint
    c. Thickest part of the nonflexed joint
    d. Cranial to the carpal joint

259. The bisecting angle principle states that the plane of an x-ray beam should be 90 degrees to the:
    a. Long axis of the tooth
    b. Plane of the film
    c. Imaginary line that bisects the angle formed by the tooth's long axis and the film plane
    d. Imaginary line that bisects the angle formed by the animal's head and the film plane

260. All of the following are components of the x-ray tube, *except:*
    a. Cathode
    b. Anode
    c. Grid
    d. Tungsten filament

261. With film-based imaging, which of the following are receptor components?
    a. Intensifying screen
    b. Cassette
    c. Film
    d. All of the above

Ⓔ *Answers and rationales available on Evolve*
http://evolve.elsevier.com/Prendergast/QAvettech/

Jody Nugent-Deal, RVT, VTS (Anesthesia, Clinical Practice—Exotic Companion Animal), Mary Ellen Goldberg, BS, LVT, CVT, SRA, CCRA, and Tasha McNerney, BS, CVT

QUESTIONS

1. Which of the following statements define regional anesthesia?
   a. Loss of sensation in a limited area of the body produced by administration of a local anesthetic or other agent in proximity to sensory nerves
   b. Loss of sensation in a small area of the body produced by administration of a local anesthetic agent in proximity to the area of interest
   c. Loss of sensation of a localized area produced by administration of a local anesthetic directly to a body surface or to a surgical or traumatic wound
   d. A drug-induced sleeplike state that impairs the ability of the patient to respond appropriately to stimuli

2. If an oxygen flowmeter uses a ball for oxygen readings, where is the reading taken from to determine flow of oxygen in the system?
   a. The top of the ball
   b. The center of the ball
   c. The bottom of the ball
   d. None of the above

3. Which of the following statements defines balanced anesthesia?
   a. The administration of two or more agents in equal volume
   b. Administration of multiple drugs concurrently in smaller quantities than would be required if each were administered alone
   c. General anesthesia in which the patient's physiological status remains stable
   d. The administration of a local and general anesthetic concurrently

4. Which of the following terms refers to a loss of sensation in a small area of the body produced by administration of a local anesthetic?
   a. Sedation
   b. General anesthesia
   c. Surgical anesthesia
   d. Local anesthesia

5. Which of these statements regarding anesthesia is incorrect?
   a. Anesthetic agents have wide therapeutic indices
   b. There is always a risk to patient safety when anesthetics are administered
   c. Most anesthetics cause significant changes in cardiopulmonary function
   d. All statements are false

6. Which of the following opioids is preferable in the patient undergoing a painful ophthalmic procedure?
   a. Morphine
   b. Methadone
   c. Diazepam
   d. Midazolam

7. Which of the following drugs is classified as an opioid?
   a. Amantadine
   b. Carprofen
   c. Ketamine
   d. Butorphanol

8. Physical examinations are an important step when assessing the patient's risk factor. Which of the following statements is incorrect, as it refers to PE findings?
   a. Dehydration increases the risk for hypotension
   b. Anemia predisposes the patient to hypoxemia
   c. Patients with bruising may be at higher risk for potentially life-threatening intraoperative and postoperative bleeding
   d. A dog with a body condition score of 8/9 will require more anesthetic per unit body weight than a dog of the same breed with a body condition score of 5/9

9. When a capnometer is combined with a continuous graphical display, the monitoring device is referred to as a:
   a. Capnometer
   b. Capnograph
   c. Pulse oximeter
   d. Capillary refill time

10. Using a Doppler for blood pressure measurement will yield which of the following readings?
    a. Systolic
    b. Mean
    c. Diastolic
    d. All of the above

11. When using the emergency oxygen flush valve, what step must the technician also do simultaneously?
    a. Disconnect the patient from the breathing circuit to avoid barotrauma
    b. Disconnect the oxygen supply
    c. Close the pop-off valve
    d. Turn off the isoflurane

12. You have a patient that looks asleep, will not respond to voice, but will respond to pain. Which of the following would describe its level of consciousness?
    a. Lethargic
    b. Obtunded
    c. Stuporous
    d. Comatose

13. Which of the following is used for direct blood pressure monitoring?
    a. Cardell
    b. Dinamap
    c. Arterial catheter
    d. Doppler

14. Which of the following products listed would be considered a colloid solution?
    a. Lactated Ringer's solution
    b. Normal saline solution
    c. Hetastarch
    d. 5% dextrose

15. What is the function of a vaporizer?
    a. To regulate flow of oxygen into the anesthetic system
    b. To deliver safe and effective levels of anesthetic gas
    c. To measure the pressure of gas in the system
    d. All of the above

16. What is the American Society of Anesthesiologists (ASA) Physical Status Classification system rating for a patient that is anemic or moderately dehydrated?
    a. Class P1
    b. Class P2
    c. Class P3
    d. Class P4

17. Which of the following fluids listed is an example of a colloid?
    a. Lactated Ringer's
    b. Normosol-R
    c. Whole blood
    d. Hypertonic saline

18. You have a calm canine patient that must be anesthetized. Which of the following conditions could present the greatest risk to anesthesia?
    a. Wheezing while breathing
    b. Lethargy
    c. Temperature of 104.1° F
    d. Sinus arrhythmia

19. Which of the following inhaled anesthetics has a very low boiling point and therefore has to be contained within an electrically heated chamber?
    a. Halothane
    b. Desflurane
    c. Isoflurane
    d. Sevoflurane

20. Which of the following patients would be of greatest concern regarding the patent airway when anesthesia is being considered?
    a. Brachiocephalic breeds
    b. Exotic breeds
    c. Cats and horses
    d. Sight hounds

21. Which of the following is often used to calculate a patient's tidal volume?
    a. 100 mL/kg
    b. 200 mL/kg
    c. 1–2 mL/kg
    d. 10–20 mL/kg

22. The width of the blood pressure cuff in a dog should be what percentage of the circumference of the leg?
    a. 40%
    b. 50%
    c. 25%
    d. 30%

23. What does the term *minute volume* mean?
    a. The volume of anesthetic agent used in 1 min
    b. The flow of oxygen through the system in 1 min
    c. The sum of all gas volumes exhaled in 1 min
    d. The volume of gas exhaled in one breath

24. Monitoring patients with IV catheters is just as critical as the techniques used to administer medications. Which of the following statements is incorrect?
    a. Choose an administration set with an injection port
    b. Provide all IV drugs slowly unless told otherwise
    c. Always follow IV injections through a catheter with sterile saline flush
    d. Choose a catheter that is small in diameter to minimize the risk of bleeding

25. What is the main component of soda lime (a substance used to absorb carbon dioxide from the breathing system)?
    a. Carbon dioxide
    b. Potassium hydroxide
    c. Calcium hydroxide
    d. Baking soda

26. Blood pressure cuff placement is common in all of the following areas *except* the:
    a. Tail
    b. Forelimb
    c. Hind limb
    d. Foot

27. What is the name given to the opening opposite of the bevel of the endotracheal tube?
    a. Pilot hole
    b. Accessory opening
    c. Murphy eye
    d. Murphy opening

28. The adult animal is composed of a large amount of fluid. Which statement about body fluids is incorrect?
    a. About 40% of the body weight is water
    b. About two thirds of the total body water resides inside the cells
    c. Blood plasma makes up about 5% of the total body weight
    d. Dogs have a larger total blood volume than cats

29. A patient is admitted to the hospital with moderate dehydration. The veterinarian has asked that the patient be rehydrated. Which of the following solutions would be considered ideal for rehydration?
    a. Colloids
    b. Hypertonic saline
    c. Isotonic crystalloids
    d. 50% dextrose

30. Which of the following is a main disadvantage for using a chamber to induce anesthesia?
    a. Patient struggling causes increased catecholamines
    b. Increased risk of cardiac arrhythmias
    c. Staff exposure to harmful waste anesthetic gases
    d. All of the above

31. All of the following factors would be indicators for placing a patient on a controlled ventilator, *except:*
    a. An open thorax thoracotomy or chest wall trauma
    b. Neuromuscular blockade
    c. Pneumothorax
    d. Intestinal foreign body

32. Which of the following administration rates describes that of a microdrip set?
    a. 10 gtt/mL
    b. 10–15 gtt/mL
    c. 20–60 gtt/mL
    d. 60 gtt/mL

33. All of the following are clinical signs used to evaluate the depth of anesthesia, *except:*
    a. Eye position
    b. Ear pinch
    c. Jaw tone
    d. Palpebral reflex

34. All of the following statements regarding fluid infusion rates are false, *except:*
    a. Standard shock doses of fluids are about the same as doses used during routine surgery
    b. Surgery patients with blood loss may require colloids instead of crystalloids
    c. Crystalloids are generally given at lower administration rates than colloids
    d. Hypertonic saline is administered in large volumes to patients in shock

35. What is the function of an esophageal stethoscope?
    a. Perform cardiac and lung auscultation via the esophagus
    b. Temperature readings via the esophagus
    c. Measures exhaled end tidal carbon dioxide
    d. Measures central venous pressure

36. Which of the following monitoring parameters is used for the measurement and numerical display of the carbon dioxide concentration in the respiratory gas?
    a. Electrocardiogram
    b. Capnometry
    c. Pulse oximeter
    d. Capillary refill time

37. Fluid overload can carry serious consequences. All of the following clinical signs are consistent with that of fluid overload, *except:*
    a. Ocular and nasal discharge
    b. Hypotension
    c. Increased lung sounds and respiratory rate
    d. Dyspnea

38. Which of the following describes capnometers where the measuring chambers are placed directly in the airway and the measurement signal is generated?
    a. Sidestream capnometer
    b. Invasive capnometer
    c. Mainstream capnometer
    d. Endstream capnometer

39. Which of the following locations would be acceptable for placement of a pulse oximeter probe?
    a. Tongue
    b. Prepuce
    c. Nonpigmented toe
    d. All of the above

40. In the equine patient, which heart rhythm is *not* normal?
    a. Normal sinus rhythm
    b. Sinus arrhythmia
    c. Second-degree AV block
    d. Third-degree AV block

41. Which of the following blood pressure measuring techniques is considered "gold standard" in terms of accurate measurements?
    a. Invasive blood pressure measurements
    b. Doppler blood pressure measurements
    c. Oscillometric blood pressure measurements
    d. All of the above

42. Which of the following terms describes the volume of gas exhaled in one breath?
    a. Tidal volume
    b. Minute volume
    c. Dead space volume
    d. Oxygen flow rate

43. What combination of drugs is in a neuroleptanalgesic cocktail?
    a. An opioid and an anticholinergic
    b. An anticholinergic and a tranquilizer
    c. An opioid and a tranquilizer
    d. An anticholinergic and a benzodiazepine

44. Where is the intravenous catheter placed for measurement of central venous pressures?
    a. Vena cava
    b. Right atrium
    c. Left ventricle
    d. Cephalic vein

45. Which of the following drugs is a phenothiazine tranquilizer most commonly used as a premedication in small animal practice?
    a. Acepromazine
    b. Midazolam
    c. Diazepam
    d. Morphine

46. Where does atropine block the release of acetylcholine?
    a. Muscarinic receptors of the parasympathetic system
    b. Nicotinic receptors of the parasympathetic system
    c. Muscarinic receptors of the sympathetic system
    d. Nicotinic receptors of the sympathetic system

47. All of the following are common side effects of acepromazine, *except:*
    a. Peripheral vasodilation
    b. Decrease in body temperature
    c. Increase in body temperature
    d. Increase in overall blood pressure

48. Which of the following is an example of an alpha-2 adrenoreceptor agonist?
    a. Dexmedetomidine
    b. Xylazine
    c. Medetomidine
    d. All of the above

49. How is it best to treat bradycardia induced by dexmedetomidine?
    a. Atropine
    b. Naloxone
    c. Epinephrine
    d. Atipamezole

50. Which of the following medications will reverse the effects of opioids?
    a. Atipamezole
    b. Naloxone
    c. Atropine
    d. Yohimbine

51. What class of drugs is not only used as premedicants, but also as a first-line intervention for animals presenting in status epilepticus?
    a. Opioids
    b. Benzodiazepines
    c. Alpha-2 adrenoreceptor agonist
    d. Antibiotics

52. Of the following drugs listed, which one *does not* have analgesic properties?
    a. Dexmedetomidine
    b. Morphine
    c. Methadone
    d. Diazepam

53. What is the indication for induction with etomidate in dogs?
    a. Severe cardiac disease
    b. Renal failure
    c. Orthopedic disease
    d. Pediatric (younger than 4 weeks)

54. Which of the following represents how a drug can be eliminated from the body?
    a. Urine excretion
    b. Digestion
    c. Biotransformation
    d. Metabolized

55. Which of the following opioids would be the best choice as a premedication in a patient with moderate to severe pain?
    a. Butorphanol
    b. Diazepam
    c. Methadone
    d. Naloxone

56. Which of the following is a dissociative anesthetic?
    a. Thiopental sodium
    b. Pentobarbital sodium
    c. Ketamine hydrochloride
    d. Propofol

57. What should the vaporizer be set at to maintain a surgical plane of anesthesia?
    a. $0.5 \times MAC$
    b. $1 \times MAC$
    c. $1.5 \times MAC$
    d. $2 \times MAC$

58. Which of the following is considered a reversal drug for all opioid agonist effects at all receptors?
    a. Butorphanol
    b. Naloxone hydrochloride
    c. Morphine
    d. Hydromorphone

59. How do local anesthetic drugs function as analgesics?
    a. By reducing inflammation
    b. By blocking impulse conduction in nerve fibers
    c. By facilitating the breakdown of arachidonic acid
    d. By acting as an antipyretic

60. What can be done to avoid transient apnea from the drug propofol?
    a. Administer by infusion only
    b. Premedicate with opioids
    c. Administer intravenously only
    d. Titrate this drug in several boluses

61. Tiletamine-zolazepam can cause what problem in dogs on recovery?
    a. Excitement
    b. Bradycardia
    c. Hypotension
    d. Laryngospasm

62. An injection of a local anesthetic into the area around a peripheral nerve to block sensory and/or motor function such as a ring block before declaw procedure is an example of what?
    a. Spinal anesthesia
    b. Regional anesthesia
    c. Topical anesthesia
    d. Subcutaneous injection

63. Which of the following drugs is not considered an NMDA receptor antagonist?
    a. Ketamine
    b. Methadone
    c. Morphine
    d. Amantadine

64. Which of the following is a common adverse effect of isoflurane?
    a. Hepatic toxicity
    b. Accumulation in body fat stores
    c. Depression of respiration
    d. Seizures during recovery

65. Which of the following opioids has been shown to have the lowest likelihood of causing vomiting in cats?
    a. Morphine
    b. Methadone
    c. Oxymorphone
    d. Hydromorphone

66. Which of the following drugs has been shown to be useful at reducing opioid-related nausea and vomiting that occur after administration of opioids when given preoperatively?
    a. Maropitant
    b. Carprofen
    c. Morphine
    d. Hydromorphone

67. What components of pain are involved in an ovariohysterectomy?
    a. Somatic pain only
    b. Visceral pain only
    c. Both somatic and visceral pain
    d. Neither somatic nor visceral pain

68. Which of the following opioids is most commonly used for epidural analgesia?
    a. Morphine
    b. Buprenorphine
    c. Bupivacaine
    d. Lidocaine

69. Rapid administration of morphine intravenously can cause release of what hormone?
    a. Testosterone
    b. Histamine
    c. Endogenous opioids
    d. Estrogen

70. Electrical signals (action potentials) are converted by thermal, mechanical, or chemical noxious stimuli during which process?
    a. Perception
    b. Modulation
    c. Transduction
    d. Transmission

71. Which of the following opioids would be best to use in cases where you want to avoid vomiting such as cases with increased intracranial pressure?
    a. Morphine
    b. Methadone
    c. Oxymorphone
    d. Hydromorphone

72. Young puppies and kittens have limited glucose reserves and are at a greater risk of what condition because of the fasting required before anesthesia?
    a. Hypothermia
    b. Hypotension
    c. Hypoglycemia
    d. Hyperglycemia

73. Pain impulses can be altered by neurons that either suppress or amplify nerve impulses in the spinal cord during which process?
    a. Perception
    b. Modulation
    c. Transduction
    d. Transmission

74. Where does "wind-up" occur?
    a. Brain
    b. Spinal cord
    c. Visceral pain receptors
    d. Peripheral pain receptors

75. Which of the following is a common side effect when opioids such as morphine and hydromorphone are used preoperatively?
    a. Vomiting
    b. Decreased mucous membrane secretions
    c. Tachycardia
    d. Hypertension

76. Which of the following is *not* a barbiturate anesthetic drug?
    a. Pentobarbital
    b. Methohexital
    c. Propofol
    d. Thiopental

77. During multimodal analgesic therapy, which of the following statements is true?
    a. The dose of each drug is decreased when several drugs are used
    b. Multiple pain receptor mechanisms are targeted by one drug
    c. Several drugs target one pain receptor mechanism
    d. Using several drugs increases side effects

78. Which of the following drugs is *not* considered a benzodiazepine?
    a. Midazolam
    b. Methadone
    c. Zolazepam
    d. Diazepam

79. The drug Telazol is a combination of which two drugs?
    a. Ketamine and diazepam
    b. Ketamine and midazolam
    c. Tiletamine and zolazepam
    d. Methadone and midazolam

80. Choose an analgesic plan that targets three different pain receptor mechanisms.
    a. Morphine IM, fentanyl CRI, lidocaine nerve block
    b. Morphine IM, fentanyl CRI, bupivacaine nerve block
    c. Morphine IM, ketamine CRI, lidocaine nerve block
    d. Ketamine CRI, lidocaine and bupivacaine nerve block

81. Which of the following is a neuroactive steroid anesthetic?
    a. Alfaxalone
    b. Telazol
    c. Propofol
    d. Etomidate

82. In what organ are most inhalant anesthetic drugs metabolized (biotransformed)?
    a. Skin
    b. Lungs
    c. Eye
    d. Liver

83. Giving analgesics before tissue injury is known as:
    a. Premedication
    b. Local analgesia
    c. Multimodal analgesia
    d. Preemptive analgesia

84. Which of the following opioids would be the best choice for a surgery that is anticipated to be moderately to severely painful?
    a. Butorphanol
    b. Propofol
    c. Hydromorphone
    d. Naloxone

85. Which of the following opioid analgesics is often used as a continuous rate infusion because of its short duration of action (approximately 30 minutes)?
    a. Morphine
    b. Ketamine
    c. Buprenorphine
    d. Fentanyl

86. Opioid administration in cats and dogs can have side effects. Which one is not a side effect from opioid administration in cats and dogs?
    a. Vomiting
    b. Dysphoria
    c. Renal failure
    d. Respiratory depression

87. Which of the following terms refers to a specific stage in general anesthesia in which there is a sufficient degree of analgesia and muscle relaxation to allow surgery to be performed without patient pain or movement?
    a. Sedation
    b. General anesthesia
    c. Surgical anesthesia
    d. Local anesthesia

88. Which of the following preoperative tests should be performed on a patient with a suspected clotting disorder?
    a. Blood glucose measurement
    b. Urine specific gravity
    c. Buccal mucosal bleeding time
    d. Schirmer tear test

89. Nonsteroidal anti-inflammatory drugs have what mechanism of action (MOA)?
    a. They block sodium channels
    b. They are alpha-2 receptor agonists
    c. They inhibit prostaglandin synthesis
    d. They are mu opioid receptor agonists

90. Which term describes the drugs given before general anesthesia?
    a. Induction agents
    b. Maintenance agents
    c. Preanesthetic medications
    d. Postanesthetic medications

91. Which of the following is the most commonly used alpha-2 agonist in dogs and cats?
    a. Dexmedetomidine
    b. Xylazine
    c. Morphine
    d. Detomidine

92. Which of the following options is not a side effect of NSAID administration?
    a. Liver damage
    b. Kidney damage
    c. Gastrointestinal ulcers
    d. Respiratory depression

93. Which of the following induction agents can cause tissue irritation and sloughing after perivascular injection?
    a. Thiopental
    b. Propofol
    c. Alfaxalone
    d. None of the above

94. What will the tank pressure gauge read when the oxygen tank is half full?
    a. 1100 psi
    b. 2000 psi
    c. 500 psi
    d. 2200 psi

95. Which of the following statements is true of isoflurane?
    a. A precision vaporizer is used to administer isoflurane
    b. Isoflurane has no analgesic properties
    c. Isoflurane is stable at room temperature
    d. All of the above

96. A tank of nitrous oxide is present in what state(s)?
    a. Liquid
    b. Gas
    c. Liquid and a gas
    d. Solid and liquid

97. All of the following sites can be used for placement of an arterial catheter used to measure arterial pressures during anesthesia, *except:*
    a. Lingual artery
    b. Medial pedal artery
    c. Auricular artery
    d. Coccygeal artery

98. Which condition causes a decrease in the requirements for general anesthesia?
    a. Hypoventilation
    b. Hyperthermia
    c. Hypothermia
    d. Hypotension

99. What shows the amount of oxygen the patient is receiving?
    a. Oxygen tank pressure gauge
    b. Flowmeter
    c. Pressure manometer
    d. Vaporizer

100. Which of the following is *not* a recommended method of actively warming a patient while under anesthesia?
    a. Circulating warm water blankets
    b. Convective warm air devices
    c. Commercial bubble wrap
    d. Radiant heat via heat lamp

101. Which of the following is an example of a monitoring parameter that would be useful during the recovery process?
    a. Continuous ECG monitoring
    b. Temperature monitoring
    c. Postoperative pain scoring
    d. All of the above

102. The reservoir bag's minimum size can be calculated as:
    a. 20 mL/kg
    b. 60 mL/kg
    c. 80 mL/kg
    d. 100 mL/kg

103. If a patient regurgitates while waking up from anesthesia, what is the best course of action?
    a. Remove the regurgitation and lavage the esophagus with saline
    b. Feed the patient a meal as quickly as possible
    c. Place the patient back on gas anesthetic
    d. No treatment is needed

104. What is the function of the pop-off valve?
    a. Vaporize the liquid anesthetic
    b. Prevent excess gas pressure from building up within the breathing circuit
    c. Keep the oxygen flowing in one direction only
    d. Prevent waste gases from reentering the vaporizer

105. Which term describes the drugs given after general anesthesia and after the surgical stimulus is finished?
    a. Induction agents
    b. Maintenance agents
    c. Preanesthetic medications
    d. Postanesthetic medications

106. Which of the following drugs is a phenothiazine tranquilizer commonly used to calm patients in the recovery period?
    a. Acepromazine
    b. Midazolam
    c. Diazepam
    d. Morphine

107. The pressure manometer reading should not exceed _____ when the small animal patient is bagged.
    a. 5 cm H_2O
    b. 10 cm H_2O
    c. 15 cm H_2O
    d. 20 cm H_2O

108. Which of the following medications would be a good choice for providing sedation and analgesia in the recovery period?
    a. Midazolam
    b. Diazepam
    c. Acepromazine
    d. Dexmedetomidine

109. Of the following drugs listed, which one would not be the best choice to use for a patient recovering from surgery as it *does not* have analgesic properties?
    a. Dexmedetomidine
    b. Morphine
    c. Methadone
    d. Diazepam

110. What is the maintenance flow rate of non-rebreathing systems?
    a. Very low (5–10 mL/kg/min)
    b. Low (20–40 mL/kg/min)
    c. Moderate (50–100 mL/kg/min)
    d. Very high (≥200 mL/kg/min)

111. Which of the following terms describes a diminished volume or a lack of air in part or all of a lung lobe?
    a. Atelectasis
    b. Hypoxia
    c. Tidal volume
    d. Functional residual capacity

112. All of the following techniques can be used to prevent laryngospasm in cats, *except:*
    a. Spraying the endotracheal tube with lidocaine
    b. Spraying the larynx with local anesthetic
    c. Ensuring adequate depth before intubation
    d. Using a gentle intubation technique

113. When is the negative pressure relief valve important?
    a. When nitrous oxide is being used
    b. If there is no scavenging system present
    c. If there is a failure of oxygen flow through the system
    d. When the carbon dioxide absorber is no longer functioning

114. Which of the following describes a reason why red rubber endotracheal tubes should no longer be used in practice?
    a. The solid color of the tube makes it impossible to detect occlusions from mucus
    b. Over time the tube can soften, making it more prone to cracking
    c. Red rubber endotracheal tubes are less likely to cause cross contamination between patients
    d. Red rubber endotracheal tubes are shorter and cannot provide adequate anesthesia delivery to the patient

115. What is the tidal volume of an anesthetized animal in mL/kg of body weight?
    a. 5
    b. 10
    c. 19
    d. 20

116. What should the pressure be between the flowmeters and breathing circuit?
    a. 5 psi
    b. 15 psi
    c. 25 psi
    d. 45 psi

117. For which of the following patients would it be advantageous to use a laryngeal mask airway?
    a. Brachycephalic dogs
    b. Rabbits
    c. Pigs
    d. All of the above

118. What is the function of a laryngoscope?
    a. To obtain tissue samples from the trachea
    b. To facilitate endotracheal intubation by allowing direct visualization of the opening to the trachea
    c. To cover the esophagus and prevent regurgitation during surgery
    d. To provide a way for anesthetic gases to be delivered

119. Which anesthetic that is used in today's practice is associated with neurologic and adverse reproductive effects?
    a. Isoflurane
    b. Halothane
    c. Methoxyflurane
    d. Nitrous oxide

120. What is the function of an endotracheal tube?
    a. To obtain tissue samples from the trachea
    b. To facilitate endotracheal intubation by allowing direct visualization of the opening to the trachea
    c. To cover the esophagus and prevent regurgitation after surgery
    d. To provide a way for oxygen and anesthetic gases to be delivered to the lungs

121. Which type of laryngoscope is composed of a straight blade with a light source on a handle?
    a. Murphy
    b. Cole
    c. Miller
    d. Magill

122. Which of the following endotracheal tubes can be heat sterilized with steam from an autoclave?
    a. Silicone tubes
    b. PVC tubes
    c. Red rubber tubes
    d. All of the above

123. In the United States, the National Institute for Occupational Safety and Health (NIOSH) recommends that the levels of waste anesthetic gases for anesthetics such as isoflurane, halothane, or methoxyflurane should not exceed ___ ppm.
    a. 0.2
    b. 2
    c. 20
    d. 200

124. Anesthesia machines function to deliver all of the following, *except:*
    a. To deliver oxygen
    b. To deliver anesthetic gas
    c. To remove oxygen
    d. To remove carbon dioxide and waste gases

125. How many ppm is halothane when a person can smell it?
    a. 5
    b. 33
    c. 200
    d. 5000

126. What is the function of a flush valve within the anesthetic circuit?
    a. To deliver oxygen to the system at a specific rate in L/min
    b. To deliver a burst of pure oxygen into the breathing system
    c. To flush more anesthetic gas into the system if the patient is in a light anesthetic plane
    d. To shut off the oxygen supply

127. Which of the following is used to effectively monitor waste anesthetic gases?
    a. Odor of waste gas
    b. Passive dosimeter badge
    c. Radiation monitor
    d. Regular preventive maintenance by qualified personnel

128. The numbers on the vaporizer dial indicate the:
    a. Concentration (in percent) delivered at the output of the vaporizer
    b. Depth of anesthesia
    c. Flow of oxygen through the system
    d. Amount of anesthetic gas left in the reservoir

129. How often is a low-pressure leak test conducted on an anesthesia machine?
    a. Each day that the machine is used
    b. At least once/week
    c. At least once/month
    d. When the anesthetist smells anesthetic gases

130. Which of the following breathing systems is made of an inspiratory tube running within an expiratory tube for the purpose of aiding in the warming and humidification of inspired gases?
    a. Mapleson
    b. Bain coaxial
    c. Modified Jackson Rees
    d. Universal F

131. What is the normal capillary refill time in veterinary patients?
    a. 1–2 seconds
    b. 3–4 seconds
    c. <1 second
    d. 10 seconds

132. If you want to transport a high-pressure O_2 tank, what is the safest way?
    a. Carrying it
    b. Rolling it along the floor
    c. Using a handcart
    d. Dragging it by the neck

133. What can pale mucous membranes indicate in a veterinary patient?
    a. Vasoconstriction because of drugs
    b. Vasodilation because of drugs
    c. Increased cardiac output
    d. Hypertension

134. If anesthetic waste gases are present in a room, how many air changes per hour should occur?
    a. 5
    b. 10
    c. 15
    d. 30

135. All of the following sites are acceptable for palpating peripheral pulses in patients under anesthesia, *except:*
    a. Femoral artery
    b. Articular artery
    c. Dorsal pedal artery
    d. Lingual artery

136. How can a technician reduce the amount of waste anesthetic gases?
    a. Use uncuffed endotracheal tubes
    b. Ensure that the anesthetic machine has been tested for leaks
    c. Use a mask or chamber
    d. Use high fresh gas flows

137. What is a Doppler device used to measure?
    a. Patient oxygenation
    b. Temperature
    c. Blood pressure
    d. End-tidal carbon dioxide

138. How would one conduct a low-pressure test on a circle system?
    a. Open the pop-off valve and occlude the end of the circuit
    b. Turn off the oxygen tank
    c. Inflate the reservoir bag
    d. Pressurize the circuit with a volume of gas

139. What should be used to clean most monitoring devices?
    a. Bleach
    b. Mild soap and water
    c. Alcohol
    d. No cleaning is needed

140. Which side effects are common with injectable and inhalant anesthetics?
    a. A period of apnea
    b. Progressive depression of the cardiovascular and respiratory function as the depth of anesthesia increases
    c. Tachycardia followed by bradycardia
    d. Hypothermia-related event

141. Which of the following terms describes the amount of air left in the lungs after normal ventilation?
    a. Functional residual capacity
    b. Atelectasis
    c. Hypoxia
    d. Tidal volume

142. Which of the following would be a cause of spontaneous ventilations not being active enough, therefore requiring controlled ventilation?
    a. Deep level of anesthesia
    b. Use of neuromuscular blockers
    c. During intrathoracic surgery
    d. All of the above

143. What is the desired anesthetic plane for surgical procedures?
    a. Stage III, plane 1
    b. Stage III, plane 2
    c. Stage III, plane 3
    d. Stage III, plane 4

144. What is the term used to express when an animal is trying to breathe against the set respiratory rhythm and volume being delivered by the mechanical ventilator?
    a. Checking
    b. Pulling
    c. Pushing
    d. Bucking

145. Which of the following drugs provides sedation but *no* analgesia?
    a. Butorphanol
    b. Dexmedetomidine
    c. Midazolam
    d. Morphine

146. What is the stage of anesthesia when you see breath holding, vocalization, and involuntary movement of the limbs?
    a. Stage I
    b. Stage II
    c. Stage III, plane 1
    d. Stage III, plane 2

147. Which of the following terms describes a state in which patients are in a trancelike state and unaware of their surroundings?
    a. Catalepsy
    b. Sedation
    c. Sleeping
    d. Nystagmus

148. What is considered anatomic dead space?
    a. Room air within the breathing circuit
    b. Air within the digestive tract
    c. Air within the trachea, pharynx, larynx, bronchi, and nasal passages
    d. Air within the alveoli

149. Which of the following techniques helps to minimize the occurrence of respiratory depression when using propofol as an induction agent?
    a. Administrating the entire dose as a fast IV bolus
    b. Slow IV administration
    c. Administrating subcutaneously
    d. Administrating intramuscularly

150. All of the following patients would be a good candidate for etomidate as the induction drug, *except* for patients that are experiencing:
    a. Cesarean section
    b. Known cardiac disease
    c. Cardiovascular instability resulting from trauma
    d. All of the above

151. What is the minimum acceptable heart rate for a large breed dog that is anesthetized?
    a. 60 bpm
    b. 70 bpm
    c. 80 bpm
    d. 100 bpm

152. Which of the following is *not* a characteristic of alpha-2 agonists?
    a. Sedation
    b. Increased heart rate
    c. Analgesia
    d. Muscle relaxation

153. An anesthetized dog that has a respiratory rate less than _____ should be reported to the veterinarian.
    a. 4 bpm
    b. 6 bpm
    c. 10 bpm
    d. 15 bpm

154. Patients given alpha-2 agonists often have pale mucous membranes and cold extremities in the initial phase because of what side effect of the drug?
    a. Peripheral vasoconstriction
    b. Hypothermia
    c. Hypoglycemia
    d. Decreased hepatic blood flow

155. Ketamine administration would be contraindicated in which of the following disease processes?
    a. Hypotrophic cardiomyopathy
    b. Congestive heart failure
    c. Healthy patients
    d. Panosteitis

156. Tachypnea is:
    a. An increase in respiratory depth (tidal volume)
    b. An increase in respiratory rate
    c. A decrease in respiratory depth (tidal volume)
    d. A decrease in respiratory rate

157. Which of the following opioids has been shown to have the highest likelihood of causing vomiting in cats?
    a. Hydromorphine
    b. Morphine
    c. Oxymorphone
    d. Methadone

158. Your patient has a pulse oximetry reading of 89%. What does this indicate?
    a. Normal value
    b. Need for supportive therapy
    c. State of hypoxemia, but no need for therapy
    d. Medical emergency

159. Which anesthetic monitoring tool is important for patients on a ventilator to verify the efficiency of gas exchange and adequate ventilation?
    a. Capnography
    b. Pulse oximeter
    c. ECG
    d. Blood pressure

160. Which of the following could be a cause of an increase in intraocular pressure (IOP) in an ophthalmology patient?
    a. Struggling and excitement in a poorly sedated pet
    b. Vomiting or gagging
    c. Pressure on the jugular vein from neck leads
    d. All of the above

161. Which of the following statements regarding body temperature is true?
    a. Body temperatures of 36° to 38° C (96.8° to 100.4° F) cause prolonged anesthetic recovery
    b. Dangerous central nervous system depression and changes in cardiac function may be seen at body temperatures <32° C (89.6° F)
    c. There is no need to warm IV fluids before administration to surgery patients
    d. Circulating warm water blankets should be set at 45° C (approximately 111° F)

162. Which of the following induction methods should be avoided in patients undergoing an ophthalmic procedure?
    a. Alfaxalone
    b. Propofol
    c. Thiopental
    d. Mask or box inductions

163. When monitoring anesthesia and nystagmus is present, which statement is correct?
    a. Nystagmus is commonly seen in horses in very light plane of anesthesia
    b. Nystagmus is a useful indicator of anesthetic depth in small animals
    c. In a cat, a "divergent eye sign" is typically associated with an adequate plane of anesthesia for surgery
    d. Ruminants often show nystagmus under anesthesia

164. Which of the following inhalant anesthetics should be avoided in the ophthalmology patient?
    a. Isoflurane
    b. Sevoflurane
    c. Nitrous oxide
    d. Desflurane

165. Pale mucous membranes are indicative of:
    a. Acidosis
    b. Hypotension
    c. Decreased perfusion
    d. Hypertension

166. Which drug class is commonly used in ophthalmology procedures to prevent movement of the eye during the procedure and to keep the eye in a central position?
    a. Inhalant anesthetics
    b. Opioids
    c. Neuromuscular blocking agents
    d. Alpha-2 agonists

167. What nerve block is commonly used to desensitize nerves and add additional analgesia to an ocular procedure?
    a. Retrobulbar block
    b. Epidural
    c. Circumferential nerve block
    d. Sacrococcygeal block

168. Which sign would a patient under stage III, plane 2 anesthesia exhibit?
    a. Very brisk palpebral reflex
    b. Irregular respiration
    c. Relaxed skeletal muscle tone
    d. Very dilated pupils

169. Use of ophthalmic local anesthetic drops in the eye before an ophthalmic examination would be an example of _____ anesthesia.
    a. Topical
    b. Surgical
    c. General
    d. Epidural

170. What is the main stimulus to breathe in the healthy awake animal?
    a. Excess oxygen concentration in the blood
    b. Excess carbon dioxide concentration in the blood
    c. Insufficient oxygen in the blood
    d. Insufficient carbon dioxide in the blood

171. Which of the following is the most common form of heart disease seen in cats?
    a. Dilated cardiomyopathy
    b. Hypertrophic cardiomyopathy
    c. Mitral valve insufficiency
    d. Low blood pressure

172. Which of the following drugs should be avoided when premedicating the cat with hypertrophic cardiomyopathy because of its likelihood of causing tachycardia and tachyarrhythmia?
    a. Hydromorphone
    b. Midazolam
    c. Atropine
    d. Etomidate

173. What is the normal tidal volume in an awake animal?
    a. 5–10 mL/kg
    b. 10–15 mL/kg
    c. 16–20 mL/kg
    d. 20–25 mL/kg

174. Which of the following factors can cause an increase in intracranial pressure?
    a. Hypercapnia
    b. Ketamine administration
    c. Pressure on the jugular vein
    d. All of the above

175. Where is nerve impulse transmission blocked with local anesthetics?
    a. Sensory neurons only
    b. Motor neurons only
    c. Sensory and motor neurons only
    d. Sensory, motor, and autonomic neurons

176. Which of the following techniques is useful for reducing intracranial pressure and therefore reducing brain size during neurosurgery?
    a. Controlled hyperventilation
    b. Controlled hypoventilation
    c. Starting a ketamine CRI
    d. Placing the patient in a head down position

177. What effect do inhalant anesthetics such as isoflurane and sevoflurane have on intracranial pressure?
    a. No change
    b. Increased intracranial pressure
    c. Decreased intracranial pressure

178. Which of the following is the mechanism of action for local anesthetics?
    a. Local anesthetics do not have a mechanism of action
    b. They interfere with the movement of sodium ions
    c. They block all impulses at the spinal cord level
    d. They affect neurotransmission within the brain

179. Which of the following opioids would be the *best* choice for emergency department patients who have experienced some sort of head trauma and may need serial neurological exams?
    a. Morphine
    b. Methadone
    c. Fentanyl
    d. Remifentanil

180. Which of the following opioids would be the best choice of analgesic for a patient with suspected head trauma for whom vomiting and/or abdominal contractions are contraindicated?
    a. Methadone
    b. Midazolam
    c. Morphine
    d. Hydromorphone

181. If a cat was receiving an epidural, what is the most caudal aspect that the epidural could be administered?
    a. T13
    b. L6
    c. L7
    d. S1

182. Which drug is often used in patients with intracranial disease because of its effect of reducing brain edema and intracranial pressure?
    a. Ketamine
    b. Isoflurane
    c. Glycopyrrolate
    d. Mannitol

183. What is the maximum subcutaneous dose of lidocaine in a dog?
    a. 1 mg/kg
    b. 4 mg/kg
    c. 10 mg/kg
    d. 15 mg/kg

184. Which inhalant anesthetic causes the most dramatic increase in cerebral blood flow and intracranial pressure?
    a. Desflurane
    b. Isoflurane
    c. Nitrous oxide
    d. Halothane

185. Which of the following terms is used to describe a tumor of the pancreas that results in excessive insulin production, leading to hypoglycemia?
    a. Pancreatitis
    b. Insulinoma
    c. Diabetes
    d. Hyperglycemia

186. To what does *atelectasis* refer?
    a. Excess fluid in the respiratory system
    b. The absence of breathing
    c. Collapse of the alveoli
    d. Bronchial constriction

187. If a specific neuromuscular blocking drug is given and you see an initial surge of muscle activity before paralysis, what drug has most likely been used?
    a. Succinylcholine
    b. Gallamine
    c. Pancuronium
    d. Cisatracurium

188. What is the treatment of choice for an insulinoma?
    a. Antibiotics
    b. Start insulin therapy
    c. Surgical removal
    d. Antifungal medications

189. Which of the following drugs may not be the best choice in a diabetic patient undergoing surgery because of its effect of increasing glucose and then a decrease in insulin that can last several hours?
    a. Dexmedetomidine
    b. Isoflurane
    c. Morphine
    d. Fentanyl

190. When using neuromuscular blocking agents, what is the most affected type of muscle?
    a. Cardiac
    b. Smooth muscle
    c. Skeletal muscle
    d. All types are equally affected

191. In preparation for an anesthetic procedure, you have drawn up a syringe of barbiturate and an identical syringe of saline. You are then called to the examination room to assist the veterinarian. About 10 minutes later you return to prepare the animal for induction. With the IV catheter in place, you are just about to inject some saline into the animal when you realize that you are not sure whether the syringe contains saline. The best thing to do is:
    a. Inject a small amount of the solution and see what effect it has
    b. Discard both syringes and begin again
    c. Ask the person who was holding the animal which syringe had saline in it
    d. Discard both syringes, label some new syringes, and begin again

192. Which of the following drug classes should be avoided in patients with renal disease?
    a. Opioids
    b. Nonsteroidal anti-inflammatory drugs
    c. Inhalant anesthetics
    d. Anticholinergics

193. Which of the following serum enzyme values are commonly used to directly evaluate liver function before an anesthetic event?
    a. Glucose and fructosamine
    b. PCV and total protein
    c. Creatinine and blood urea nitrogen
    d. Alanine aminotransferase (ALT) and alkaline phosphatase

194. What should you do if you are monitoring an anesthetic patient and you notice that the O₂ tank is empty?
    a. Disconnect the patient from the circuit, put on a new oxygen tank, and then reconnect the patient to the circuit
    b. Remove the circuit from the patient to allow it to breathe room air for the remainder of the procedure
    c. Resuscitate the patient with an Ambu bag
    d. Switch to an injectable anesthetic

195. Which of the following drug classes is not commonly used in pediatric patients because of its side effect of bradycardia?
    a. Alpha-2 agonists
    b. Anticholinergics
    c. Opioids
    d. Benzodiazepines

196. Which of the following methods is considered the least suitable choice for anesthetic induction in the pediatric canine and feline patient?
    a. IV injection of propofol
    b. IV injection of ketamine/diazepam mixture
    c. IM injection of alfaxalone
    d. Chamber induction with isoflurane

197. Inadequate oxygenation of the tissues for longer than_____ minutes could result in brain damage.
    a. 2
    b. 4
    c. 6
    d. 8

198. Which type of breathing system is commonly used in the pediatric patient because of lower resistance to breathing and minimal apparatus dead space?
    a. Non-rebreathing system
    b. Flow by oxygen via facemask
    c. Rebreathing system
    d. Ventilator

199. Which of the following fluids is an example of a crystalloid?
    a. Dextrans
    b. Hetastarch
    c. Plasma-Lyte 148
    d. Plasma

200. What is a reason to suspect that the pop-off valve has been closed or that it is malfunctioning?
    a. The anesthetist smells isoflurane
    b. Patient has difficulty exhaling
    c. Patient wakes up
    d. Flow rate starts to drop

201. Which fluid type should be used with caution in patients with blood clotting abnormalities?
    a. Plasma-Lyte
    b. Normosol-R
    c. Hetastarch
    d. Lactated Ringer's

202. Which of the following procedures can be completed to reduce the risk of anesthesia for a brachycephalic dog?
    a. Use dexmedetomidine as part of the anesthetic protocol
    b. Preoxygenate the animal before administering any anesthetic
    c. Chamber induce the dog
    d. Use a laryngeal mask airway

203. Crystalloid solutions are considered balanced when they have a fluid composition that closely resembles the patient's extracellular fluid. Which of the following crystalloids is *not* considered a balanced solution?
    a. Normal 0.9% saline
    b. Lactated Ringer's solution
    c. Normosol-R
    d. Plasma-Lyte 148

204. What would the approximate tidal volume be for a 40-kg canine patient?
    a. 40–80 mL
    b. 400–800 mL
    c. 4–8 mL
    d. 10 mL

205. If a patient has cardiovascular disease, what anesthetic agents or drugs might you want to avoid?
    a. Lidocaine
    b. Isoflurane
    c. Xylazine
    d. Opioids

206. What is the formula to calculate minute volume?
    a. Tidal volume multiplied by respiration rate
    b. % of inhaled anesthetic multiplied by respiration rate
    c. Tidal volume multiplied by % of inhaled anesthetic
    d. There is no formula to calculate minute volume

207. Which of the following patients would *not* be a good candidate for premedication with acepromazine?
    a. A 2-year-old mixed breed canine here for ovariohysterectomy
    b. A 6-year-old German shepherd presenting after being hit by a car
    c. A 1-year-old male cat presenting for castration
    d. All of the above are good candidates for premedication with acepromazine

208. What might cause tachypnea?
    a. Increased levels of arterial oxygen
    b. Increased levels of arterial CO_2
    c. The use of ketamine
    d. Too high a plane of anesthesia

209. Consider the following scenario: You are performing a procedure on a canine patient that you feel is at an appropriate anesthetic depth. Which of the following settings would be most appropriate if using sevoflurane in this patient?
    a. 2.5%
    b. 2 L/min
    c. 5%
    d. 8 mL/min

210. Which of the following drugs is *not* considered an alpha-2 adrenoreceptor agonist?
    a. Dexmedetomidine
    b. Xylazine
    c. Medetomidine
    d. Yohimbine

211. When inducing anesthesia in a young healthy patient by using an IV agent such as thiopental or propofol, which statement is false?
    a. If the patient is not adequately anesthetized to allow intubation after giving the initial amount, give the rest of the calculated dose
    b. Draw up the calculated dose, give about $\frac{1}{4}$ to $\frac{1}{2}$ first, and give the rest to effect anesthetization
    c. You must be sure the drug gets in the vein
    d. Old, sick, or debilitated patients often require less

212. In what organ are most drugs metabolized (biotransformed) in the patient?
    a. Skin
    b. Liver
    c. Eye
    d. Intestines

213. Which of the following terms refers to a drug-induced central nervous system depression and drowsiness that vary in intensity from light to deep?
    a. Sedation
    b. General anesthesia
    c. Surgical anesthesia
    d. Local anesthesia

214. When giving IV induction agents, which statement is false?
    a. Ketamine-diazepam takes slightly longer to act and lasts somewhat longer than propofol
    b. When using propofol, provide about 25%–50% of the calculated dose every 30 seconds to effect
    c. Significantly lower doses of thiopental sodium must be used in sick, old, or debilitated patients
    d. Thiopental sodium is generally given intravenously but can be given intramuscularly in uncooperative patients

215. Which of the following is *not* a recommended method of actively warming a patient during the recovery period?
    a. Circulating warm water blankets
    b. Convective warm air devices
    c. Commercial bubble wrap
    d. Electric heating blankets

216. Which of the following terms describes impaired oxygen delivery as a result of systemic delivery issues?
    a. Atelectasis
    b. Hypoxia
    c. Tidal volume
    d. Functional residual capacity

217. If you want to maintain anesthesia with a barbiturate and not have a prolonged recovery, which drug should be used?
    a. Pentobarbital
    b. Methohexital
    c. Thiopental sodium
    d. Phenobarbital

218. Which of the following are symptoms experienced by veterinary personnel who are exposed to waste anesthetic agents on a short-term basis?
    a. Headache
    b. Excitement
    c. Increased energy
    d. Happiness

219. Which of the following statements are false?
    a. Choosing a tube that is too short may cause increased mechanical dead space
    b. Choosing a tube that is too small may result in increased resistance to breathing
    c. Choosing a tube that is too long may result in hypoxemia
    d. Failure to cuff the tube may result in aspiration of foreign material

220. All of the following conditions are known health issues that result from long-term exposure to waste anesthetic gases, *except:*
    a. Reproductive disorders
    b. Liver damage
    c. Hyperexcitability
    d. Kidney damage

221. How can you tell the endotracheal tube has been placed in the esophagus?
    a. The patient coughs when the tube is placed
    b. The unidirectional valves do not move
    c. The pressure manometer indicates 0–2 cm H_2O while the patient is spontaneously breathing
    d. Only one firm structure in the neck is palpated

222. All of the following are mechanisms to decrease the amount of waste anesthetic gases in the veterinary facility, *except:*
    a. Anesthetic machine maintenance
    b. Scavenger system(s)
    c. Anesthetic technique used
    d. Using only inhalant gases

223. When should a dog be extubated after anesthesia?
    a. Right after you turn off the vaporizer
    b. About 10 minutes after turning off the vaporizer
    c. When the animal begins to swallow
    d. Any time that is convenient

224. Which of the following best describes a passive scavenger system?
    a. Uses suction created by a vacuum pump or fan to draw gas into the scavenger
    b. Uses positive pressure of the gas in the anesthetic machine to push gas into the scavenger
    c. Uses positive pressure created by a vacuum to draw gas out of the anesthetic machine
    d. Uses negative pressure of the gas in the anesthetic machine to push gas into the scavenger

225. What does the term *hypostatic congestion* mean?
    a. Accumulation of mucus in the trachea
    b. Pooling of blood in the dependent lung
    c. Leakage of fluid into the chest
    d. Pooling of ingesta in one area of the gastrointestinal tract

226. The advantages of a non-rebreathing system, as compared with a circle breathing system, include all of the following, *except:*
    a. Reduced resistance to breathing
    b. Greater potential for hypothermia caused by high flows needed
    c. Reduced mechanical dead space
    d. No soda lime required

227. Which anesthetic plan will give the fastest induction time and the best control over anesthetic depth?
    a. IM induction and maintenance
    b. IV induction with an ultra–short-acting agent and maintenance with bolus injections of the same
    c. Inhalant induction and maintenance
    d. IV induction with an ultra–short-acting agent and maintenance with an inhalant

228. An intravenous catheter should be:
    a. Large enough to allow adequate fluid delivery in the event of an emergency
    b. As small as possible to avoid pain
    c. Placed in critically ill patients only
    d. Left in place for at least 3 days after surgery

229. Pulse oximetry monitoring devices give an estimate of:
    a. Respiratory rate
    b. Cardiac output
    c. Percentage of hemoglobin saturation with oxygen in arterial blood
    d. Oxygen content of arterial blood

230. Of the techniques listed, which is used most often in general small animal practices?
    a. General anesthesia and sedation
    b. Sedatives and local techniques
    c. Neuromuscular blockade and neuroleptanalgesia
    d. Local and general anesthesia

231. Nitrous oxide cylinders are painted what color?
    a. Green
    b. Gray
    c. Blue
    d. Yellow

232. Activated charcoal devices absorb all inhalation agents *except:*
    a. Isoflurane
    b. Halothane
    c. Sevoflurane
    d. Nitrous oxide

233. What endotracheal tube would an 18 kg Labrador Retriever require?
    a. 7–7.5 mm
    b. 8–8.5 mm
    c. 9–9.5 mm
    d. 11 mm

234. Which animal is most likely to experience laryngospasm during endotracheal intubation?
    a. Thoroughbred mare
    b. Hereford cow
    c. Persian cat
    d. Dalmatian dog

235. The best method for determining the proper inflation of an endotracheal tube cuff is:
    a. Use 1 mL of air for each mm of internal diameter of the tube.
    b. Inject air while applying pressure from the reservoir bag until no air escapes around the tube.
    c. Inject air until the bulb on the cuff tubing is too hard to collapse.
    d. Use a 12-mL syringe and inject 12 mL of air into the cuff.

236. What is the purpose of an endotracheal tube?
    a. Increase dead space
    b. Maintain a patent airway
    c. Protect the patient from reflex tachycardia
    d. Allow the anesthetist to monitor the patient

237. The preferred method for treating a cat with laryngospasm is to:
    a. Use a sharp stylet to insert the endotracheal tube between the vocal cords
    b. Return the animal to its cage and wait 20 minutes before trying again
    c. Place a drop of a topical anesthetic onto each arytenoid, wait several seconds, and then intubate the animal
    d. Use a stiffer endotracheal tube that can force the vocal cords open

238. In a pug, the endotracheal tube should be removed:
    a. As soon as the surgery or diagnostic technique is completed
    b. Only after the animal is fully conscious and able to maintain a free airway
    c. When the animal is taken off of the anesthesia machine
    d. As soon as the animal begins to swallow and cough

239. When monitoring the vital signs of an anesthetized patient, you must observe and record all of the following, *except:*
    a. Mucous membrane color and capillary refill time
    b. Heart rate and respiratory rate and depth
    c. Reflexes
    d. Pulse quality and strength

240. What could be a complication from improper intubation?
    a. Increased dead space
    b. Pressure necrosis of the tracheal mucosa
    c. Intubation of alveoli
    d. Atelectasis

241. The responsibilities of the anesthetist during a surgical procedure include continuous monitoring of the patient's vital signs and recording observations at approximately:
    a. 10-min intervals
    b. 5-min intervals
    c. 2-min intervals
    d. 15-min intervals

242. It is recommended in patients with which of the following characteristics to wait longer before extubation because of the likelihood of an airway obstruction:
    a. Dolichocephalic
    b. Prognathism
    c. Brachycephalic
    d. Cleft palate

243. When performing maintenance anesthesia:
    a. The patient should be monitored every 30 minutes
    b. The patient should be placed on an electric heating pad to prevent hypothermia
    c. If a patient has one diseased lung, it should be positioned with the diseased side down
    d. The anesthetist should avoid any more than a 5-degree elevation of the rear quarters

244. Use of an indwelling catheter in an artery to monitor blood pressure is termed:
    a. Direct monitoring
    b. Central venous pressure
    c. Indirect monitoring
    d. Peripheral venous pressure

245. What can influence the anesthetic recovery period?
    a. Body temperature
    b. Patient condition
    c. The length of time the patient was under
    d. The breed of the patient
    e. All of the above

246. The most accurate way to evaluate the effectiveness of respiration is by:
    a. Observing abdominal and chest movements during respiration
    b. Counting the respiratory rate
    c. Feeling air move through the endotracheal tube or nostrils
    d. Measuring the arterial blood oxygen and carbon dioxide partial pressures

247. What is not a normal sign during recovery?
    a. Head bobbing
    b. Mydriasis
    c. Seizures
    d. Rapid limb paddling

248. Kidney function can be assessed by all of the following preanesthetic screening tests, *except:*
    a. Blood urea nitrogen
    b. ALT
    c. Urinalysis
    d. Creatinine

249. A preanesthetic check of the anesthesia machine should include all of the following, *except:*
    a. Leak testing
    b. Weighing the charcoal canister
    c. Calibrating the vaporizer
    d. Filling the vaporizer with anesthetic gas agent

250. Please choose the appropriate action for anesthetic recovery.
    a. Administer oxygen at a high flow rate for 5 minutes after discontinuation of the anesthetic or until extubation
    b. Leave the cage door open so you can monitor the patient from across the room
    c. Turn the patient about every 45 minutes
    d. Use cooling methods to prevent hyperthermia

251. A patient in ASA class I physical status is:
    a. A normal patient with no organic disease
    b. A moribund patient
    c. An adult animal with no signs of evident disease on physical examination
    d. In absolutely no danger while under anesthesia

252. Treatment for hypotension during anesthesia includes:
    a. Turning up the anesthetic gas
    b. Increasing the drip rate of the IV fluids
    c. Increasing the flow of oxygen
    d. Giving ventilating breaths

253. When performing surgery on a horse and administrating a standing chemical restraint, which statement is true?
    a. Horses must be intubated for standing chemical restraint
    b. Risk of myopathy or neuropathy is higher with standing chemical restraint
    c. The head must be supported in a normal position to avoid nasal congestion
    d. Hypoxemia is a common complication of standing chemical restraint

254. It is generally safe to extubate a canine or a feline when the patient:
    a. Vocalizes
    b. Swallows
    c. Stands
    d. Can rest in a sternal position

255. An epidural agent is most commonly administered where in a dog?
    a. Between L7 and the sacrum
    b. Just cranial to C1
    c. Immediately caudal to T13
    d. Directly into the spinal cord at T1

256. What is the next step for the anesthetist if a horse becomes excited after it has been premedicated with xylazine intravenously before general anesthesia?
    a. Allow the horse time to calm down before proceeding
    b. Physically restrain the horse using ropes
    c. Induce anesthesia with acepromazine
    d. Induce anesthesia with ketamine

257. Epidural anesthesia could be appropriately used for all procedures *except:*
    a. Tail amputation
    b. Cesarean section
    c. Eye enucleation
    d. Femur fracture repair

258. What is prevented by appropriate positioning and padding of the horse on the surgery table?
    a. Hypoxemia and hypotension positions would not help this
    b. Myopathies and neuropathies
    c. Hypoventilation and hypertension positions would not help this
    d. Regurgitation and aspiration padding would not help this

259. Propofol is a/an:
    a. Neuroactive steroid
    b. Ultra–short-acting barbiturate
    c. Ketaminelike dissociative
    d. Short-acting hypnotic agent

260. Some anesthesiologists suggest that acepromazine be avoided in:
    a. Patients with a history of seizures
    b. Aggressive patients
    c. All senior dogs
    d. All Dobermans

261. In dogs, normal doses of opioids generally produce all of the following *except:*
    a. Respiratory depression
    b. Decreased heart rate
    c. Analgesia
    d. Excitement

262. What is the function of guaifenesin when added to an induction protocol in horses?
    a. Muscle relaxation
    b. Analgesia
    c. Sedation
    d. All of the above

263. The oxygen flush valve:
    a. Allows oxygen to flow into the breathing system without going through the vaporizer
    b. Increases the anesthetic concentration within the circuit
    c. Causes the patient to breathe deeper
    d. Is used primarily to keep the reservoir bag deflated

264. The minimum fresh gas flow in a semiclosed circle system is correctly determined by:
    a. Patient's metabolic rate
    b. Patient's respiratory rate
    c. Drugs used for premedication
    d. Size of the soda lime canister

265. When would an inhalant induction via nasotracheal tube be appropriate?
    a. A 2-year-old Arabian stallion undergoing arthroscopy
    b. A 25-year-old thoroughbred mare undergoing sinus surgery
    c. A 3-week-old foal undergoing colic surgery
    d. A 6-month-old foal undergoing umbilical hernia repair

266. All inhalant anesthetic machines should have:
    a. A nitrous oxide flowmeter
    b. Blood pressure monitors
    c. Respiratory monitors
    d. An anesthetic waste gas scavenging system

267. In a Siamese cat, the endotracheal tube should be removed:
    a. As soon as the surgery or diagnostic procedure is completed
    b. Only after the animal is fully conscious and able to maintain a free airway
    c. When the animal is taken off of the anesthesia machine
    d. As soon as the animal begins to swallow and cough

268. What best describes endotracheal intubation in the horse?
    a. Intubation is performed blindly with the head and neck extended
    b. It is not advised to rinse the horse's mouth out before intubation
    c. A laryngoscope is useful for visualization of the larynx
    d. An endoscope is commonly used to facilitate intubation

269. What is the best technique for securing an endotracheal tube to an animal?
    a. It is best not to secure the tube to the animal, so that it can move freely if the animal starts to wake up
    b. It should be secured by a gauze tie or IV tubing around the maxilla, mandible, or behind the ears
    c. It can be secured with several wraps of cloth and tape around the animal's nose and the tube
    d. A rubber band can be looped tightly around the tube and the animal's nose

270. Hypoventilation that occurs in the anesthetized patient is characterized by:
    a. Reduced tidal volume and respiratory rate followed by increased carbon dioxide levels
    b. Decreased carbon dioxide levels and decreased oxygen levels
    c. Increased tidal volume and oxygen levels followed by decreased carbon dioxide levels
    d. Increased respiratory rate and hypocarbia followed by hypotension

271. During maintenance of anesthesia in horses with inhalant anesthetics, what are the most common complications?
    a. Hypoxemia, hypertension, and bradycardia
    b. Hypoxemia, hypotension, and bradycardia
    c. Hypoxemia, hypertension, and hypoventilation
    d. Hypoxemia, hypotension, and hypoventilation

272. For which patients should mask induction with isoflurane be avoided?
    a. Patients with impaired liver function
    b. Patients with impaired cardiac function
    c. Patients with impaired respiratory function
    d. Patients with impaired gastrointestinal function

273. What anesthetic agent does the cat kidney excrete largely intact?
    a. Atropine
    b. Ketamine
    c. Sevoflurane
    d. Acepromazine

274. When treating hypotension in the anesthetized horse, what drug is commonly used?
    a. Dextrose
    b. Digoxin
    c. Dobutamine
    d. Doxycycline

275. Ideally, in a patient under anesthesia:
    a. The PaO_2 should be high, and the $PaCO_2$ should be low
    b. The PaO_2 should be high, and the $PaCO_2$ should be high
    c. The PaO_2 should be low, and the $PaCO_2$ should be low
    d. The PaO_2 should be low, and the $PaCO_2$ should be high

276. The approximate volume of oxygen in an E cylinder is:
    a. 65 L
    b. 650 L
    c. 6500 L
    d. 2000 L

277. The approximate volume of oxygen in an H cylinder is:
    a. 69 L
    b. 690 L
    c. 6900 L
    d. 2200 L

278. Which phase of anesthesia is the greatest risk for horses?
    a. Preanesthesia
    b. Induction
    c. Maintenance
    d. Recovery

279. In cattle, an epidural block is most commonly performed by inserting a spinal needle between which vertebrae?
    a. T13 and L1
    b. L7 and the sacrum
    c. The sacrum and C1
    d. Cy1 and Cy2

280. What is the most likely diagnosis in a horse that has recovered from anesthesia for arthroscopy and shows the following symptoms: hard, swollen gluteal muscles, stiff gait, and reluctance to walk?
    a. Colic
    b. Myopathy
    c. Neuropathy
    d. Nephropathy

281. You have been asked to perform low-flow anesthesia on a 40-kg canine patient needing repair of a fractured femur. Which of the following flow rates would be appropriate for this patient?
    a. 80–280 mL/kg/min
    b. 500–1000 mL/kg/min
    c. 10–20 mL/kg/min
    d. 600–800 mL/kg/min

282. Which of the following offers a continuous, noninvasive way to estimate the partial pressure of carbon dioxide in arterial blood?
    a. Pulse oximetry
    b. Direct arterial blood pressure
    c. Central venous pressure
    d. Capnometry

283. What is the best choice when comparing cattle, horses, and swine with xylazine usage?
    a. Cattle are more sensitive than horses, which are more sensitive than swine
    b. Cattle are more sensitive than swine, which are more sensitive than horses
    c. Horses are more sensitive than cattle, which are more sensitive than swine
    d. Swine are more sensitive than cattle, which are more sensitive than horses

284. A blood pH of 7.2 is referred to as:
    a. Alkalemia
    b. Acidemia
    c. Hypoxemia
    d. Hyponatremia

285. Blood flow to the major organs is jeopardized when mean arterial blood pressure drops below:
    a. 60 mm Hg
    b. 100 mm Hg
    c. 80 mm Hg
    d. 90 mm Hg

286. Which drug is normally used in premedication in cattle?
    a. Anticholinergic
    b. Local anesthetic
    c. Alpha-2 adrenoceptor agonist
    d. Inhalation agent

287. An increased or rising central venous pressure (CVP) is caused by:
    a. Hypovolemia
    b. Increased cardiac output
    c. Hypertension
    d. Fluid overload

288. What are the 2 main components of "double drip"?
    a. Guaifenesin and dobutamine
    b. Guaifenesin and ketamine
    c. Xylazine and ketamine
    d. Acepromazine and ketamine

289. Which of the following drugs cannot be safely administered via an intravenous bolus?
    a. Butorphanol
    b. Morphine
    c. Methadone
    d. Hydromorphone

290. Which of the following drugs is classified as a full mu opioid?
    a. Butorphanol
    b. Buprenorphine
    c. Dexmedetomidine
    d. Hydromorphone

291. You have been tasked to anesthetize a 1000-kg bull and maintain anesthesia by using an inhalant technique. Which is the correct statement regarding intubation of this patient?
    a. The inhalant can be safely delivered via a facemask
    b. The tube does not need to be lubricated before intubation
    c. You will have to manually intubate the bull
    d. All of the above

292. Which of the following drugs produces the most profound analgesia in dogs and cats?
    a. Methadone
    b. Midazolam
    c. Ketamine
    d. Butorphanol

293. Mu agonist opioids cause which of the following?
    a. Miosis in both dogs and cats
    b. Miosis in cats and mydriasis in dogs
    c. Mydriasis in cats and miosis in dogs
    d. Mydriasis in both dogs and cats

294. Which of the following inhalants cannot be used safely in ruminants?
    a. Nitrous oxide
    b. Isoflurane
    c. Halothane
    d. Sevoflurane

295. Which of the following drugs is used to reverse the effects of mu agonist opioids?
    a. Flumazenil
    b. Remifentanil
    c. Atipamezole
    d. Naloxone

296. Which of the following is *not* a contraindication for the use of NSAIDs?
    a. Pulmonary disease
    b. Impaired renal or hepatic function
    c. Coagulopathies
    d. Dehydration and hypovolemia

297. If you position the head of an anesthetized ruminant with the pharynx higher than the mouth, what can this help to prevent?
    a. Hyperventilation
    b. Hypotension
    c. Aspiration
    d. Hypoxemia

298. An infraorbital dental nerve block is used to block the sensation of pain to which of the following areas?
    a. The lower dental arcade and hard palate
    b. The rostral maxilla
    c. The rostral mandible
    d. The upper dental arcade and tongue

299. Why should ruminants be placed in sternal recumbency during recovery?
    a. Eructate
    b. Regurgitate
    c. Salivate
    d. Hyperventilate

300. You have been asked to perform an epidural in a canine patient that requires repair of a fractured ilium. This procedure is estimated to take at least 3 to 4 hours. The veterinarian would like you to use a combination of a local anesthetic and an opioid. Which of the following drug combinations would be the most appropriate on the basis of the time frame and extent of the procedure?
    a. Lidocaine and morphine
    b. Bupivacaine and morphine
    c. Lidocaine only
    d. Bupivicaine only

301. All of the following items make it easier to intubate swine, *except:*
    a. Speculum
    b. Laryngoscope
    c. Stylet
    d. Epiglotoscope

302. Unlike other domestic species, the spinal cord in the dog ends at which of the following vertebra?
    a. S1
    b. L6
    c. L7
    d. T13

303. In the feline patient, the spinal cord ends at the level of which of the following vertebra?
    a. S1
    b. L6
    c. L7
    d. T13

304. Which statement regarding swine anesthesia is true?
    a. Oscillometric blood pressure monitors work well in pigs
    b. All pigs should have complete blood work before anesthesia
    c. Pigs are very sensitive to alpha-2 agonists
    d. Intravenous sedation is virtually impossible in healthy pigs

305. Which of the following is *not* a contraindication for epidural administration?
    a. Pyoderma
    b. Coagulopathy
    c. Breed
    d. Septicemia

306. Which of the following drug combinations is considered neuroleptanalgesia?
    a. Atropine and morphine
    b. Midazolam and etomidate
    c. Hydromorphone and acepromazine
    d. Butorphanol and oxymorphone

307. Which of the following conditions does not occur in porcine stress syndrome?
    a. Hypothermia
    b. Hyperthermia
    c. Hyperkalemia
    d. Hypercapnia

308. Which of the following fluids is considered a synthetic colloid?
    a. Lactated Ringer's solution
    b. Hetastarch
    c. Fresh frozen plasma
    d. 0.9% saline

309. Why should glycopyrrolate be used in rabbits instead of atropine?
    a. Atropine is highly toxic in rabbits
    b. Many rabbits have high levels of atropinase, so atropine is relatively ineffective
    c. Rabbits are unable to metabolize atropine
    d. Atropine causes marked bradycardia in rabbits

310. Which of the following is *not* a consideration for blood administration during surgery?
    a. Type of procedure and blood loss anticipated
    b. Age and breed of patient
    c. Hemoglobin content of the patient's blood
    d. Hematocrit of the patient's blood

311. Why might you not get an accurate reading from a pulse oximeter in small mammals?
    a. The heart rate of the animal may exceed the upper range of the instrument
    b. The hemoglobin absorption characteristics are different in rodents and dogs and cats
    c. Pulse oximeters do not function on animals that have dark fur
    d. Small rodents have a rapid respiratory rate

312. Which of the following drugs should likely be avoided in patients requiring ocular surgery because it causes an increase in intraocular pressure?
    a. Propofol
    b. Isoflurane
    c. Fentanyl
    d. Ketamine

313. Why can't you use the position of the eyes to assess depth of anesthesia in rodents?
    a. The eye is too small to assess its position accurately
    b. The position of the eye does not change during anesthesia
    c. The eye rotates downward in very light planes of anesthesia
    d. The eyelids remain closed throughout anesthesia

314. You have been asked to anesthetize a patient with a suspected brain tumor. This patient is at risk for increased intracranial pressure. Which of the following drugs does not contribute in any way to increasing intracranial pressure and is thus "safe" for this patient?
    a. Propofol
    b. Ketamine
    c. Morphine
    d. Hydromorphone

315. What is an advantage of using medetomidine combined with ketamine for anesthesia of rodents and rabbits?
    a. It is readily absorbed from body fat
    b. It can be given by mouth to produce anesthesia
    c. It promotes gut motility and so reduces the occurrence of postoperative inappetence
    d. It can be partially reversed by using atipamezole, allowing faster recovery

316. Because of the enlarged fleshy tongue and a narrowed upper airway, which of the following statements is correct when dealing with neonatal and pediatric patients undergoing general anesthesia?
    a. Neonatal and pediatric patients should be induced and maintained via an anesthetic mask and inhalant
    b. Neonatal and pediatric patients should not be preoxygenated because it increases the risk of obstruction
    c. Neonatal and pediatric patients should be intubated for all procedures requiring general anesthesia because they are at risk for upper airway obstruction
    d. Neonatal and pediatric patients are at no more risk for airway obstruction compared with adult patients

317. What will the approximate blood volume of a 40-g adult mouse be?
    a. 10 mL
    b. 3 mL
    c. 50 mL
    d. 0.2 mL

318. Which of the following drugs is most likely the safest to give as part of an anesthetic protocol for a healthy, 1-year-old Labrador cesarean section?
    a. Dexmedetomidine
    b. Propofol
    c. Midazolam
    d. Acepromazine

319. Which of the following statements is correct?
    a. Arteries carry blood to the heart
    b. Veins carry blood to the heart
    c. Both veins and arteries carry blood away from the heart
    d. Both veins and arteries carry blood to the heart

320. What should be done to fluids such as lactated Ringer's solution when they are given to small mammals?
    a. Used at about 4° C so that they are rapidly absorbed
    b. Administered orally because it is not possible to use any other route
    c. Warmed to body temperature before administration to avoid causing hypothermia
    d. Given only postoperatively to avoid overloading the circulation

321. The P wave in the electrocardiograph represents which of the following?
    a. Ventricular depolarization
    b. Ventricular repolarization
    c. Atrial depolarization
    d. Atrial repolarization

322. The T wave in the electrocardiograph represents which of the following?
    a. Ventricular depolarization
    b. Ventricular repolarization
    c. Atrial depolarization
    d. Atrial repolarization

323. When using an anesthetic breathing circuit in a small rabbit, which of the following is the most accurate statement?
    a. Be constructed of only plastic components because rabbits are allergic to latex
    b. Have low equipment dead space
    c. Have high equipment dead space
    d. Always include soda lime to prevent rebreathing

324. The QRS complex in the electrocardiograph represents which of the following?
    a. Ventricular depolarization
    b. Ventricular repolarization
    c. Atrial depolarization
    d. Atrial repolarization

325. When giving postoperative analgesics to rodents and rabbits to alleviate pain, which of the following statements is true precaution?
    a. NSAIDs cannot be used because they cause gastric ulceration at normal therapeutic doses in these species
    b. Opioids (narcotics) cause severe respiratory depression and so must never be used
    c. Opioids must be given with care if a neuroleptanalgesic mixture has been used for anesthesia
    d. Local anesthetics cannot be used because they produce cardiac arrest even at low doses in these species

326. Which of the following best represents systolic blood pressure?
    a. The pressure measured when the left ventricle relaxes
    b. The pressure measured when the right ventricle relaxes
    c. The pressure measured when the left ventricle contracts
    d. The pressure measured when the right ventricle contracts

327. What is the tidal volume range for a 20-kg beagle mix?
    a. 200–400 mL
    b. 20–40 mL
    c. 2000–4000 mL
    d. 2–4 mL

328. What will happen if postoperative pain is not alleviated in rabbits?
    a. They will not eat or drink normally
    b. They will recover much faster from anesthesia
    c. They will spend a great deal of time grooming themselves
    d. Porphyrin staining will appear around their eyes

329. Which of the following patients should have coagulation profile submitted before anesthetizing for an elective hernia repair?
    a. Doberman
    b. Labrador
    c. Domestic shorthair
    d. Chihuahua

330. Common locations for pulse palpation in the dog include all of the following *except:*
    a. Femoral
    b. Dorsopedal
    c. Auricular
    d. Palmar digital

331. What will pulse oximetry often allow you to estimate?
    a. Arterial blood pressure
    b. Pulse pressure
    c. PaO_2
    d. Percent saturation of hemoglobin with oxygen

332. In relation to anesthesia, a patient with moderate risk that has systemic changes and some clinical alterations would be classified into which of the following categories?
    a. ASA I
    b. ASA II
    c. ASA III
    d. ASA IV

333. How many micrograms are in 1 milligram?
    a. 100
    b. 1000
    c. 10
    d. 1

334. A 2% solution of lidocaine has a mg/mL concentration of:
    a. 2 mg/mL
    b. 0.2 mg/mL
    c. 200 mg/mL
    d. 20 mg/mL

335. The drug xylazine is best described as an:
    a. Anti-inflammatory
    b. Analgesic and sedative
    c. Antiemetic
    d. Anesthetic

336. When pressure checking a rebreathing circuit, why is it important to keep your thumb over the end of the hose until the pressure is fully released from the system?
    a. Releasing your thumb before releasing the pressure in the circuit can create a vacuum effect causing some of the carbon dioxide absorbent to be sucked into the circuit
    b. Releasing your thumb before releasing the pressure in the circuit can cause the pop-off valve to become stuck in the closed position
    c. Releasing your thumb before releasing the pressure in the circuit can cause the scavenge system to malfunction
    d. Releasing your thumb before releasing the pressure in the circuit can lead to a malfunction of the one-way valves

337. The carbon dioxide absorbent should be changed when how much of the canister has changed to violet?
    a. $\frac{1}{2}$ of the canister
    b. $\frac{1}{4}$ of the canister
    c. $\frac{2}{3}$ of the canister
    d. $\frac{1}{8}$ of the canister

338. An endotracheal tube should be checked and left inflated for about how many minutes before use?
    a. 2–4 min
    b. 1–2 min
    c. 1–15 min
    d. 5–10 min

339. Detomidine is approved for use in:
    a. Dogs
    b. Cats
    c. Horses
    d. Cattle

340. The benefits of placing an arterial catheter include all of the following *except:*
    a. Ability to obtain central venous pressure
    b. Ability to obtain direct blood pressure
    c. Provides access to quick blood sample collection
    d. Ability to obtain and monitor blood gas samples

341. Hypothermia in the anesthetized patient can cause all of the following complications *except:*
    a. MAC reduction
    b. Decreased tissue perfusion
    c. Bradycardia
    d. Hypertension

342. Butorphanol is best described as a/an:
    a. Anti-inflammatory
    b. Analgesic
    c. Anesthetic
    d. Diuretic

343. Which of the following is not an advantage to endotracheal intubation in an anesthetized patient?
    a. Allows for complete control of the airway
    b. Oxygen and inhalant are delivered close to the lungs
    c. Increases anatomic dead space compared with a facemask
    d. Helps prevent aspiration of foreign material into the lungs

344. One disadvantage of an endotracheal tube that has a low-volume high-pressure cuff is:
    a. The endotracheal tube is hard to clean and sanitize
    b. A tight seal cannot be obtained without a large volume of air placed into the cuff
    c. A stylet must be used to advance these endotracheal tubes
    d. The high pressure in the cuff can cause tracheal necrosis over time

345. Diazepam is considered a good choice in patients when which body system is compromised?
    a. Hepatic
    b. Renal
    c. Cardiovascular
    d. All body systems

346. Placing an endotracheal tube that is too small compared with the diameter of the trachea can cause:
    a. Increase in airway resistance
    b. Decrease in tidal volume
    c. Increase in dead space
    d. Decrease in peak inspiratory pressure

347. Before anesthetic induction, it is ideal to preoxygenate the patient for:
    a. 1–2 min
    b. 10 min
    c. 3–5 min
    d. Preoxygenation is not necessary

348. In the United States, xylazine is not approved for use in:
    a. Dogs
    b. Cats
    c. Horses
    d. Cattle

349. You have just induced and intubated a canine patient. The patient has normal chest excursions, but the capnograph is reading zero. What has likely happened?
    a. The patient is not completely anesthetized
    b. The endotracheal tube has been inserted too deeply
    c. The oxygen flow rate is too high, thus flushing the system
    d. The endotracheal tube is likely in the esophagus

350. The small oxygen tank that attaches to the anesthesia machine is labeled as what type of tank?
    a. "E"
    b. "H"
    c. "J"
    d. "G"

351. Guaifenesin is most often used in horses and cattle to provide:
    a. Analgesia
    b. Muscle relaxation
    c. Anesthesia
    d. Diuresis

352. You have been asked to provide inhalant anesthesia to a patient by using low-flow anesthetic rates. Which of the following rates would you use to calculate low-flow anesthesia?
    a. 4–7 mL/kg/min
    b. 5–10 mL/kg/min
    c. 10–15 mL/kg/min
    d. 15–25 mL/kg/min

353. What is the purpose for higher flow rates when using a non-rebreathing system?
    a. To eliminate rebreathing of carbon dioxide
    b. To ensure the patient receives the proper percentage of inhalant
    c. To help keep the patient warm
    d. To provide humidity to the respiratory system

354. Which of the following ECG leads is most commonly used to monitor patients under general anesthesia?
    a. Lead I
    b. Lead II
    c. Lead III
    d. Lead IV

355. Your patient's ECG strip is showing a fast, regular rhythm with normal morphology. Which of the following do you suspect?
    a. 1st degree AV block
    b. Atrial fibrillation
    c. Premature ventricular contractions
    d. Sinus tachycardia

356. The combination of xylazine and butorphanol is used to:
    a. Provide greater analgesia and muscle relaxation than either drug can alone
    b. Cause central nervous system (CNS) excitement
    c. Increase the dose of butorphanol
    d. Increase the dose of xylazine

357. Which of the following drugs is used to treat bradycardia in the anesthetized patient?
    a. Doxapram
    b. Glycopyrrolate
    c. Alfaxalone
    d. Ketamine

358. Which of the following arrhythmias is characterized by a prolonged P-R interval?
    a. 1st degree AV block
    b. 2nd degree AV block
    c. 3rd degree AV block
    d. AV dissociation

359. Which drug is the most potent sedative?
    a. Xylazine
    b. Detomidine
    c. Acepromazine
    d. Diazepam

360. Which of the following arrhythmias is characterized by a P wave that lacks a QRS complex to follow?
    a. 1st degree AV block
    b. 2nd degree AV block
    c. 3rd degree AV block
    d. AV dissociation

361. Which drug is most likely to cause hypotension in normal doses?
    a. Diazepam
    b. Butorphanol
    c. Acepromazine
    d. Flunixin meglumine

362. Which of the following arrhythmias is characterized by a fast, irregular rhythm with wide and bizarre QRS complexes?
    a. 3rd degree AV block
    b. Atrial premature complexes
    c. Ventricular tachycardia
    d. Sinus bradycardia

363. You are monitoring a 12-year-old dog for a humeral fracture repair. You notice that the complexes on the ECG are intermittently wide and bizarre; otherwise, the rhythm is normal. Which arrhythmia is most likely occurring?
    a. Atrial fibrillation
    b. Ventricular fibrillation
    c. Atrial premature complexes
    d. Ventricular premature complexes

364. The combination drug Telazol contains:
    a. Diazepam and ketamine
    b. Diazepam and xylazine
    c. Zolazepam and tiletamine
    d. Xylazine and tiletamine

365. Which of the following drugs would most likely be the cause of atrioventricular block in a patient under anesthesia?
    a. Propofol
    b. Ketamine
    c. Dexmedetomidine
    d. Alfaxalone

366. All of the following cross the placental barrier in significant amounts *except*:
    a. Acepromazine
    b. Diazepam
    c. Isoflurane
    d. Neuromuscular blocking agents

367. Which of the following drugs is used to treat ventricular premature contractions (VPCs)?
    a. Lidocaine
    b. Doxapram
    c. Dopamine
    d. Phenylephrine

368. Which drug is not classified as a barbiturate?
    a. Phenobarbital
    b. Thiopental
    c. Pentobarbital
    d. Propofol

369. Common causes of ventricular premature contractions include all of the following *except*:
    a. Hypoxia
    b. Pain
    c. Gastric dilation and volvulus
    d. Anemia

370. Glycopyrrolate is an anticholinergic with all of the following advantages over atropine *except*:
    a. It has a longer duration of action
    b. It crosses the placental barrier
    c. It is less likely to cause cardiac arrhythmias
    d. It has a smaller dose volume

371. A patient breathing 100% oxygen should have a pulse oximetry reading of what percentage?
    a. 95%–100%
    b. 90%–100%
    c. 93%–100%
    d. 90%–95%

372. Which of the following drugs is most likely to affect a pulse oximetry reading?
    a. Ketamine
    b. Fentanyl
    c. Oxymorphone
    d. Dexmedetomidine

373. Which of the following is not a side effect of hypothermia under anesthesia?
    a. Impaired platelet function
    b. Death
    c. Anemia
    d. Coagulopathy

374. Which of the following reflexes should *always* be present in patients under anesthesia?
    a. Palpebral reflex
    b. Corneal reflex
    c. Withdrawal reflex
    d. Swallowing reflex

375. Normal capillary refill time in mammals is how long?
    a. 1 second
    b. 1–3 seconds
    c. Less than 1–2 seconds
    d. Greater than 2 seconds

376. At normal doses, what effect does atropine have on the heart rate?
    a. Decreases
    b. No effect
    c. Increases
    d. Depends on the species

377. Anesthetic drugs that cause vasoconstriction often cause the mucous membranes to become:
    a. Pink
    b. Red
    c. Blue
    d. Pale

378. Opioid drugs are used in anesthetic protocols primarily as:
    a. Anesthetics
    b. Analgesics
    c. Anti-inflammatories
    d. Antihistamines

379. The advantage of xylazine over acepromazine is that it:
    a. Does not cause cardiac arrhythmias
    b. Produces a short period of analgesia
    c. Has antiemetic properties
    d. Is an anti-inflammatory

380. Routine use of atropine in horses should be avoided because it may:
    a. Cause colic
    b. Slow the heart rate
    c. Cause excitement
    d. Increase salivation

381. Which drug should be avoided in the stallion because it may cause permanent prolapse of the penis?
    a. Glycopyrrolate
    b. Acepromazine
    c. Xylazine
    d. Diazepam

382. Anesthetic drugs that cause vasodilation often cause the mucous membranes to become:
    a. Pink
    b. Red
    c. Blue
    d. Pale

383. Which drug is a narcotic antagonist?
    a. Naloxone
    b. Atropine
    c. Pancuronium
    d. Droperidol

384. The width of the blood pressure cuff in a cat should be what percentage of the circumference of the leg?
    a. 20%
    b. 30%
    c. 65%
    d. 70%

385. The audible sound coming from the Doppler probe is produced by red blood cells circulating though the:
    a. Vein
    b. Artery
    c. Capillaries
    d. Mucous membranes

386. Depressant preanesthetic medication may have what effect on the anesthesia procedure?
    a. Shorten the recovery time
    b. Prolong the recovery time
    c. Leave the recovery time unaltered
    d. Necessitate increasing the dose of induction agent

387. The use of oscillometric blood pressure monitoring should be reserved for patients more than how many kg because of inaccuracies in smaller patients?
    a. 2 kg
    b. 3 kg
    c. 4 kg
    d. 5 kg

388. Which of the following provides a noninvasive method for assessing ventilation, cardiac output, pulmonary perfusion, and systemic metabolism?
    a. Electrocardiograph
    b. Capnograph
    c. Central venous pressure
    d. Arterial blood gas

389. Which drug is an antagonist of xylazine?
    a. Butorphanol
    b. Detomidine
    c. Yohimbine
    d. Pentazocine

390. Which of the following is considered mechanical dead space?
    a. Excessively long endotracheal tube
    b. Air in the nasal passages
    c. Air in the trachea
    d. Air in the mouth

391. Which of the following fluids is considered a colloid?
    a. Lactated Ringer's solution
    b. Plasma-Lyte
    c. 0.9% saline
    d. Hetastarch

392. Diazepam is used to produce:
    a. Analgesia
    b. Hypnosis
    c. Muscle relaxation
    d. Vomiting

393. Epinephrine:
    a. Increases the heart rate
    b. Decreases the heart rate
    c. Decreases the blood pressure
    d. Should be used to reverse the effects of acepromazine

394. The use of nitrous oxide in anesthesia:
    a. Increases the amount of inhalation anesthetic required
    b. Decreases the amount of inhalation anesthetic required
    c. Slows the induction process
    d. Has no effect on the time or amount of anesthetic required

395. Which of the following have a similar sodium and chloride concentration to that of the extracellular fluid as well as a similar osmolarity?
    a. Hypertonic fluids
    b. Hypotonic fluids
    c. Isotonic fluids
    d. None of the above

396. Which of the following fluids is considered an unbalanced solution?
    a. Lactated Ringer's solution
    b. Normosol-R
    c. Plasma-Lyte 148
    d. 0.9% saline

397. A disadvantage of breathing 50% nitrous oxide is that it:
    a. Decreases the arterial oxygenation
    b. Increases the arterial oxygenation
    c. Slows the induction time
    d. Prolongs the recovery time

398. Which of the following fluids is *not* a colloid?
    a. Whole blood
    b. Plasma-Lyte 148
    c. Hetastarch
    d. Hextend

399. Which of the following are considered sensible losses?
    a. Urine output
    b. Fecal waste
    c. Loss of fluid through the skin
    d. Loss of fluid through the respiratory tract

400. How many milligrams per milliliter (mg/mL) does a 2% lidocaine solution contain?
    a. 5
    b. 10
    c. 20
    d. 30

401. You must anesthetize a patient that will require a whole blood transfusion. To avoid contamination, blood products should be given within how many hours after collection?
    a. 2 hr
    b. 4 hr
    c. 8 hr
    d. 12 hr

402. Apneustic breathing patterns are frequently seen in cats when high doses of _____ are used.
    a. Pentobarbital
    b. Thiamylal
    c. Ketamine
    d. Guaifenesin

403. If 180 mL of a 5% solution of guaifenesin is administered to a 150-kg foal, how many mg/kg would be administered?
    a. 30
    b. 60
    c. 90
    d. 15

404. Which of the following are tranquilizers that cause muscle relaxation, and in some young healthy animals, this can also cause excitation?
    a. Alpha-2 agonists
    b. Opioids
    c. Dissociates
    d. Benzodiazepines

405. Which of the following premedication drugs would be contraindicated in patients that are tachycardic?
    a. Morphine
    b. Atropine
    c. Methadone
    d. Midazolam

406. Caudal epidural administration of lidocaine in the dog is:
    a. Useful to prevent movement
    b. Not to be used for cesarean section
    c. An excellent caudal analgesic
    d. An old procedure with little value in veterinary anesthesia today

407. Because diazepam is not water soluble, it should only be administered via which routes:
    a. Intravenously and orally
    b. Subcutaneously and intramuscularly
    c. Intramuscularly and intravenously
    d. Intramuscularly only

408. Which of the following opioids is *not* appropriate for a fracture repair in a dog or cat?
    a. Methadone
    b. Oxymorphone
    c. Hydromorphone
    d. Butorphanol

409. Mask inductions are:
    a. Best used in dogs and cats with airway obstruction
    b. Best used in aggressive dogs and cats
    c. Absolutely the best way to induce anesthesia in all dogs and cats
    d. More appropriately used in calm dogs and cats

410. Which of the following drugs reverses the effects of a full mu opioid?
    a. Flumazenil
    b. Atipamezole
    c. Alfaxalone
    d. Naloxone

411. Which of the following drugs is a partial agonist?
    a. Butorphanol
    b. Buprenorphine
    c. Morphine
    d. Naloxone

412. Which of the following is not an effect associated with atropine administration?
    a. Tachycardia
    b. Excessive salivation
    c. Mydriasis
    d. Decreased gastrointestinal motility

413. Which of the following drugs can cause the release of histamine when administered intravenously?
    a. Buprenorphine
    b. Hydromorphone
    c. Butorphanol
    d. Morphine

414. Which of the following induction drugs causes the palpebral reflex to be retained, increases the heart rate and blood pressure, causes the eyes to stay centrally located, and maintains a fair amount of jaw tone?
    a. Propofol
    b. Alfaxalone
    c. Fentanyl
    d. Ketamine

415. The dosage of acepromazine is 0.1 mg/kg, and the maximum dose is 4 mg. How many milligrams would you administer to a 60-kg dog?
    a. 2 mg
    b. 4 mg
    c. 6 mg
    d. 8 mg

416. Which drug is a dissociative anesthetic?
    a. Propofol
    b. Ketamine
    c. Alfaxalone
    d. Etomidate

417. The adverse effects of anesthetic compounds are:
    a. Nothing to worry about
    b. Never present with smaller doses
    c. Dose dependent
    d. Not dose dependent

418. Heinz body formation, lethargy, vomiting, diarrhea, and anorexia can occur in cats given which of the following drugs repeatedly over a short period?
    a. Propofol
    b. Midazolam
    c. Ketamine
    d. Alfaxalone

419. Which of the following drugs should be avoided in cats with renal failure?
    a. Propofol
    b. Ketamine
    c. Alfaxalone
    d. Fentanyl

420. Which of the following factors do not influence minimum alveolar concentration (MAC)?
    a. Age
    b. Temperature
    c. Sex
    d. Stress

421. The definition for the rate at which a liquid will turn into a gas at a given temperature is:
    a. Sublimation
    b. Vapor pressure
    c. Evaporation
    d. Deposition

422. Which of the following statements is correct?
    a. The higher the solubility of the anesthetic, the more rapid gas anesthetics will go from the alveoli into the blood
    b. The higher the solubility of the anesthetic the more rapid the gas anesthetics will go from the blood into the alveoli
    c. The lower the solubility of the anesthetic, the less rapid gas anesthetics will go from the alveoli into the blood
    d. The lower the solubility of the anesthetic, the more rapid gas anesthetics will go from the alveoli into the blood

423. Which of the following statements about inhalant anesthetics is incorrect?
    a. Inhalant anesthetics affect the CNS
    b. The primary method of excretion of inhalant anesthesia is via hepatic metabolism
    c. Inhalants cause dose-dependent vasodilation
    d. Most inhalants decrease the rate a depth of respiration

424. What is the MAC value of isoflurane in the dog?
    a. 1.28
    b. 1.65
    c. 1.77
    d. 1.17

425. What is the MAC value of isoflurane in the cat?
    a. 1.35
    b. 1.63
    c. 2.60
    d. 2.10

426. What is the MAC value of sevoflurane in the dog?
    a. 2.70
    b. 1.82
    c. 2.10
    d. 1.61

427. What is the MAC value of sevoflurane in the cat?
    a. 2.60
    b. 1.81
    c. 2.25
    d. 1.69

428. Which of the following affects the solubility coefficient of an inhalant anesthetic?
    a. Patient weight
    b. Age
    c. Body temperature
    d. Anesthetic drug protocol

429. Which of the following inhalants is twice as soluble as sevoflurane?
    a. Isoflurane
    b. Halothane
    c. Desflurane
    d. Nitrous oxide

430. Which of the following inhalant anesthetics does not need to be vaporized for administration?
    a. Halothane
    b. Isoflurane
    c. Sevoflurane
    d. Nitrous oxide

431. Which of the following drugs causes a dose-dependent vasodilation?
    a. Fentanyl
    b. Thiopental
    c. Isoflurane
    d. Midazolam

432. Which of the following contributes to a prolonged recovery?
    a. Hypothermia
    b. Breed of dog or cat
    c. Sex of patient
    d. Hyperthermia

433. Ideally, vital signs should be monitored in all patients recovering from anesthesia how often?
    a. Every 45 min
    b. Every hour
    c. Every 15 min
    d. Every 1–2 hr

434. Respiratory acidosis is most often caused by:
    a. Hyperventilation
    b. Hypoventilation
    c. Hypercarbia
    d. Eupnea

435. A complete blockage of the endotracheal tube will cause which of the following?
    a. Eupnea
    b. Regurgitation
    c. Aspiration
    d. Respiratory acidosis

436. Which of the following drugs can cause excitation in healthy patients when used as a premedication or induction agent?
    a. Midazolam
    b. Fentanyl
    c. Morphine
    d. Alfaxalone

437. Which of the following is a potential side effect of administering propofol too quickly?
    a. Tachycardia
    b. Apnea
    c. Hypertension
    d. Hypothermia

438. When is airway obstruction most likely to occur in a surgical patient?
    a. During the surgical procedure
    b. During the preanesthetic and recovery period
    c. During surgery and postoperatively
    d. During recovery as the patient is awakening

439. Using which of the following drugs can prevent laryngospasm?
    a. Isoflurane
    b. Oxymorphone
    c. Lidocaine
    d. Diazepam

440. Which term best describes the following definition: "Reduced minute volume due to a reduction in tidal volume and/or respiratory rate"?
    a. Hypoventilation
    b. Dyspnea
    c. Tachypnea
    d. Hyperventilation

441. All of the following contribute to hypoventilation *except:*
    a. Hyperthermia
    b. Pulmonary disease
    c. Accidental endobronchial intubation
    d. Restrictive chest bandage

442. All of the following contribute to hyperventilation *except:*
a. Inadequate anesthetic depth
b. Pain
c. Hypoxia
d. Hypothermia

443. You have anesthetized a 9-year-old male, castrated mixed-breed dog for a right hind limb amputation. What would be the lowest acceptable mean arterial blood pressure for this patient?
a. 40 mm Hg
b. 60 mm Hg
c. 80 mm Hg
d. 100 mm Hg

444. Which of the following terms best describes the following definition: "Sudden cessation of functional ventilation and systemic perfusion"?
a. Bradycardia
b. Cardiopulmonary arrest
c. Ventricular tachycardia
d. Hypercapnia

445. How long does it take after cardiopulmonary arrest before irreversible neurological damage can occur?
a. 5 min
b. 10 min
c. 7 min
d. 3 min

446. During CPCR what is the preferred order of routes for drug administration?
a. Central venous, intraosseous, peripheral venous, intratracheal
b. Peripheral venous, central venous, intraosseous, intratracheal
c. Peripheral venous, central venous, intratracheal, intraosseous
d. Central venous, peripheral venous, intraosseous, intratracheal

447. Which of the following is a direct response of epinephrine administration?
a. Vasoconstriction
b. Vasodilation
c. Hypoventilation
d. Hyperventilation

448. Which of the following drugs is used to treat ventricular tachycardia?
a. Thiopental
b. Lidocaine
c. Alfaxalone
d. Dopamine

449. Which of the following drugs is most commonly used to treat bradycardia?
a. Lidocaine
b. Dobutamine
c. Alfaxalone
d. Atropine

450. Which of the following devices is essential to monitor the heart rate and rhythm?
a. Capnograph
b. Doppler
c. Electrocardiogram
d. Pulse oximeter

451. Why is placing alcohol onto ECG leads contraindicated in patients requiring CPCR?
a. Alcohol can cause skin irritation
b. Alcohol can cool the patient
c. Alcohol can cause a fire if defibrillation is performed
d. Alcohol is actually not contraindicated in these patients

452. Which of the following best describes the term *multimodal anesthesia*?
a. The use of one single drug to achieve analgesia
b. The use of multiple drugs to help reduce the doses of each agent, thus decreasing negative side effects
c. An anesthetic protocol that does not use a premedication in an attempt to decrease the negative side effects of anesthetic drugs
d. The use of opioids only to decrease anesthetic requirements

453. Which of the following is the best technique for providing effective preoxygenation in a dog or cat before anesthetic induction?
a. Using flow-by oxygen via the breathing circuit
b. Using a mask without the diaphragm
c. Using a mask with a fitted diaphragm
d. Oxygen is not necessary before anesthetic induction

454. Which of the following best describes the inability to move blood forward effectively enough to meet metabolic needs?
a. Liver failure
b. Heart failure
c. Renal failure
d. Pulmonary failure

455. The normal peak inspiratory pressure delivered during mechanical ventilation should range between:
a. 10–15 cm H_2O
b. 10–20 cm H_2O
c. 20–25 cm H_2O
d. 15–20 cm H_2O

456. The normal respiratory rate in the anesthetized dog and cat ranges between:
   a. 4–6 breaths/min
   b. 8–12 breaths/min
   c. 6–10 breaths/min
   d. 10–15 breaths/min

457. An intact thoracic cavity is under _____.
   a. Negative pressure
   b. Positive pressure
   c. Both negative and positive pressure
   d. Neutral pressure

458. What percent decrease in renal function must be present before seeing any abnormalities on a blood chemistry panel?
   a. 40%–50%
   b. 25%–40%
   c. 60%–65%
   d. 70%–75%

459. Which of the following drugs is contraindicated in cats presenting with renal failure?
   a. Ketamine
   b. Propofol
   c. Oxymorphone
   d. Isoflurane

460. Which of the following organs plays a crucial role in the metabolism and clearance of most anesthetic drugs?
   a. Lungs
   b. Kidneys
   c. Pancreas
   d. Liver

461. Which of the following can result in decreased drug binding, prolonged recoveries, and relative overdose from highly protein-bound drugs?
   a. Low total protein and low albumin
   b. Low total protein and low blood urea nitrogen
   c. Low total protein and high creatinine
   d. Low total protein and high packed cell volume

462. Of the following drug protocols, which is most commonly used in ruminant patients undergoing minor surgical procedures?
   a. Premedicate with butorphanol and mask down with isoflurane
   b. Premedicate with atropine and morphine and induce with alfaxalone
   c. Premedicate with acepromazine and induce with propofol
   d. Premedicate with butorphanol and use a standing position with local blocks

463. To decrease regurgitation in ruminants undergoing anesthesia, food should be withheld for how many hours before induction?
   a. 12 hr
   b. 6 hr
   c. 48 hr
   d. 24 hr

464. Why is the neck of ruminants elevated with the head placed in a downward position during general anesthesia?
   a. This position helps decrease intracranial pressure
   b. This position helps keep the endotracheal tube in place
   c. This position helps facilitate drainage of saliva and regurgitation
   d. This position is not necessary in ruminants

465. Which of the following nerve blocks is used for dehorning ruminants?
   a. Auriculopalpebral nerve block
   b. Cornual nerve block
   c. Peroneal nerve block
   d. Digital nerve block

466. Which of the following local blocks would provide additional anesthesia/analgesia to a sheep undergoing a large abdominal surgery?
   a. Epidural block
   b. Caudal block
   c. Peroneal block
   d. Cornual block

467. Improper administration or an overdose of a local anesthetic into the epidural space can lead to all of the following *except:*
   a. Seizures
   b. Hypertension
   c. Paralysis of the respiratory system
   d. Unconsciousness

468. Which of the following is safe to use in animals that will be slaughtered?
   a. Xylazine
   b. Ketamine
   c. Romifidine
   d. None of the above

469. Which of the following drugs is not generally suggested for use in ruminants?
   a. Ketamine
   b. Butorphanol
   c. Propofol
   d. Atropine

470. Which of the following vessels is most commonly used for intravenous catheter placement in cattle undergoing anesthesia?
    a. Jugular
    b. Cephalic
    c. Lateral saphenous
    d. Auricular

471. You have been asked to anesthetize a horse for a laceration repair. You just administered xylazine to the patient and realized it has been overdosed by 10 times. Which of the following drugs is used to reverse the effects of xylazine?
    a. Flumazenil
    b. Naloxone
    c. Dexmedetomidine
    d. Yohimbine

472. The MAC of isoflurane in the equine patient is:
    a. 1.7%–2.1%
    b. 1.31%–1.64%
    c. 2.11%–2.34%
    d. 1.12%–1.54%

473. In the horse, which of the following is considered unreliable when assessing anesthetic depth?
    a. Respiratory rate
    b. Swallow reflex
    c. Heart rate
    d. Lateral nystagmus

474. Which of the following is the ideal way to assess ventilation in the horse?
    a. Assessing mucous membrane color
    b. Blood gas analysis
    c. ETCO$_2$
    d. Pulse oximetry

475. The average oxygen flow rate used for inhalant anesthetic induction in horses ranges between:
    a. 5–10 mL/kg/min
    b. 10–15 mL/kg/min
    c. 15–20 mL/kg/min
    d. 20–25 mL/kg/min

476. The average oxygen flow rate used for maintenance anesthesia in the horse ranges between:
    a. 2–4 mL/kg/min
    b. 5–10 mL/kg/min
    c. 4–8 mL/kg/min
    d. 1–2 mL/kg/min

477. Which of the following is a potential problem with maintaining a patient on room air during an anesthetic procedure?
    a. Hypertension
    b. Hyperthermia
    c. Apnea
    d. Hypoxemia

478. NSAIDs should not be administered in conjunction with corticosteroids because of:
    a. Increased risk of liver failure
    b. Increased risk of renal failure
    c. Effects of the two drugs cancel each other
    d. Increased risk of GI ulceration

479. Which of the following drugs used for post op analgesia is not a true opioid, nor produces opioid effects?
    a. Oxymorphone
    b. Meperidine
    c. Tramadol
    d. Deracoxib

480. Which of the following opioids is an NMDA antagonist?
    a. Morphine
    b. Methadone
    c. Butorphanol
    d. Fentanyl

481. Which of the following is an example of chronic pain?
    a. Osteoarthritis
    b. Fractured leg after being hit by a car 12 hours earlier
    c. Fresh laceration
    d. Bite wound from a dogfight earlier the same day

482. Which of the following is *not* an example of maladaptive pain?
    a. Cancer
    b. Fresh laceration
    c. Osteoarthritis
    d. Profound gingivitis

483. Which of the following types of pain dissipates as the initial source of pain resolves?
    a. Chronic pain
    b. Acute pain
    c. Maladaptive pain
    d. Wind-up pain

484. Which of the following types of pain is most associated with trauma or surgery?
    a. Adaptive pain
    b. Maladaptive pain
    c. Chronic pain
    d. Neuropathic pain

485. Which of the following drugs drastically reduces cardiac output?
    a. Morphine
    b. Meloxicam
    c. Dexmedetomidine
    d. Ketamine

486. You have been asked to anesthetize a 1-year-old Labrador for removal of a foreign body in the GI tract. This is a painful procedure, and you want to provide an opioid that will not induce vomiting. Which of the following would be the best choice for this?
    a. Morphine
    b. Oxymorphone
    c. Hydromorphone
    d. Methadone

487. Which of the following drugs acts by preventing painful signals from reaching the spinal cord?
    a. Morphine
    b. Alfaxalone
    c. Propofol
    d. Bupivacaine

488. To avoid the risk of GI ulceration, NSAIDs should be stopped for how many days before starting a different NSAID?
    a. 30 days
    b. 15–30 days
    c. 1–3 days
    d. 4–10 days

489. Which of the following are considered adjuncts for pain management?
    a. Weight loss
    b. Laser therapy
    c. Physical rehabilitation
    d. All of the above

490. Which of the following is not a normal sign of pain in the dog?
    a. Dilated pupils
    b. Increased grooming
    c. Lack of appetite
    d. Licking wound or surgery site

491. Which of the following terms best describes: "An unpleasant sensory and emotional experience individuals have when they perceive actual or potential tissue damage to their body"?
    a. Dysphoria
    b. Pain
    c. Anxiety
    d. Aggression

492. Which of the following is best characterized by visceral pain?
    a. Dull, diffuse pain in the kidneys
    b. Chronic, deep, burning sensation in the bone
    c. Superficial pain originating in the dermis
    d. A throbbing pain originating in the mucous membranes

493. Which of the following types of pain is considered a protective pain?
    a. Chronic pain
    b. Acute pain
    c. Neuropathic pain
    d. Wind-up pain

494. Which of the following is best described as somatic pain?
    a. Dull, diffuse pain in the liver
    b. Achy pain in the bladder
    c. Spasmlike pain in the intestines
    d. Superficial pain originating in the skin

495. It is believed that the viscera may contain more kappa receptors than mu receptors. If this is correct, which of the following drugs would provide better analgesia for visceral pain?
    a. Morphine
    b. Oxymorphone
    c. Hydromorphone
    d. Butorphanol

496. You have been asked to anesthetize a ferret for a small mass removal on the flank. How long should this patient be fasted before induction?
    a. No fasting time is required
    b. 1–2 hr
    c. 2–4 hr
    d. 4–6 hr

497. Premedications in the ferret are most often administered into which of the following sites?
    a. Caudal thigh
    b. Forelimbs
    c. Caudal lumbar
    d. Cephalic vein

498. Which of the following drugs is used to help prevent laryngospasm in the ferret before endotracheal intubation?
    a. Ketamine
    b. Lidocaine
    c. Alfaxalone
    d. Propofol

499. What is the most common site for an IO catheter in a rat?
a. Femur
b. Tibia
c. Fibula
d. Radius

500. You have anesthetized a patient that presented with a gastric dilatation-volvulus (GDV). After induction, you notice tachycardia, hypotension, prolonged capillary refill time, and pale mucous membranes. What is likely the cause of this?
a. Hyperthermia
b. Hypovolemic shock
c. Light plane of anesthesia
d. Hypocapnia

501. Which of the following crystalloid fluids would likely be a better choice for a patient with hyperkalemia currently undergoing a surgical procedure?
a. Lactated Ringer's solution
b. Normosol-R
c. 0.9% sodium chloride
d. D5W

502. An anesthetic patient has metabolic acidosis and a blood pH of 7.122. Which of the following drugs can be administered to help increase pH?
a. Dopamine
b. Sodium bicarbonate
c. Etomidate
d. Doxapram

503. You are preparing for an emergency German shepherd patient presenting with a suspected GDV. It will likely require emergency surgery soon after arrival. In preparing for the procedure, where are you going to place the IV catheter?
a. Large-bore catheter in the jugular vein
b. Large-bore catheter in the lateral saphenous vein
c. Large-bore catheter in the auricular vein
d. Large-bore catheter in the medial saphenous vein

504. Which of the following preanesthetic drugs should be avoided in the GDV patient?
a. Hydromorphone
b. Methadone
c. Oxymorphone
d. Morphine

505. Which of the following is *not* an anticipated problem of a patient undergoing anesthesia for the repair of a GDV?
a. Arrhythmias
b. Electrolyte imbalances
c. Pain
d. Severe blood loss

506. Which of the following would be considered a complication of recovery for a patient that had a foreign body removed from the trachea?
a. Severe pain
b. Airway obstruction resulting from swelling
c. Aspiration
d. Hypovolemic shock

507. Which of the following is a potential complication for a patient anesthetized for a myelogram?
a. Hyperthermia
b. Seizures
c. Pain
d. Bleeding

508. A cat with a urethral obstruction presents to the hospital on emergency. This patient needs to be anesthetized for a urethrotomy. Before induction you decide to place an ECG on the patient. You immediately notice wide QRS complexes with a lack of P waves. What does this indicate?
a. Hypernatremia
b. Hyperchloremia
c. Hypophosphatemia
d. Hyperkalemia

509. A 10-year-old mixed-breed intact male dog presents to the clinic after being rescued from a house fire. He is tachycardiac, dyspneic, and has a large wound on his left hind limb. This patient is compromised. Which of the following would be the better premedication protocol?
a. Midazolam and butorphanol
b. Oxymorphone and dexmedetomidine
c. Midazolam and methadone
d. Buprenorphine only

510. A 10-year-old mixed-breed intact male dog presents to the clinic after being rescued from a house fire. He is tachycardiac, dyspneic, and has a large wound on his left hind limb. This patient is compromised. Which of the following would be the better anesthetic induction protocol?
a. Etomidate and midazolam
b. Propofol
c. Mask induction
d. Any of the above would be acceptable for this patient

511. Which of the following drugs best fits this description: "Class IV controlled substance that acts as an anxiolytic, muscle relaxant, hypnotic, and anticonvulsant"?
a. Propofol
b. Midazolam
c. Fentanyl
d. Thiopental

512. How many hours after thoracic trauma does it take to show the full extent of pulmonary lesions via radiographs?
    a. 12–16 hr
    b. 12–24 hr
    c. 20–25 hr
    d. 24–36 hr

513. Which of the following statements about anesthesia for a cesarean section is true?
    a. Mask induction is the safest means of anesthetic induction
    b. GI transit time and lower esophageal sphincter tone are decreased, leading to increased risk of regurgitation and aspiration
    c. PCV and plasma protein levels are often increased in these patients
    d. Urine specific gravity is decreased in these patients

514. Because of the increase in cerebral oxygen demand, which of the following drugs is no longer recommended to stimulate respiration in the newborn after cesarean section?
    a. Dobutamine
    b. Dopamine
    c. Doxapram
    d. Naloxone

515. Which of the following techniques can be considered for use in a cesarean section to help reduce the need for larger doses of other more detrimental drugs?
    a. Epidural
    b. Constant rate infusion of morphine
    c. Bier block
    d. Constant rate infusion of ketamine

516. Why are uncuffed endotracheal tubes suggested for use in birds undergoing anesthesia?
    a. The trachea in birds is too small for a cuffed endotracheal tube
    b. The trachea is made up of a mixture of complete and incomplete tracheal rings
    c. The trachea is made up of complete tracheal rings that lack elasticity
    d. The trachea is made up of incomplete tracheal rings only

517. Which of the following structures makes it possible for birds to vocalize even after they have been properly intubated?
    a. Choana
    b. Syrinx
    c. Larynx
    d. Operculum

518. Which of the following bones are pneumatic in birds and should therefore *not* be used for intraosseous catheter placement?
    a. Ulna and radius
    b. Femur and radius
    c. Humerus and tibiotarsus
    d. Femur and humerus

519. Guinea pigs are difficult to intubate because of which of the following anatomic structures?
    a. Enlarged nasopharynx
    b. Hyperplastic oropharynx
    c. Palatal ostium
    d. Nasopharyngeal diverticula

520. Nasotracheal intubation is possible in which of the following species?
    a. Chinchilla
    b. Ferret
    c. Rabbit
    d. Guinea pig

521. A sidestream capnograph samples approximately how much gas from the attachment site?
    a. 200–300 mL/min
    b. 100–400 mL/min
    c. 50–150 mL/min
    d. Sidestream capnography does not sample gas

522. Intramuscular injections are most commonly administered into which of the following muscles in the avian patient?
    a. Quadriceps muscle
    b. Biceps muscle
    c. Pectoral muscle
    d. Gastrocnemius muscle

523. Which of the following is the most commonly used drug for maintenance anesthesia in the fish and amphibian patient?
    a. MS-222
    b. Propofol
    c. Isoflurane
    d. Ketamine

524. A blood sample is needed to run a PCV and total solids before anesthetic induction in a small frog. What site is most commonly used for blood collection in amphibians?
    a. Cephalic vein
    b. Ventral abdominal vein
    c. Lingual venous plexus
    d. Lateral saphenous

525. Which of the following drugs may decrease the heart rate of a neonatal patient?
    a. Midazolam
    b. Glycopyrrolate
    c. Morphine
    d. Dexmetetomidine

526. Reptiles have a three-chambered heart consisting of the following:
    a. One atrium and two ventricles
    b. One atrium, one ventricle, and a cavum venosum
    c. Two atria and one ventricle
    d. Reptiles actually have a four-chambered heart similar to birds

527. Which of the following can profoundly affect cardiac output and blood pressure in the neonate?
    a. Tachycardia
    b. Bradycardia
    c. Apnea
    d. Hyperthermia

528. Because pediatric patients have less functional contractile tissue, limited cardiac reserve, low ventricular compliance, and a reduced ability to increase stroke volume, they are highly dependent on heart rate to maintain which of the following?
    a. Cardiac output and blood pressure
    b. Body temperature and systemic vascular resistance
    c. Myocardial oxygen consumption and pulmonary reserve
    d. Glycogen storage and hepatic blood flow

529. Which of the following statements is correct regarding sedation and anesthesia in the pediatric patient?
    a. Because of an increased metabolic rate, drug doses need to be higher compared with that in adults
    b. Pediatric patients are prone to hyperglycemia; therefore it should be monitored throughout the anesthetic period
    c. Drug doses often need to be reduced because of slow metabolism, biotransformation, and excretion of drugs
    d. Oxygen consumption is 10 times that in an adult because of a high metabolic rate

530. The pliable rib cage of pediatric patients can lead to which of the following for efficient ventilation?
    a. More
    b. Less
    c. The pliable rib cage does not affect ventilation under anesthesia
    d. The rib cage is actually less pliable compared with adult dogs

531. You have been asked to induce and monitor anesthesia in an unweaned kitten presenting for wound care after being stepped on by a child. How long should you fast this patient before anesthetic induction?
    a. 1–2 hr
    b. 2–4 hr
    c. 4–6 hr
    d. Fasting is not suggested in these patients

532. You have been asked to induce and monitor anesthesia in a 7-week-old puppy for a GI foreign-body removal from the stomach. How long should this patient be fasted before anesthetic induction?
    a. 1–3 hr
    b. 3–6 hr
    c. 6–9 hr
    d. Fasting is not suggested in these patients

533. Water should be withheld from neonatal and pediatric patients for how long before anesthetic induction?
    a. Water is never withheld from these patients
    b. 1–2 hr
    c. 2–4 hr
    d. 4–6 hr

534. Minimum laboratory tests that should be evaluated before induction of a pediatric patient includes which of the following?
    a. BUN, creatinine, PCV, TP
    b. PCV, TP, BUN, blood glucose
    c. PCV, TP, blood glucose
    d. BUN, PCV, TP, WBC count

535. Which of the following drugs is generally avoided in the pediatric patient because of negative side effects such as severe bradycardia, respiratory depression, and extensive hepatic metabolism?
    a. Midazolam
    b. Morphine
    c. Glycopyrrolate
    d. Dexmedetomidine

536. Shivering during anesthetic recovery leads to which of the following?
    a. Increase in metabolic oxygen demand
    b. Decrease in metabolic oxygen demand
    c. Increase in glyconeogenesis
    d. Decrease in glyconeogenesis

537. Peak airway pressure in the pediatric patient should range between:
    a. 10–20 cm H_2O
    b. 5–10 cm H_2O
    c. 15–20 cm H_2O
    d. 5–15 cm H_2O

538. Which of the following methods is the most accurate way to assess blood pressure in the pediatric patient?
    a. Oscillometric
    b. Doppler
    c. Palpation of pulse
    d. Direct

539. Fasting time in the geriatric patient should be limited to how many hours before anesthetic induction?
    a. 8 hr
    b. 12 hr
    c. 24 hr
    d. 1–2 hr

540. Which of the following anesthetic drugs is not reversible?
    a. Acepromazine
    b. Diazepam
    c. Methadone
    d. Dexmedetomidine

541. You have been asked to induce and maintain a geriatric poodle with Addison's disease. Which of the following anesthetic drugs should be avoided?
    a. Fentanyl
    b. Midazolam
    c. Etomidate
    d. Alfaxalone

542. Which of the following is defined as the delivery of specific drugs for analgesia, sedation, amnesia, and muscle relaxation?
    a. Regional anesthesia
    b. Epidural anesthesia
    c. Balanced anesthesia
    d. Premedication

543. To help prevent artificially low or high blood pressure readings, the blood pressure cuff width should be approximately what percentage of the circumference of the limb where it will be placed?
    a. 25 percent
    b. 30 percent
    c. 40 percent
    d. 50 percent

544. Basic anesthetic patient parameters should be monitored and recorded in a permanent record every _____ minutes.
    a. 5
    b. 10
    c. 15
    d. 20

545. All of the following are signs of hypotension *except:*
    a. Vasoconstriction
    b. Poor pulses
    c. Increasing heart rate
    d. Increasing $ETCO_2$

546. Hypotension is most often caused by which of the following?
    a. Hypovolemia and anesthetic drugs
    b. Hyperthermia and toxemia
    c. Cardiac arrhythmias and opioid administration
    d. Hypercarbia and increased central venous pressure

547. All of the following are potential signs of pain *except:*
    a. Vocalization
    b. Decreased heart rate
    c. Inappetence
    d. Increased temperature

548. Which of the following opioids can be used effectively in the feline patient when administered via the transmucosal route?
    a. Butorphanol
    b. Morphine
    c. Methadone
    d. Buprenorphine

549. You have been asked to anesthetize a 5-year-old mixed breed, female spayed dog for a severe degloving injury of the left forelimb. Which of the following drugs might be beneficial in helping deal with the acute neuropathic pain this patient may be undergoing?
    a. Ketamine
    b. Propofol
    c. Alfaxalone
    d. Oxymorphone

550. Which of the following drugs should be used with caution in cats because of the potential for severe cardiotoxic effects?
    a. Ketamine
    b. Dexmedetomidine
    c. Lidocaine
    d. Morphine

551. You are recovering a canine patient from a surgical procedure. On extubation, it is howling, paddling, and swaying from side to side. After a quick assessment, it has been determined that he is dysphoric and not painful. What can be done to help a patient that is experiencing opioid-induced dysphoria?
a. Administer an additional dose of opioids to help calm the patient
b. Hold the patient tightly until he calms down
c. Induce anesthesia and try waking him up again
d. Slowly titrate a dose of naloxone to effect

552. During anesthesia, why is administering a constant rate infusion advantageous over providing intermittent boluses of a drug(s)?
a. You can administer higher doses when using a CRI
b. You can use multiple different drugs in a CRI
c. A CRI allows for continuous low doses of various analgesics
d. It is not advantageous. Intermittent boluses are safer and more effective

553. A patient undergoing which of the following procedures would likely benefit from an epidural?
a. Femoral head osteotomy
b. Humeral fracture repair
c. Total ear canal ablation
d. Glossectomy

554. Which of the following blocks a particular opioid receptor?
a. An agonist
b. An antagonist
c. COX-2 inhibition
d. COX-1 inhibition

555. All of the following are primary goals of anesthesia *except:*
a. Provide immobilization
b. Ensure amnesia
c. Eliminate pain
d. Having a standard anesthetic protocol

556. Which of the following drugs causes Heinz body formation with repeated dosing in cats?
a. Ketamine
b. Propofol
c. Alfaxalone
d. Etomidate

557. Which of the following is the best indicator of anesthetic depth?
a. Palpebral reflex
b. Toe pinch
c. Jaw tone
d. Blood pressure

558. Which of the following is not an advantage of low-flow anesthesia?
a. Less moisture is lost from the airways
b. Less heat is lost because of low oxygen flow rates
c. Low-flow is more economical
d. Low-flow anesthesia can be used on any anesthetic circuit

559. Overventilation of a patient can lead to all of the following *except:*
a. Decreased preload
b. Decreased blood pressure
c. Decreased cardiac output
d. Decreased core body temperature

560. Which of the following statements is true regarding carbon dioxide absorbents?
a. Storage of absorbent should consist of a sealable pail, canister, carton, or bag
b. High temperatures greatly affect absorbent, even when properly sealed
c. Freezing temperatures aid in the longevity of the absorbent
d. Absorbents are respiratory irritants but are not caustic to the skin

561. Why are unidirectional valves an important part of the anesthesia machine?
a. They are directly involved with scavenging waste gases
b. They play a large role in helping warm the anesthetic gases before being delivered to the patient
c. They ensure that gases flow toward the patient in one breathing tube and away from the patient in the other breathing tube
d. They act as a safety mechanism, ensuring the patient does not receive a tidal volume larger than 20 cm H_2O

562. A respirometer is used for which of the following purposes?
a. To measure respiratory rate
b. To measure ventilatory volume
c. To measure $ETCO_2$
d. To measure the amount of moisture in the breathing circuit

563. Which of the following is false regarding a Mapleson breathing system?
a. Unidirectional valves are present
b. Fresh gas flow must remain high to flush out carbon dioxide
c. There is no device for absorbing carbon dioxide
d. Mapleson systems are less economical compared with circle systems

564. Why is the pin index safety system (PISS) an important feature for anesthetic cylinders?
    a. The PISS ensures that the cylinders are properly identified by specific colors (i.e., green/oxygen, yellow/medical air, etc.)
    b. The PISS ensures that waste gas is properly collected and removed from the surgical area
    c. The PISS aids in the delivery of oxygen from the house gas supply
    d. The PISS ensures that the correct cylinder is mounted into the correct yoke for delivery of the proper anesthetic gas

565. What is the purpose for the vaporizer interlock device?
    a. It prevents the vaporizer from becoming detached from the anesthesia machine during transport
    b. It reduces the amount of waste gases from entering the environment
    c. It prevents two vaporizers on the same machine from being turned on at the same time
    d. This device alarms when the vaporizer becomes dangerously low on inhalant gases

566. You are examining the capnography waveform of the patient under anesthesia. You notice that the baseline is elevated (not going back to zero), but the waveform otherwise looks normal. Why might this be happening?
    a. The patient is hyperventilating
    b. The patient is hypoventilating
    c. The patient has been intubated into the esophagus
    d. The patient is rebreathing carbon dioxide

567. Monitoring carbon dioxide allows for analysis of all of the following *except:*
    a. Ventilation
    b. Circulation
    c. Equipment malfunction
    d. Core body temperature

568. What is the purpose of the common gas outlet?
    a. The common gas outlet is the area where the APL valve connects to the machine
    b. The common gas outlet connects anesthetic machine to the breathing systems, ventilator or oxygen supply device
    c. The common gas outlet connects the fresh gas to the scavenge system
    d. The common gas outlet connects the oxygen flowmeter to the vaporizer

569. Which of the following receives oxygen directly from the cylinder, or pipeline, and bypasses the vaporizer?
    a. Oxygen flush
    b. Oxygen flowmeter
    c. Rebreathing circuit
    d. Non-rebreathing circuit

570. Which of the following is the volume of the breathing system occupied by gases that are rebreathed without any change in composition?
    a. Tidal volume
    b. Apparatus dead space
    c. Peak inspiratory pressure
    d. Minute volume

571. You have been asked to help prepare an anesthetic protocol for a glaucoma patient that needs multiple dental extractions. The patient is otherwise systemically healthy. Which of the following induction agents should be avoided in this patient?
    a. Ketamine
    b. Propofol
    c. Diazepam
    d. Alfaxalone

572. All of the following drugs have the potential to raise both intraocular and intracranial pressure *except:*
    a. Morphine
    b. Dexmedetomidine
    c. Hydromorphone
    d. Methadone

573. You are monitoring anesthesia on a patient undergoing an enucleation. The patient suddenly becomes severely bradycardiac during manipulation of the globe. What is likely occurring?
    a. The patient is in a light plane of anesthesia and can feel the surgical stimulation
    b. The patient has an underlying heart condition that went unrecognized until now
    c. This is likely a result of the oculocardiac reflex
    d. The patient is in too deep of an anesthetic plane and should be turned down

574. Which of the following is a common side effect of opioid administration in the cat?
    a. Miosis
    b. Mydriasis
    c. Meiosis
    d. Mitosis

575. A dog you are monitoring under anesthesia has lost a significant amount of blood during the surgical procedure. You must estimate current blood loss by assessing the sponges and suction canister volume. Before estimating volume deficit, you must first know what is normal for a dog. What is the normal blood volume in a canine patient?
    a. 50–60 mL/kg
    b. 10–20 mL/kg
    c. 80–90 mL/kg
    d. 30–50 mL/kg

576. Which solution has the same proportion of particles and water as that found in plasma?
    a. A hypertonic solution
    b. An isotonic solution
    c. A hypotonic solution
    d. A buffered solution

577. You must extract multiple molars and premolars on the lower left and right dental arcade. Which of the following local blocks can be used to provide pain relief both during and after the procedure?
    a. Infraorbital block
    b. Inferior alveolar block
    c. RUMM block
    d. Auriculotemporal block

578. Which of the following block the generation and conduction of nerve impulses by inhibiting voltage-gated sodium channels within neuronal membranes?
    a. Local anesthetics
    b. Full mu opioids
    c. Alpha-2 agonists
    d. Kappa agonists

579. Which of the following local blocks could be used to help manage pain in patients undergoing a lateral thoracotomy or in those that have rib fractures?
    a. RUMM block
    b. Paravertebral block
    c. Intercostal block
    d. Epidural block

580. Common side effects of acepromazine include all of the following *except:*
    a. Decreasing body temperature
    b. Antiemetic properties
    c. Antiarrhythmic
    d. Respiratory depressant

581. Which of the following drugs when administered alone produces minimal sedation in healthy dogs and cats?
    a. Acepromazine
    b. Midazolam
    c. Dexmedetomidine
    d. Morphine

582. A cat you are monitoring under anesthesia has lost a significant amount of blood during the surgical procedure. You must estimate current blood loss by assessing the sponges and suction canister volume. Before estimating volume deficit, you must first know what is normal for a cat. What is the normal blood volume in a feline patient?
    a. 60–70 mL/kg
    b. 10–20 mL/kg
    c. 80–90 mL/kg
    d. 30–50 mL/kg

583. You must anesthetize a patient that was hit by a car and has suspected head trauma. This patient may have increased intracranial pressure as a result of the trauma. All of the following are techniques that can help reduce intracranial pressure *except:*
    a. Keeping head at a 30-degree angle
    b. Administering mannitol to decrease blood viscosity and increase blood volume
    c. Ventilating patient to provide normocapnia
    d. Only drawing blood from the jugular vein

584. During CPR, adequate cardiac massage is present when:
    a. The electrocardiogram (ECG) is normal
    b. The heart rate is 60 beats/min
    c. A peripheral pulse can be palpated
    d. The end-tidal CO_2 is normal

585. No more than what percentage nitrous oxide should be delivered to an anesthetized patient?
    a. 45%
    b. 30%
    c. 65%
    d. 75%

586. Which of the following is a concern when recovering a patient from anesthesia when nitrous oxide has been used?
    a. Solubility
    b. Diffusion hypoxia
    c. Biotransformation
    d. Inflammation

587. Local anesthetics:
    a. Cause increased release of inhibitory neurotransmitters
    b. Block transmission of the impulse along the nerve fiber
    c. Work by acting on GABA receptors
    d. Block catecholamine release

588. In nonbrachycephalic breeds of dogs recovering from anesthesia, the endotracheal tube should be removed when:
    a. Palpebral reflex returns
    b. Swallowing reflex returns
    c. The eyes resume a central position
    d. Animal shows voluntary movement of the limbs

589. What agent should be avoided in geriatric patients?
    a. Atropine
    b. Dexmedetomidine
    c. Isoflurane
    d. Midazolam

590. A capillary refill time that is over 3 seconds is indicative of:
    a. Renal failure
    b. Poor tissue perfusion
    c. Increased ventilation
    d. Hypertension

591. Normal urinary output in canine and feline patients is 1–2 mL/kg/hr. Why is normal urinary output important in patients under general anesthesia?
    a. Normal urinary output is directly related to liver function
    b. Normal urinary output is directly related to pulmonary function
    c. Normal urinary output reflects cardiovascular status and normal renal perfusion
    d. Normal urinary output reflects appropriate central venous pressure and ventilation status

592. Cardiac output in the pediatric patient is primarily dependent on which of the following?
    a. Respiratory rate
    b. Heart rate
    c. Pulse quality
    d. Fluid rate

593. Which of the following is *not* a cause of barotrauma in patients undergoing anesthesia?
    a. Closed pop-off valve
    b. Excessive peak inspiratory pressure with positive pressure ventilation
    c. Repetitive collapse and re-expansion of normal or diseased lung during positive pressure ventilation
    d. Providing a ventilatory rate in excess of 25 breaths/min

594. Which of the following is the intrinsic pacemaker of the heart?
    a. Sinoatrial node
    b. Atrioventricular node
    c. Purkinje fibers
    d. Bundle of His

595. Spirometers are used to measure which of the following?
    a. Central venous pressure and respiratory rate
    b. Minute volume and tidal volume
    c. Respiratory rate and effort
    d. Pulmonary ventilation and mechanical dead space

596. The normal pH range of blood is 7.35–7.45. If a patient has a blood pH of 7.25, this patient is considered to have:
    a. Acidosis
    b. Alkalosis
    c. Ketoacidosis
    d. Ketoalkalosis

597. Which of the following drugs is not generally suggested for use in ruminants?
    a. Ketamine
    b. Butorphanol
    c. Propofol
    d. Atropine

ⓔ *Answers and rationales available on Evolve*
http://evolve.elsevier.com/Prendergast/QAvettech/

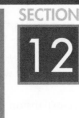
Emergency and Critical Care

Brandy Tabor, BS, CVT, VTS (ECC)

QUESTIONS

1. Which of the following is least useful when resuscitating a dog in shock?
   a. D5W
   b. Hetastarch
   c. Hypertonic saline
   d. Plasma-Lyte 48

2. The first drug of choice for a cat that experiences status epilepticus is:
   a. Diazepam
   b. Pentobarbital
   c. Potassium bromide
   d. Propofol

3. Tension pneumothorax occurs when pressure in the thoracic cavity is:
   a. Less than atmospheric pressure
   b. Equal to atmospheric pressure
   c. Greater than atmospheric pressure
   d. Constant as animal breathes in and out

4. Emesis should not be induced in patients that have ingested:
   a. Anticholinergics
   b. Hydrocarbons
   c. Organophosphates
   d. Salicylates

5. The mucous membranes of a dog in septic shock are:
   a. Cyanotic
   b. Hyperemic
   c. Icteric
   d. Pale

6. The most desirable induction agent for an emergency cesarean section in a dog is:
   a. Etomidate
   b. Diazepam
   c. Propofol
   d. Thiopental

7. The underlying disease for most cases of feline aortic thromboembolism is _____ in origin.
   a. Cardiac
   b. Hepatic
   c. Renal
   d. Respiratory

8. To reduce intracranial pressure that results from trauma, _____ may be administered every 4 to 8 hours.
   a. Atropine
   b. Dexamethasone
   c. Diazepam
   d. Mannitol

9. Four patients present at the same time with emergency conditions. In which order should the patients be triaged?
   a. Dyspnea, dystocia, proptosis, laceration
   b. Proptosis, dyspnea, dystocia, laceration
   c. Laceration, dystocia, dyspnea, proptosis
   d. Dystocia, proptosis, laceration, dyspnea

10. Which of the following conditions heals best through first intention?
    a. Abscess
    b. Degloving
    c. Simple laceration
    d. Puncture wound

11. A patient is experiencing cardiopulmonary arrest. The most desirable route of drug administration is:
    a. Intratracheal
    b. Intracardiac
    c. Intravenous
    d. Intraosseous

12. A patient that has been hit by a car and has no palpable pulse or detectable heartbeat requires chest compressions. These compressions should be performed at a rate (per minute) of:
    a. 60–80 compressions per minute
    b. 80–100 compressions per minute
    c. 100–120 compressions per minute
    d. 120–140 compressions per minute

13. To minimize hemorrhage to the head of a canine trauma patient, where should pressure be applied?
    a. At the thoracic inlet in both jugular grooves
    b. At the thoracic inlet of the left jugular groove
    c. To the area adjacent and ventral to the mandible
    d. To the lateral points of the temporomandibular joint

14. In emergency care cases in which it is not possible to administer large volumes of desired fluids, it may be beneficial to properly administer:
    a. D5W
    b. Hypertonic saline
    c. Hypotonic saline
    d. Isotonic saline

15. During emergency intubation, the cranial nerve _____ may be stimulated, resulting in _____.
    a. I; bradycardia
    b. IV; tachycardia
    c. X; bradycardia
    d. XII; tachycardia

16. A man phones the veterinary practice to say that he has just hit a dog with his car and it is now lying on the side of the road. It appears to be breathing with minimal distress; however, there is blood coming from both nostrils and there is a small river of dark blood coming from a laceration on the lateral side of its hind leg. The dog can raise its head and is attempting to stand. In advising the man, your recommendation is to do all of the following *except:*
    a. Be aware for any signs of aggression
    b. Tie the mouth securely closed with your shoelace
    c. Transport the dog on a board lying on its side
    d. Apply direct pressure to the wound

17. A normal central venous pressure (CVP) range is:
    a. 0–5 cm H2O
    b. 5–10 cm H2O
    c. 10–15 cm H2O
    d. 15–20 cm H2O

18. When monitoring patients on fluids and/or patients that undergo diuresis, urine output is an important consideration. The normal urine production for a healthy dog or cat is approximately:
    a. 0–1 mL/kg/hr
    b. 1–2 mL/kg/hr
    c. 2–3 mL/kg/hr
    d. 3–4 mL/kg/hr

19. Multiple parameters are measured to determine a category of shock that an animal might be experiencing. The central venous pressure is high in which of the following types of shock?
    a. Cardiogenic
    b. Distributive
    c. Hypovolemic
    d. Septic

20. Hypoglycemia is most common in patients that experience:
    a. Anaphylactic shock
    b. Cardiogenic shock
    c. Neurogenic shock
    d. Septic shock

21. A patient has increased muscular tone in the thoracic limbs and flaccid paralysis in the pelvic limbs when lying on his side. He is able to ambulate when placed on his feet and has a normal mentation. What posture do these clinical signs indicate?
    a. Decerebellate
    b. Decerebrate
    c. Opisthotonus
    d. Schiff-Sherrington

22. The Schiff-Sherrington posture is indicative of injury to which part of the spine?
    a. Cranial-C_6
    b. C_6-T_2
    c. T_1-T_3
    d. T_3-L_3

23. NSAIDs are also referred to as:
    a. Anti-prostaglandins
    b. Neoprostaglandins
    c. Pro-prostaglandins
    d. Prostaglandoids

24. Which of the following is a colloid solution?
    a. Hetastarch
    b. Lactated Ringer's
    c. Normosol-R
    d. Plasma-Lyte 148

25. Defibrillation is the passing of an electrical current through the heart to:
    a. Cause the already depolarized cardiac cells to repolarize in a uniform manner
    b. Cause the cardiac cells to depolarize and then repolarize in a uniform manner
    c. Prevent the cardiac cells from depolarizing, thus maintaining rhythm
    d. Prevent any contractile activity of the cardiac cells temporarily

26. Which of the following is least likely to be seen in a patient suffering from shock?
    a. Hyperthermia
    b. Hypotension
    c. Tachycardia
    d. Tachypnea

27. Gastric dilatation/volvulus (GDV) is a life-threatening emergency. Which of the following veins becomes obstructed as a result of GDV?
    a. Femoral vein
    b. Gastroduodenal vein
    c. Portal vein
    d. Renal vein

28. The unit of measurement for insulin is:
    a. Milliliters
    b. Microliters
    c. Milligrams
    d. International units

29. Dystocia in the dog or cat may be defined as active straining without delivery of a fetus for more than _____ minutes.
    a. 20 minutes
    b. 30 minutes
    c. 40 minutes
    d. 60 minutes

30. When approaching an animal that requires emergency treatment, which direction should one approach the patient?
    a. Caudal
    b. Lateral
    c. Rostral
    d. Let the animal try to come to you

31. Ocular exposure to a toxin has occurred in a dog. On examination, it is discovered that there is possible damage to the corneal epithelium. Which of the following procedures is contraindicated?
    a. Continuous flushing with physiologic saline
    b. Provision of mild sedative or analgesic or both
    c. Corticosteroid administration to prevent inflammation
    d. Use of antibiotic cream after flushing

32. A client calls the veterinary practice indicating that her cat drank ethylene glycol 6 hours earlier. Everyone is at lunch, and you immediately page the veterinarian; however, the client wants to make her cat vomit to rid it of the toxin. What should you advise her?
    a. To use 3% hydrogen peroxide at 1 Tbl/20 lb
    b. To use salt on the back of the tongue
    c. To use dry mustard powder only
    d. Not to induce vomiting and to bring in the cat immediately

33. Eclampsia produces elevated body temperatures as a result of:
    a. Increased levels of endotoxins that are present
    b. A large fetal mass that is present
    c. Heat produced through muscle movement
    d. Eclampsia does not result in elevated body temperature

34. To place a nasal oxygenation catheter in a dog, a veterinary technician would measure to the:
    a. Beginning of the thoracic inlet
    b. Medial canthus of the eye
    c. Pharynx
    d. No measurement is needed; a standard catheter that is 1.5 inches in length is used

35. A client calls to say she has come home to find her cat lying with the lamp cord in its mouth. The first thing you should advise her to do is:
    a. Immediately place the cat in a carrier, and bring it to clinic
    b. Explain how to perform CPR
    c. Immediately disconnect the plug of the lamp cord from the wall socket
    d. Take note of the amperage of the lamp

36. The most common artery to use when assessing the pulse of a dog or cat is the:
    a. Jugular
    b. Femoral
    c. Carpal
    d. Tarsal

37. A healthy, adult, small-breed dog is presented to the veterinary practice for a wellness exam. At what point does one become concerned about an elevated heart rate?
    a. 175 beats/min
    b. 250 beats/min
    c. 300 beats/min
    d. 350 beats/min

38. A pulse deficit occurs when the pulse:
    a. Occurs before the heartbeat
    b. Occurs with the heartbeat
    c. Occurs after the heartbeat
    d. Does not occur

39. A normal sinus arrhythmia occurs when heart rate:
    a. Increases with expiration
    b. Decreases with expiration
    c. May increase or decrease with expiration
    d. Does not increase or decrease with expiration

40. An abnormal increase in the depth and rate of respirations is called:
    a. Dyspnea
    b. Hypernea
    c. Orthopnea
    d. Tachypnea

41. An 18-gauge needle would be most appropriate for administering SQ fluids to which patient?
    a. Cockatiel
    b. Labrador retriever
    c. Kitten
    d. Rat

42. The proper site for an intraperitoneal injection is:
    a. On the lateral abdominal wall just caudal to the rib cage
    b. Caudal to the umbilicus to the midline
    c. At the level of the umbilicus to the right or left of the midline
    d. Cranial to the umbilicus

43. Which of the following statements is true regarding the administration of liquids via the oral cavity in a dog?
    a. Flush a large bolus of fluid directly into the mouth
    b. Flush a very small bolus of fluid directly into pharyngeal area
    c. Place fluid between the teeth and the cheek, and allow the patient to swallow on its own accord
    d. Place the fluid between the teeth and the cheek in large enough amounts so that the patient will be forced to swallow

44. Which area of the body is best to assess skin turgor in a canine patient?
    a. Lateral aspect of the neck
    b. Caudal abdomen
    c. Base of the tail
    d. Axillary region

45. Knuckling is an abnormality of which system?
    a. Cardiac
    b. Neurologic
    c. Respiratory
    d. Urinary

46. The rapid intravenous administration of large amounts of potassium can result in:
    a. Respiratory arrest
    b. Cardiac arrest
    c. Polyuria
    d. Polydipsia

47. Which of the following route(s) can potassium solutions be administered to dogs and cats without causing severe pain?
    a. Intravenous only
    b. Subcutaneous only
    c. Intramuscular only
    d. Intravenous and subcutaneous

48. Which of the following is not a contraindication for crystalloid fluid therapy?
    a. Pulmonary edema
    b. Cerebral edema
    c. Pitting of the soft tissues
    d. Swollen soft tissue from bruising caused by trauma

49. Which of the following is the *easiest* method for monitoring fluid therapy?
    a. Central venous pressure (CVP)
    b. Packed-cell volume/total protein (PCV/TP)
    c. Urine output (UOP)
    d. Weight

50. What part of the eye can be used to indicate fluid overload?
    a. Conjunctiva
    b. Lens
    c. Pupil
    d. Nictitating membrane

51. Rapid fluid replacement with crystalloids is contraindicated in conditions of:
    a. Severe dehydration
    b. Shock
    c. Cerebral edema
    d. Renal failure

52. Which of the following is a common colloid preparation that is administered intravenously?
    a. Lactated Ringer's solution
    b. Normosol-R solution
    c. Sodium chloride 9%
    d. Vetstarch

53. Fluid-therapy solutions administered subcutaneously are:
    a. Colloids
    b. Hypertonic
    c. Hypotonic
    d. Isotonic

54. The best route for rapid fluid administration of large amounts of fluids to patients with poor venous access is:
    a. Intraosseous
    b. Intraperitoneal
    c. Oral
    d. Subcutaneous

55. In trauma cases, fluid therapy should be used with caution in which of the following scenarios?
    a. Severe shock
    b. Mild shock
    c. Pulmonary contusions
    d. Severe skin damage

56. When a critical patient arrives at the veterinary practice, which body system should be evaluated first?
    a. Cardiac
    b. Neurologic
    c. Respiratory
    d. Urinary

57. Which of the following is the safest and most effective first aid for frostbite?
    a. Apply warm towels and massage the area
    b. Immerse the affected area in hot water
    c. Immerse the affected area in lukewarm water
    d. Rub the affected area with snow

58. Which of the following methods for controlling hemorrhage from a traumatic wound is least likely to cause further damage to the animal?
    a. Clamping the wound with a hemostat
    b. Direct pressure
    c. Tourniquet
    d. Applying silver nitrate

59. Which would be considered the least important physical measure evaluated during triage of a patient?
    a. Heart rate
    b. Respiratory rate
    c. Capillary refill time
    d. Weight

60. Which of the following statements is true regarding a patient that is in shock?
    a. An initial decrease in heart rate that then increases as the patient nears death
    b. A decreased heart rate
    c. An initial increase in heart rate that then decreases as the patient nears death
    d. An increased heart rate

61. The mucous membranes of patients in hemorrhagic shock are:
    a. Cyanotic
    b. Hyperemic
    c. Icteric
    d. Pale or white

62. What is the minimum concentration of hemoglobin required to detect cyanosis?
    a. 3 g/dL
    b. 4 g/dL
    c. 5 g/dL
    d. 6 g/dL

63. According to the principles of triage, which patient should the veterinarian see first?
    a. Cat with a closed fracture
    b. Dog in respiratory distress
    c. Dog with otitis externa
    d. Cat with a small laceration on a paw pad

64. Which of the following would petechiation on the mucous membranes indicate?
    a. Hemoglobinemia
    b. Methemoglobinemia
    c. Myoglobinemia
    d. Thrombocytopenia

65. Which of the following is not a characteristic of compensatory shock?
    a. Normal blood pressure
    b. Cool extremities
    c. Capillary refill time <1 second
    d. Tachycardia

66. According to the principles of triage, which patient should a veterinarian see first?
    a. Dog with a small laceration on a pinna
    b. Dog with acute gastric dilatation/volvulus
    c. Cat with dystocia, not in shock, no kitten in birth canal
    d. Cat with possible linear foreign body in the bowel

67. Which of these signs is not an indication of dystocia?
    a. Green or black vulvar discharge
    b. Profuse vulvar hemorrhage
    c. Pup or kitten in the birth canal for 5 minutes
    d. More than 1 hour of vigorous contractions with no pup or kitten produced

68. What is not usually a sign of acute gastric dilatation/ volvulus?
    a. Unproductive vomiting
    b. Hypersalivation
    c. Abdominal distention
    d. Profuse diarrhea

69. Crackles on thoracic auscultation indicate:
    a. Asthma
    b. Pleural effusion
    c. Pneumothorax
    d. Pulmonary edema

70. A client describes his male cat as lethargic and constipated; he has observed the cat straining in the litter box. You suspect that the cat is actually suffering from:
    a. Peritonitis
    b. Urethral obstruction
    c. Intestinal obstruction
    d. An upper respiratory viral infection

71. If the hindquarters were elevated in a dog with a severe diaphragmatic hernia, what effect would this have on respiration?
    a. There is no change in respiratory rate or labor of respirations
    b. Respiratory rate decreases and respiration becomes less labored
    c. Respiratory rate increases and respiration becomes more labored
    d. A cough is induced

72. A veterinarian is assessing a cat with a spinal injury. When the doctor pinches the cat's toe, a positive response to deep pain would be indicated by:
    a. Kicking of the foot without vocalizing
    b. Kicking of the foot while vocalizing
    c. Withdrawal of the foot without vocalizing
    d. Withdrawal of the foot while vocalizing

73. Signs of cardiopulmonary arrest include all of the following *except:*
    a. Alertness
    b. Dilated pupils
    c. Agonal breathing
    d. No femoral pulse

74. A patient that was hit by a car and has multiple pelvic fractures has not urinated in more than 24 hours. One may suspect the cause of anuria to be:
    a. A ruptured urinary bladder
    b. Severe dehydration
    c. Renal failure
    d. Urethral calculi

75. A free-roaming dog is brought to the hospital for listlessness and dyspnea. While performing venipuncture, you notice that the animal seems to have a prolonged clotting time. A possible cause of prolonged clotting times would be the ingestion of

    _____.
    a. Anticoagulant rodenticide
    b. Ethylene glycol
    c. Organophosphate insecticide
    d. Strychnine

76. Which statement concerning status epilepticus is accurate?
    a. It occurs in geriatric animals only
    b. It is a life-threatening medical emergency
    c. It is treated by the administration of acepromazine
    d. It will resolve spontaneously

77. Signs of organophosphate toxicity include all of the following *except:*
    a. Bradycardia
    b. Lacrimation
    c. Mydriasis
    d. Salivation

78. Normal capillary refill time in dogs is:
    a. <1 second
    b. 1 to 2 seconds
    c. 2 to 4 seconds
    d. 4 to 6 seconds

79. A client calls the hospital and indicates that a car has just hit his cat. The recommendations that should be made include:
    a. Immediately bring the cat in to be examined by a veterinarian
    b. Observe the cat at home for an hour, and call back if problems occur
    c. Bring the cat in for an examination by a veterinarian the following day
    d. Bring the cat to you for initial examination, so you can determine whether the animal needs to be seen by a veterinarian

80. A client calls the hospital and advises that his puppy has walked through motor oil and is licking its paws. What should be recommended?
    a. Do not induce emesis, and immediately bring the pet to the clinic for examination and treatment
    b. Induce emesis and then immediately bring the pet to the clinic for examination and treatment
    c. Induce emesis; no further treatment is required
    d. Induce emesis and then bring the pet to the clinic only if it shows signs of toxicity

81. A client calls the practice and states that his dog has just ingested sugar-free gum. He is 90 minutes from the practice. What should be recommended?
    a. Do not induce emesis and immediately bring the pet to the clinic for examination and treatment
    b. Induce emesis then immediately bring the pet to the clinic for examination and treatment
    c. Induce emesis; no further treatment is required
    d. Induce emesis then bring the pet to the clinic only if it shows signs of toxicity

82. A client owning a diabetic cat calls the practice and says that her cat has just had a seizure and collapsed. She gave the cat its usual dose of insulin that morning, but the animal has not eaten anything during the day. What should the next recommendation entail?
    a. Another dose of insulin, then bring the cat to the clinic for medical attention
    b. Some corn syrup or sugar solution on the gums, then observe the cat at home
    c. Some corn syrup or sugar solution on the gums, then bring the cat to the clinic for medical attention
    d. Another dose of insulin, then observe the cat at home

83. A client has just treated his 5-week-old kitten with a flea dip that contains lindane. The cat is acting slightly lethargic, and the client then notices that the label on the dip reads "for dogs only." The client calls the practice. What advice should be given?
    a. Observe the kitten at home
    b. Wash the kitten with mild dish soap, rinse well, and then bring the animal to the clinic for examination
    c. Wash the kitten with mild dish soap, rinse well, and then administer acetaminophen for discomfort
    d. Induce emesis and observe the kitten at home

84. A client calls the hospital because he has noticed that his cat has a string protruding from under the tongue. The client should be advised to:
    a. Gently attempt to pull out the string
    b. Induce emesis
    c. Cut the string and administer laxatives at home
    d. Bring the cat to the clinic for examination

85. A client calls the hospital because she has noticed a barbed fishhook embedded in her dog's lower lip. The client should be advised to:
    a. Gently attempt to pull out the fishhook
    b. Observe the dog at home; most fishhooks fall out spontaneously within 24 hours
    c. Bring the animal to see the veterinarian as soon as possible
    d. Administer aspirin for discomfort and see the veterinarian right away

86. A dog has a lacerated paw pad. The client has placed a small bandage over the wound, but blood is soaking through. The appropriate treatment is to:
    a. Remove the bandage and apply digital pressure to the wound
    b. Apply another bandage over the client's original bandage
    c. Remove the bandage and apply a tourniquet to the limb
    d. Do nothing; no further treatment is required if the bleeding is not excessive

87. An extremely upset client calls the hospital. Her small poodle has stopped breathing and she cannot feel a heartbeat. What should the next recommendation be?
    a. Attempt no treatment; immediately transport the pet to the hospital
    b. Attempt mouth-to-mouth resuscitation and chest compressions; immediately transport the pet to the hospital
    c. Start chest compression immediately and provide mouth-to-snout breaths while closing the dog's mouth at a 30 compression to 2 breaths ratio, and immediately transport the pet to the hospital
    d. Attempt resuscitation; transport the pet to the hospital if attempts at resuscitation are unsuccessful

88. How should a patient with a potential spinal injury be transported to the hospital?
    a. Sitting
    b. Standing
    c. Lying on a flat board
    d. Moving as it wishes

89. A patient with a possible herniated intervertebral disk should be:
    a. Allowed to move freely, and if no improvement is evident after 24 hours, see the veterinarian
    b. Allowed to move freely; immediately see the veterinarian
    c. Kept strictly quiet and confined; if no improvement is evident in 24 hours, see the veterinarian
    d. Kept strictly quiet and confined; see the veterinarian immediately

90. Which of these items would be least useful on a crash cart used for emergency situations?
    a. Laryngoscope
    b. Intravenous catheter
    c. Otoscope
    d. Ambu bag

91. A patient who is apneic and cyanotic enters the practice. A quick oral examination shows a hard ball lodged in the glottal opening. Which of the following options should be performed next?
    a. Place the patient in an oxygen cage
    b. Attempt to pass a nasal oxygen catheter
    c. Attempt to pass an endotracheal tube
    d. Perform the Heimlich maneuver; if unsuccessful, prepare the patient for tracheotomy

92. A 16-year-old, 3-kg poodle is presented to the hospital with cyanosis, agonal respirations, and frothy fluid coming from the nose and mouth. Knowing the treatments that the doctor is likely to order, you prepare to:
    a. Administer intravenous fluids at 90 mL/kg/hr
    b. Administer furosemide intramuscularly, and place the patient in an oxygen cage
    c. Suction the airway and initiate cardiopulmonary resuscitation
    d. Assist with an immediate tracheostomy

93. The veterinarian has authorized you to start infusing intravenous fluids in a 0.25-kg Yorkshire terrier puppy that is critically ill. You are unable to insert a catheter into a jugular or cephalic vein. An alternate site that can be used to administer large volumes of fluids is the:
    a. Medullary cavity of the femur
    b. Carotid artery
    c. Lingual vein
    d. Ear vein

94. The veterinarian has directed you to give a whole blood transfusion to a 0.3-kg kitten with severe anemia from flea infestation. You are unable to insert an intravenous or intraosseous catheter. Which of the following would be the most effective alternate route to administer the blood effectively?
    a. Subcutaneous injection
    b. Intramuscular injection
    c. Intraperitoneal injection
    d. Per os

95. You are instructing a client to apply an emergency muzzle to his injured dog. Which of these is the least appropriate material for the muzzle?
    a. Rope
    b. Metal chain dog leash
    c. Pantyhose
    d. Necktie

96. Which of the following is least likely to be available for at-home induction of emesis?
    a. Apomorphine
    b. Syrup of ipecac
    c. Hydrogen peroxide
    d. Salt

97. Which of the following is not performed when treating acute gastric dilatation/volvulus?
    a. Induction of emesis
    b. Placement of an intravenous catheter
    c. Passing of a gastric tube
    d. Trocharization of the stomach

98. All of the following might be included in emergency treatment for epistaxis, *except:*
    a. Placing dilute epinephrine into the nares
    b. Fresh frozen plasma transfusion
    c. Applying a warm compress to the nose
    d. Keep the patient quiet

99. Which statement concerning the administration of activated charcoal via stomach tube is least accurate?
    a. Check tube placement by administering a small amount of water; listen for coughing or gagging
    b. Measure the tube from the tip of the nose to the 13th rib
    c. Measure the tube from the tip of the nose to the thoracic inlet
    d. Use a roll of tape as a speculum to keep the mouth open and to prevent the animal from biting the tube

100. Oxygen can be administered to a patient via any of the following routes, *except:*
    a. Chest tube
    b. Endotracheal tube
    c. Nasal oxygen catheter
    d. Tracheotomy tube

101. Which of the following is the most important goal when treating a patient with heat stroke?
    a. Cooling
    b. Infection control
    c. Oxygen therapy
    d. Pain control

102. All of the following are recommended treatments for a dog experiencing paraphimosis, *except:*
     a. Lubricating the penis
     b. Cleaning the penis
     c. Applying hypertonic solutions to the penis
     d. Applying a warm compress to the penis

103. Initial treatment for a dog with an open fracture includes all of the following, *except:*
     a. Copiously cleaning and flushing the wound
     b. Covering the wound
     c. Applying a temporary splint to the limb
     d. Taking radiographs of the fracture

104. Which statement concerning a dog having a seizure is most correct?
     a. Grasp the dog's tongue and pull it forward to prevent airway obstruction
     b. Administer oral anticonvulsants
     c. Prevent the dog from injuring itself
     d. Immediately start infusion of intravenous fluids

105. A client calls the hospital to say that his Pekingese has suffered an eye proptosis. Your advice to the client should include all of the following, *except:*
     a. Apply pressure to the globe to replace it in the socket
     b. Protect the globe from further trauma
     c. Keep the globe moist
     d. Immediately bring the dog to the veterinarian

106. A client calls and says that his Rottweiler has been shot in the abdomen with a BB gun but appears perfectly fine. What should be recommended?
     a. Observe the animal at home for vomiting or abdominal pain
     b. See the veterinarian immediately
     c. See the veterinarian at your earliest convenience
     d. Observe the animal for hemorrhage

107. Initial treatment for a cat with an open pneumothorax may include all of the following, *except:*
     a. Thoracocentesis
     b. Oxygen administration
     c. Covering the wound
     d. Radiographic examination

108. Which statement is least accurate concerning the emergency treatment of cats with urethral obstruction?
     a. Cats must always be sedated to have a urinary catheter passed
     b. Massaging the tip of the penis can relieve the obstruction
     c. Cats with a slow, irregular heart rate probably have a high serum potassium level
     d. If the obstruction is not relieved, the cat will die

109. What procedure is not routinely performed to resuscitate neonates following cesarean section?
     a. Clean the nose and mouth of secretions
     b. Rub the neonate with a towel to stimulate breathing
     c. Administer a drop of oxytocin under the tongue
     d. Ligate the umbilical cord

110. Inducing emesis after ingestion of a solid toxin is imperative. However, emesis has little value if induced more than _____ hours after ingestion.
     a. 0.5 hours
     b. 1.5 hours
     c. 4 hours
     d. 8 hours

111. Which is not an immediate consideration in cardiopulmonary resuscitation?
     a. Airway
     b. Analgesia
     c. Breathing
     d. Circulation

112. At what rate (breaths per minute) should respirations be administered to a patient in cardiopulmonary arrest?
     a. 4–8 breaths per minute
     b. 8–12 breaths per minute
     c. 12–26 breaths per minute
     d. 16–20 breaths per minute

113. All of the following are signs of end-stage decompensatory shock, *except:*
     a. Hypothermia
     b. Vasodilation
     c. Prolonged capillary refill time
     d. Tachycardia

114. Central venous pressure is used to guide:
     a. Rewarming measures
     b. Oxygen therapy
     c. Fluid therapy
     d. Pain management

115. Each of the following can be used to check mucous membrane color, *except* the:
     a. Sclera
     b. Gingiva
     c. Lining of vulva
     d. Lining of prepuce

116. Dehydration is assessed by all of the following, *except:*
     a. Moistness of mucous membranes
     b. Skin turgor
     c. Packed-cell volume and total plasma protein
     d. Nasal discharge

117. A 20-kg Springer spaniel is brought to the hospital because of anorexia and lethargy. Dehydration is estimated at 8%. The maintenance requirement of fluids is 66 mL/kg/day. To correct this dog's dehydration, how much fluid should it receive during the first 24 hours?
    a. 2920 mL
    b. 1600 mL
    c. 1320 mL
    d. 1336 mL

118. A 32-kg golden retriever is brought to the hospital because of anorexia and lethargy. Dehydration is estimated at 8%. The maintenance requirement of fluids is 66 mL/kg/day. To provide two times the daily maintenance requirements, what is the hourly rate of fluid infusion?
    a. 55 mL
    b. 176 mL
    c. 235 mL
    d. 1320 mL

119. Placement of a jugular catheter is contraindicated in which of the following situations?
    a. Vomiting
    b. Pancreatitis
    c. Thrombocytopenia
    d. Renal failure

120. Which of the following is not included in basic life support of CPR?
    a. Chest compressions
    b. Intubation
    c. Ventilation
    d. Medications

121. Tissue perfusion can be assessed by all of the following, *except:*
    a. Capillary refill time
    b. Rectal temperature
    c. Mucous membrane color
    d. Mentation

122. During triage, which patient should be attended to first?
    a. Dog with a penetrating wound of the abdomen
    b. Cat in respiratory arrest
    c. Cat with an intestinal foreign body
    d. Dog with gastric dilatation/volvulus

123. What is the main determinant of the treatment of a hyperthermic patient?
    a. Age of patient
    b. Duration of hyperthermia
    c. Cause of hyperthermia
    d. Breed of patient

124. What is the recommended dosage for intratracheal drug administration during cardiac arrest?
    a. Half the intravenous dosage
    b. Same as the intravenous dosage
    c. 1.5 times the intravenous dosage
    d. Double the intravenous dosage

125. A client calls the practice and is worried about her Irish wolfhound. The dog ran loose in the neighborhood, and it is now retching without bringing anything up and pacing the floor. The abdomen looks a little distended. What advice should be given?
    a. Record the client's phone number and tell her the doctor will call her back
    b. Tell the client to bring the dog in for examination immediately
    c. Advise the client to give 3% hydrogen peroxide to induce vomiting
    d. Tell the client that the dog may have eaten garbage and to call the hospital in the morning if the animal is not feeling better

126. A 6-year-old mongrel is brought to the hospital with ataxia and mydriasis. On presentation, you notice the dog is dribbling urine and seems overly sensitive to movement and sound. What toxin is the most likely cause of these signs?
    a. Chocolate
    b. Grapes
    c. Marijuana
    d. Xylitol

127. When advising a client to move an injured animal, all of the following scenarios are appropriate, *except:*
    a. If a back injury is suspected, place the animal on a board to move it
    b. Muzzle the injured animal, because it may bite when being moved
    c. Call the veterinary hospital to notify of your expected arrival time
    d. Give a baby aspirin to reduce pain before moving the animal

128. Intraosseous catheters can be used in all of the following cases, *except:*
    a. In septic animals
    b. When epinephrine and atropine must be administered during an arrest
    c. In young and/or debilitated animals
    d. When rapid access to the circulatory system is needed in hypovolemic animals

129. What is the preferred route of fluid administration in a critically ill animal?
    a. Intravenous
    b. Subcutaneous
    c. Oral
    d. Intramuscular

130. Which of the following products is a crystalloid?
    a. Packed red blood cells
    b. Lactated Ringer's solution
    c. Hetastarch
    d. Oxyglobin

131. In which of the following cases is whole blood indicated over packed red blood cells?
    a. Hemorrhage during surgery
    b. Hemorrhage secondary to an anticoagulant rodenticide
    c. Autoimmune hemolytic anemia
    d. Hemorrhage caused by trauma

132. Nutritional support can be administered in several ways. What is the preferred method?
    a. Enteral nutrition
    b. Partial parenteral nutrition
    c. Total parenteral nutrition
    d. Per rectum

133. Which of the following is the most common sign of a blood transfusion reaction?
    a. Fever
    b. Vomiting
    c. Tachycardia
    d. Seizure

134. The normal blood pH for a dog is:
    a. 6.4
    b. 7.0
    c. 7.4
    d. 8.0

135. What electrolyte imbalance is most likely to be found in a cat with total urethral obstruction?
    a. Hyperkalemia
    b. Hyperchloremia
    c. Hypernatremia
    d. Hypercalcemia

136. The heart rate of an unanesthetized patient can be determined (and monitored) using all of the following options, *except*:
    a. Stethoscope
    b. Electrocardiographic monitor
    c. Pulse rate
    d. Esophageal stethoscope

137. All of the following are noninvasive ways of monitoring a critically ill patient, *except:*
    a. Respiratory rate using a stethoscope
    b. Temperature using a tympanic thermometer
    c. Blood pressure using an arterial catheter
    d. Heart rate using an EKG

138. Which of the following options takes the lowest priority when preparing to treat a critical patient?
    a. Oxygen source
    b. Endotracheal tubes
    c. Heating pad
    d. Intravenous catheters

139. A dog presents with irregular movements over the surface of the muscle near his shoulder. This type of muscle movement is called:
    a. Dyskinesia
    b. Fasciculation
    c. Myoclonus
    d. Tremors

140. A dehydrated patient presents. Which of the following solutions would be the most appropriate fluid choice?
    a. Fresh frozen plasma
    b. Hetastarch
    c. Packed red blood cells
    d. Plasma-Lyte 48

141. A fellow veterinary technician is triaging a patient and notes the mucous membranes look brown in color. What might be the cause?
    a. Anemia
    b. Bilirubinemia
    c. Hyperthermia
    d. Methemoglobinemia

142. Which toxicity will cause salivation, lacrimation, urination, and defecation?
    a. Acetaminophen
    b. Grapes
    c. Lilies
    d. Organophosphates

143. The bandage layer that comes in contact with the wound is the:
    a. Primary layer
    b. Secondary layer
    c. Tertiary layer
    d. Quaternary layer

144. At what temperature must cooling measures be taken in a hyperthermic patient?
    a. 105° F
    b. 106° F
    c. 107° F
    d. 108° F

145. A dog presents to the practice with a history of waxing and waning vomiting, lethargy, and decreased appetite for several months. Bloodwork shows 122 mmoL/L sodium and 7.8 mmoL/L potassium. What disease can cause these symptoms and electrolyte changes?
    a. Diabetic insipidus
    b. Diabetic ketoacidosis
    c. Hypoadrenocorticism
    d. Thyroid storm

146. Which of the following bacteria is responsible for kennel cough?
    a. *Bordetella bronchiseptica*
    b. *Clostridium tetani*
    c. *Neospora caninum*
    d. *Toxoplasmosis gondii*

147. Which of the following medications should not be used to control seizures in a patient with liver disease?
    a. Levetiracetam
    b. Phenobarbital
    c. Potassium bromide
    d. Propofol

148. A dog presents 30 minutes after the owner saw him lacerate himself on a dirty nail. How would this wound be classified?
    a. Clean
    b. Clean-contaminated
    c. Contaminated
    d. Dirty-infected

149. Which insulin is a quick-acting and short-lasting insulin, making it appropriate for use as a CRI?
    a. NPH
    b. Regular
    c. Glargine
    d. PZI

150. A hospitalized patient is receiving intravenous fluids with a potassium supplementation; however, the potassium blood value continues to drop. What other blood value should be discussed with the veterinarian?
    a. Calcium
    b. Magnesium
    c. Sodium
    d. Chloride

151. Which of the following conditions can cause ventroflexion in cats?
    a. Hypokalemia
    b. Hyponatremia
    c. Hypocalcemia
    d. Hypomagnesemia

152. Which of the following options controls breathing in dogs and cats?
    a. The level of carbon dioxide in the blood
    b. The level of oxygen in the blood
    c. The level of oxygen in the airway
    d. The level of humidity in the airway

153. Which of the following blood tests can be diagnostic for anticoagulant rodenticide ingestion?
    a. Activated clotting time (ACT)
    b. Activated partial thromboplastin time (aPTT)
    c. Buccal mucosal bleeding time (BMBT)
    d. Prothrombin time (PT)

154. Which blood value will be elevated when a patient is experiencing decreased perfusion?
    a. Creatinine
    b. Glucose
    c. Lactate
    d. Sodium

155. The veterinarian has requested bloodwork on a patient. When reviewing the results, you notice that the patient has an elevated blood lactate level. What change would you expect to see on a blood gas?
    a. Normal pH
    b. Elevated pH
    c. Decreased pH
    d. No change in pH

156. Which of the following options is not a ketone?
    a. Acetone
    b. Acetoacetate
    c. Beta-hydroxybutyrate
    d. Ketoacetone

157. Which of the following options is not a goal of oxygen therapy?
    a. To decrease the work of breathing
    b. To decrease myocardial work
    c. To improve mentation
    d. To treat hypoxemia

158. The stretch (or load) placed on the myocardial fibers right before the heart contracts is known as:
    a. Afterload
    b. Contractility
    c. Preload
    d. Resistance

159. A patient presents with a history of collapse. While obtaining vitals, you notice the pulses become weaker with inspiration and stronger with expiration. The heart sounds are muffled and the height of the QRS complex on the patient's EKG changes with each beat. Which of the following conditions may be the cause of these clinical signs?
    a. Heart failure
    b. Hypovolemia
    c. Pericardial effusion
    d. Pneumothorax

160. What coagulation factors are tested by a prothrombin time?
    a. I, II, V, VII, X
    b. I, II, III, IV
    c. V, VII, X, XII
    d. V, XI, XII, XIII

161. At what point should a veterinary technician become concerned that the mean arterial pressure of a patient is becoming too low and that perfusion to the brain, heart, and kidneys will be compromised if it continues to fall?
    a. 40 mm Hg
    b. 50 mm Hg
    c. 60 mm Hg
    d. 70 mm Hg

162. Which of the following rodenticides will cause neurological signs when ingested?
    a. Bromethalin
    b. Bromadiolone
    c. Brodifacoum
    d. Warfarin

163. A patient presents with a respiratory pattern consisting of periods of apnea alternating with periods of hypernea. What is this respiratory pattern known as?
    a. Cheyne-Stokes
    b. Kussmaul's
    c. Paradoxical
    d. Orthopnea

164. How many days after a tick attaches itself to a dog will one see neurological signs associated with tick paralysis?
    a. 1
    b. 3
    c. 7
    d. 11

165. Which of the following is not a cause of hypoglycemia in a septic patient?
    a. Decreased dietary intake
    b. Increase release of insulin
    c. Increased consumption of glucose by the body
    d. Decreased production of glucose by the body

166. Which of the following medications can cause abortions?
    a. Clavamox
    b. Misoprostol
    c. Metronidazole
    d. Metoclopramide

167. A Doppler is used to measure:
    a. Blood pressure
    b. Central venous pressure
    c. SpO2
    d. End-tidal CO_2

168. _____ is a disease that causes damage to the optic nerve resulting in blindness, and it can be diagnosed by an increase in intraocular pressure.
    a. Blepharitis
    b. Glaucoma
    c. Uveitis
    d. Ulcerative keratitis

169. What is the initial cause of blepharospasm?
    a. Ocular discharge
    b. Increased intraocular pressure
    c. Lacrimation
    d. Irritation to the eye

170. What is the most common cause of hypercalcemia in dogs?
    a. Cancer
    b. Pregnancy
    c. Vomiting
    d. Diarrhea

171. Which is the correct order of changes in mentation from best to worst?
    a. Obtunded, comatose, quiet, stuporous
    b. Quiet, obtunded, stuporous, comatose
    c. Comatose, stuporous, quiet, obtunded
    d. Quiet stuporous, obtunded, comatose

172. When falling from a building, at what height (story) will a cat's injuries be less likely to be life threatening?
    a. 3 stories
    b. 5 stories
    c. 7 stories
    d. 9 stories

173. What is the expected difference between a patient's end-tidal CO_2 ($EtCO_2$) and the actual $PaCO_2$ (carbon dioxide in the arterial blood)?
    a. $EtCO_2$ 2–5 mm Hg less than the $PaCO_2$
    b. $EtCO_2$ 5–7 mm Hg less than the $PaCO_2$
    c. $PaCO_2$ 2–5 mm Hg less than the $EtCO_2$
    d. $PaCO_2$ 5–7 mm Hg less than the $EtCO_2$

174. A young, healthy patient is on intravenous fluids before a routine spay. Immediately after the fluids are started, the patient goes into cardiorespiratory arrest. What may have been the cause?
    a. Fluid rate too high
    b. The intravenous catheter was not patent
    c. There was air in the fluid line
    d. Unknown underlying disease

175. Which of the following tests can be used to diagnosis panleukopenia in a cat?
    a. Complete blood count
    b. Blood gas
    c. Electrolytes
    d. Canine Parvovirus snap test

176. What coagulation factors are tested with an activated partial thromboplastin time (aPTT)?
    a. I, II, V, VII, X
    b. I, II, V, VIII, IX, X, XI, XII
    c. V, VII, IX
    d. VIII, IX, X, XI

177. What is the correct formula when discussing cerebral perfusion pressure (CPP)?
    a. CPP = ICP (intracranial pressure) − MAP (mean arterial pressure)
    b. CPP = ICP + MAP
    c. CPP = MAP − ICP
    d. CPP = MAP + ICP

178. What type of hypersensitivity occurs when antibodies destroy the body's own, normal cells?
    a. Type I
    b. Type II
    c. Type III
    d. Type IV

179. Which patient will experience more damage from an electrical shock?
    a. A dry dog
    b. A wet dog
    c. A dog with his hair shaved
    d. A dog wearing metal tags

180. Which of these metabolites contributes more to ketoacidosis but is least detectable on a urine ketone strip?
    a. Acetone
    b. Acetoacetate
    c. Beta-hydroxybutyrate
    d. Ketoacetone

181. A dog presents to the practice after being hit by a car, and it has numerous injuries including a flail chest. How should the patient be positioned on the treatment table to minimize pain and maximize respiratory function?
    a. Affected side up
    b. Affected side down
    c. Sternal
    d. Dorsal

182. Metoclopramide is contraindicated in which of the following conditions?
    a. Postoperative gastrotomy
    b. Postoperative GDV
    c. Pancreatitis
    d. Gastrointestinal obstruction

183. A dog presents with pericardial effusion. Where should a veterinary technician shave the patient for a pericardiocentesis?
    a. Left side from the 3rd to the 7th ribs
    b. Left side from the 8th to the 12th ribs
    c. Right side from the 3rd to the 7th ribs
    d. Right side from the 8th to the 12 ribs

184. At what temperature (related to hypothermia) will a patient become comatose and develop muscular rigidity as well as cardiac arrhythmias?
    a. <83° F
    b. 83°–86° F
    c. 86°–93° F
    d. 93°–98° F

185. A patient receives chemotherapy for lymphoma and 6 hours later you notice the patient is vomiting, having diarrhea, and seems depressed. When you examine the patient more closely you note pale mucous membranes, a prolonged CRT, and bradycardia. What do you suspect is happening?
    a. Extravasation of the chemotherapeutic agent
    b. Heart failure
    c. Tumor lysis syndrome
    d. Sterile hemorrhagic cystitis

186. The oncology department brings a dog to the emergency department after vincristine (a vinca alkaloid) extravasation. Which of the following procedures is not recommended?
    a. Administration of the remainder of the medication
    b. Inject saline, dexamethasone sodium phosphate, and sodium bicarbonate around the site
    c. Withdrawal as much of the medication as possible
    d. Apply a warm compress

187. Which of the following is not a determinant of stroke volume?
    a. Afterload
    b. Contractility
    c. Heart rate
    d. Preload

188. A patient arrives at the emergency department with a presenting complaint of vomiting and diarrhea. He received chemotherapy a week earlier and was doing well until today. When obtaining his vital signs you note the dog has a temperature of 104.0° F. The veterinarian asks you to draw blood and run a complete blood count. What do you expect the results to show?
    a. Anemia
    b. Monocytosis
    c. Neutropenia
    d. Thrombocytopenia

189. A 3-year-old boxer comes into the veterinary practice and the owner states they were on a walk when the dog suddenly appeared weak, then fell over. He was unresponsive for 10–15 seconds and then recovered and seemed normal. The owner states that the dog did not thrash or lose control of his bladder or bowels. What condition may have occurred?
    a. Anaphylaxis
    b. Cardiac arrest
    c. Seizure
    d. Syncope

190. An owner calls the veterinary practice and states his dog cut his paw at the barn several days previously. The dog seemed to be fine and the cut was healing, but he started acting strangely yesterday. This morning he found the dog lying on his side with his head and neck extended backwards over his back. He was salivating heavily, and when the owner tried to open his mouth he was unable to because the dog's jaw was so stiff. Which of the following conditions might the history and clinical signs indicate?
    a. Botulism
    b. Bromethalin toxicity
    c. Seizure activity
    d. Tetanus

191. A patient with a history of megaesophagus presents to the veterinary clinic with a complaint of weakness associated with exercise. The owner says the dog seems fine for a short period and then is unable to walk. If he rests, he recovers and is normal for a few minutes, but then it happens again. What condition do you suspect is the cause?
    a. Myasthenia gravis
    b. Myopathy
    c. Polyradiculoneuritis
    d. Tick paralysis

192. While triaging a patient, you notice an increased respiratory effort on inspiration. What disease might this indicate?
    a. Upper airway disease
    b. Lower airway disease
    c. Lung disease
    d. Pleural space disease

193. A cat presents after being hit by a car. The veterinarian notes abdominal effusion, performs an abdominocentesis to obtain a sample, and asks you to run electrolytes on the abdominal fluid and compare it to serum electrolytes. Which of the following conditions is he trying to eliminate?
    a. Hemoabdomen
    b. Uroabdomen
    c. Peritonitis
    d. Septic abdomen

194. What is the cause of polyuria/polydipsia in dogs with a pyometra?
    a. Increased thirst resulting from fever
    b. Release of prostaglandin
    c. Dehydration
    d. Release of endotoxin

195. Which of the following drugs is the preferred antidote for ethylene glycol toxicity?
    a. Acetylcysteine
    b. Calcium EDTA
    c. Deferoxamine
    d. 4-methylprazole

196. When obtaining an EKG, how should the patient be positioned?
    a. Standing
    b. Right lateral
    c. Left lateral
    d. Sternal

197. With what is the P wave associated on an EKG?
    a. Depolarization of the ventricles
    b. Depolarization of the atria
    c. Repolarization of the ventricles
    d. Repolarization of the atria

198. While monitoring a patient you note the EKG suddenly flatlines. You immediately:
    a. Start CPR
    b. Auscult the heart with your stethoscope
    c. Do nothing, it is probably incorrect
    d. Check the EKG leads

199. When setting up direct arterial blood pressure monitoring, where should the transducer be placed?
    a. At the level of the heart
    b. At the level of the arterial catheter
    c. At the level of the fluid bag
    d. At the level of the monitor

200. The difference between the systolic and diastolic blood pressures is called:
    a. Mean arterial pressure
    b. Pulse pressure
    c. Blood pressure
    d. Central venous pressure

201. When measuring central venous pressure, where should the zero on the manometer be positioned?
    a. At the level of the jugular catheter
    b. At the level of the dorsal pedal artery
    c. At the level of the left atrium
    d. At the level of the right atrium

202. What is a patient's expected PaO_2 when breathing room air?
    a. 21 mm Hg
    b. 40 mm Hg
    c. 75 mm Hg
    d. 100 mm Hg

203. When preparing a patient for a temporary tracheostomy, where should the patient be shaved and scrubbed?
    a. Mandible to manubrium
    b. Between the cricoid and thyroid cartilages
    c. The thyroid cartilage to the thoracic inlet
    d. Caudal to the manubrium

204. How should a patient be positioned for a temporary tracheostomy?
    a. Laterally with the legs pulled caudally
    b. Laterally with the legs pulled cranially
    c. Dorsally with the legs pulled caudally
    d. Dorsally with the legs pulled cranially

205. When performing a thoracocentesis, the needle should be placed:
    a. Cranial to the rib with the bevel up
    b. Caudal to the rib with the bevel down
    c. Caudal to the rib with the bevel up
    d. Cranial to the rib with the bevel down

206. When performing a diagnostic peritoneal lavage, how much fluid is infused into the abdomen?
    a. 10 mL/kg
    b. 15 mL/kg
    c. 20 mL/kg
    d. 25 mL/kg

207. When passing a nasogastric tube, where should the tube be measured?
    a. From the nares to the thoracic inlet
    b. From the nares to the last rib
    c. From the nares inlet to the 10th rib
    d. From the nares to the 5th rib

208. Which is the most important measure that can be taken to control nosocomial infections?
    a. Antibiotics
    b. Barrier nursing
    c. Cleaning
    d. Handwashing

209. Which of the following medications requires a filter when administering?
    a. Cerenia
    b. Enrofloxacin
    c. Mannitol
    d. Propofol

210. A 10-kg dog requires a metoclopramide CRI at a rate of 2 mg/kg/day. The veterinarian asks that it be added to a new 1-L bag of Normosol-R. His fluid rate is 100 mL/hr, and the metoclopramide is 5 mg/mL. How many mL of metoclopramide should be added to the bag?
    a. 0.8 mL
    b. 1.7 mL
    c. 3.2 mL
    d. 4.1 mL

211. A dog presents to the hospital after being removed from a house fire. His skin shows areas that are yellow/black in color, dry, and only mildly painful. How would this burn be classified?
    a. Superficial
    b. Superficial partial-thickness
    c. Deep partial-thickness
    d. Full-thickness

212. Which of the following procedures should not be used to cool a heatstroke patient?
    a. Tepid water
    b. A fan
    c. Ice
    d. Intravenous fluids

213. While writing in a patient's medical record you make a mistake. What should you do?
    a. Scratch it out
    b. Erase it
    c. Draw a line through it
    d. Black it out

214. What is the most likely cause of respiratory distress in a dog that has suffered from a choking episode?
    a. Noncardiogenic pulmonary edema
    b. Pneumothorax
    c. Heart failure
    d. Upper airway obstruction

215. Which of the following conditions is not a cause of central vestibular disease?
    a. Neoplasia
    b. Otitis interna
    c. Infection
    d. Inflammation

216. Which of the following techniques is appropriate for a radius fracture?
    a. Robert Jones
    b. Elmer sling
    c. Spica splint
    d. Velpeau sling

217. Where would a veterinary technician shave and surgically prep a patient that requires placement of an esophagostomy tube?
    a. Left side of the neck
    b. Right side of the neck
    c. Left side of the abdomen
    d. Right side of the abdomen

218. A patient with von Willebrand's disease requires surgery. Which product can be administered to prevent hemorrhage?
    a. Cryoprecipitate
    b. Fresh whole blood
    c. Fresh frozen plasma
    d. Packed red blood cells

219. A patient receives a packed red blood cell transfusion. How many days can pass before he will require a crossmatch for a second transfusion?
    a. 2
    b. 5
    c. 8
    d. 12

220. How many square meters of surface area are contained in one gram of activated charcoal?
    a. 10
    b. 100
    c. 1000
    d. 10,000

221. A patient will develop idiogenic osmoles in response to which condition?
    a. Hypernatremia
    b. Hyperkalemia
    c. Hyperchloremia
    d. Hyponatremia

222. What changes will be seen on the pulse oximeter of a patient with carbon dioxide poisoning?
    a. It will be high
    b. It will be low
    c. No change
    d. Normal

223. The veterinarian is concerned that a patient's platelets are not functioning properly. Which test will the doctor request?
    a. Activated clotting time
    b. Activated partial thromboplastin time
    c. Buccal mucosal bleeding time
    d. Prothrombin time

224. Which of the following bacteria is responsible for tetanus?
    a. *Bordetella bronchiseptica*
    b. *Clostridium tetani*
    c. *Neospora caninum*
    d. *Toxoplasmosis gondii*

225. Which of the following drugs would be used to treat organophosphate poisoning?
    a. Atropine
    b. Diazepam
    c. Dexamethazone
    d. Mannitol

e *Answers and rationales available on Evolve* http://evolve.elsevier.com/Prendergast/QAvettech/

SECTION 13

Pain Management and Analgesia

Mary Ellen Goldberg, BS, LVT, CVT, SRA, CCRA and Tasha McNerney, BS, CVT

QUESTIONS

1. The veterinary technician can play an important role in pain management by:
   a. Monitoring urine and fecal output
   b. Changing the medication when it is ineffective
   c. Communicating directly with the clinician about particular concerns
   d. Directing the veterinary assistant to provide medications

2. Which of the following characteristics do cats exhibit when they are experiencing pain?
   a. Sleeping continuously, overeating, and attention-seeking behaviors
   b. Resentment of being handled, aggression, and abnormal posture
   c. Hyperactivity, pupillary enlargement, and tail swishing
   d. Hypotension, hypocapnia, hypopnea, and bradycardia

3. During hospitalization, how often should a pain assessment be performed?
   a. Every 4–6 hours
   b. Every 30 minutes to 1 hour
   c. Every 12–24 hours
   d. Every 8 hours

4. When a veterinary technician is trying to distinguish pain from dysphoria, which of the following would the technician do?
   a. Place the patient on comfortable blankets
   b. Speak in low tones and interacting with the animal makes the patient feel better, but behaviors resume when interaction stops
   c. Move the animal to a different ward
   d. Reverse the analgesic medication

5. Which guidelines have elevated pain to the fourth vital sign?
   a. American College of Veterinary Anesthesiologist's Pain Management Guidelines
   b. The International Veterinary Academy of Pain Management's Guidelines
   c. AAHA/AAFP Pain Management Guidelines for Dogs and Cats
   d. The AVMA Pain Management Guidelines

6. Nociception is defined as:
   a. The activity in the peripheral pathway that transmits and processes information about the stimulus to the brain
   b. A normal response to tissue damage
   c. Pain without apparent biological origin that has persisted beyond the normal tissue healing time
   d. Any stimuli to the affected area that would normally be innocuous that become noxious

7. What is the correct sequence of steps to the pain pathway?
   a. Transduction, transmission, modulation, perception
   b. Modulation, transduction, perception, transmission
   c. Transduction, modulation, transmission, perception
   d. Transmission, transduction, modulation, perception

8. Which of the following describes "wind-up"?
   a. An increase in the excitability of spinal neurons, mediated in part by the activation of NMDA receptors in dorsal horn neurons
   b. It occurs when tissue inflammation leads to the release of a complex array of chemical mediators, resulting in reduced nociceptor thresholds
   c. When brief trauma or noxious stimulus result in physiological pain
   d. The perceived increase in pain intensity with time when a given painful stimulus is delivered repeatedly in excess of a critical rate

9. Which of the following is an example of an opioid agonist?
   a. Butorphanol
   b. Naloxone
   c. Morphine
   d. Buprenorphine

10. Prostaglandins play an important role in:
    a. Production of endorphins
    b. Mammalian cardiovascular physiology
    c. Production of leukotrienes
    d. Mammalian renal physiology

11. Which of the following is an NMDA antagonist medication?
    a. Ketamine
    b. Lidocaine
    c. Meperidine
    d. Dexmedetomidine

12. Which of the following classes of drugs would include gabapentin?
    a. Corticosteroids
    b. Sodium channel blockers
    c. Antiepileptics
    d. Nutraceuticals

13. An example of an agent that is only administered topically and provides analgesia is:
    a. Buprenorphine
    b. EMLA cream
    c. Bupivicaine
    d. Fentanyl

14. Which of the following statements can apply to an intratesticular block?
    a. Intratesticular blocks can only be used in large animal patients
    b. Intratesticular blocks can be used in canine and feline orchiectomies
    c. Intratesticular blocks require the use of a vaporizer
    d. Intratesticular blocks should never been performed on veterinary patients

15. Many veterinary technicians are asked to calculate and administer constant rate infusions, as patients can benefit immensely. Which of the following statements is *not* a benefit of a CRI?
    a. CRIs provide a more stable plane of analgesia with less incidence of breakthrough pain
    b. CRIs provide greater control over drug administration
    c. CRIs allow a lower dose of drug to be delivered at any given time, resulting in a lower incidence of dose-related side effects
    d. CRIs allow the veterinary technician to leave the practice for the evening while administrating medication continuously

16. Massage is an example of which type of rehabilitation technique?
    a. Manual therapy
    b. Effleurage techniques
    c. Physical modalities
    d. Therapeutic exercise

17. What is a benefit of cryotherapy?
    a. Decreased metabolism so patient is less hungry
    b. Decreased production of pain mediators, leading to analgesia
    c. Prevention of hyperthermia
    d. Useful 2–3 weeks postinjury

18. Which of the following describes a myofascial trigger point?
    a. A point in the muscle at which a reflex can be elicited
    b. A transcutaneous electrical nerve stimulation
    c. A painful area of sustained muscle contraction that cannot easily self-release
    d. A technique where needles are used to pierce the skin at certain points to bring about a physiologic change to treat or prevent disease

19. Visceral pain is quite common among companion animals. Which of the following is *not* an example of visceral pain?
    a. Pancreatitis
    b. Gastroenteritis
    c. Bowel ischemia
    d. Osteosarcoma

20. Which of the following are three examples that are *all* considered chronic pain diseases?
    a. Lymphoma, diabetes, GDV
    b. Osteoarthritis, IVDD, cancer
    c. Respiratory infection, cardiac disease, blocked cat
    d. Broken leg, bronchitis, hypertension

21. Veterinary technicians that advocate for pain management are most closely compared to what group of nurses?
    a. Orthopedic nurses
    b. Psychiatric nurses
    c. Human neonatal and pediatric nurses
    d. Emergency and critical care nurses

22. Which of the following is essential for good communication between veterinarians and veterinary technicians who are working in pain management?
    a. Knowing each other's routine and what is regularly done for patients
    b. Knowledge of the physiology of pain and the pharmacology of analgesics
    c. Veterinarians *and* Veterinary Technicians should have attained the Certified Veterinary Pain Practitioner status from IVAPM
    d. Communication is not an essential skill, and veterinary technicians should just do as the attending veterinarian tells them

23. Why are the differences in expression among dogs and cats of all ages, and variations among certain breeds, important for pain assessment?
    a. Certain breeds vocalize and appear more sensitive to pain whereas others seem to remain stoic in the face of pain
    b. Only cats exhibit facial expressions; dogs do not
    c. No comprehensive pain scale has been developed for companion animals
    d. Expressions are insignificant; physiological parameters are what should be used to determine pain

24. The role of the veterinary technician in pain management includes:
    a. Patient assessment
    b. Differentiating pain from other stress
    c. Monitoring and treating drug effects
    d. All of the above

25. Which of the following might a dysphoric or delirious animal experience because of opioid overdose?
    a. Thrashing and yowling continuously
    b. Claustrophobia
    c. Only rare response to soothing interaction
    d. Chewing on cage doors

26. Which of the following behaviors are commonly associated with clinical signs of pain in dogs?
    a. Vocalization and increased appetite
    b. Playful actions and excessive licking of the owners
    c. Panting, anorexia, and depression
    d. Increased attention to the environment

27. It is sometimes difficult to distinguish normal from pain-associated behaviors in cats and dogs. Which of the following behaviors is most likely to be a normal, nonpainful behavior?
    a. Decreased appetite
    b. Unusual aggression
    c. Stretching all four legs when the abdomen is touched
    d. Decreased social interaction

28. Which of the following statements regarding pain assessment in dogs is true?
    a. Physiological parameters, such as heart rate and blood pressure, are sensitive tools for assessing pain in dogs
    b. A visual analog scale is a type of multidimensional pain scale and is useful for assessing pain in dogs
    c. Multidimensional pain scales yield better interobserver agreement than unidimensional pain scales
    d. Multidimensional pain scales correlate closely with vocalization and serum cortisol levels in chronically painful dogs

29. Which of the following is the most common sign of osteoarthritic pain in cats?
    a. Hiding from company
    b. Eating fewer meals
    c. Reduced frequency of jumping up to high places
    d. Sleeping all day

30. The observer's subjective interpretation of behavior and assessment of physiologic pain can be described using a pain-rating instrument such as:
    a. Visual analog scale
    b. Force plate gait analysis
    c. Health-related quality-of-life instrument
    d. Serum cortisol levels

31. Regarding the use of pain scales in hospitalized animals, which of the following statements is *false*?
    a. Pain scales may encourage routine evaluation of hospitalized animals
    b. Pain scales can be used to determine whether analgesic therapy should be discontinued
    c. Effective analgesic therapy should result in an animal with a low pain score
    d. A low pain score indicates that analgesic therapy is sufficient, even if an animal is exhibiting some questionable behaviors

32. In cats, some diseases cause behavioral changes that are often been ascribed to "old age" rather than pain. Examples include all of the following, *except*:
    a. Facet pain of spondylosis
    b. Intervertebral disc disease
    c. Osteoarthritis
    d. Basal cell tumor

33. Frequency of pain assessment depends on the situation. Which of the following is the most appropriate guideline for frequency of chronic pain assessment?
    a. Every 8 hours during the postoperative period
    b. A minimum of every 3 months for an animal with chronic pain
    c. Every 12 hours for animals with traumatic injuries
    d. Yearly for an animal with chronic pain

34. The "gold standard" to assess pain is:
    a. A physiological assessment
    b. A clinical pathological assessment
    c. A behavioral assessment
    d. There is none

35. The purpose of any pain scale is to:
    a. Help guide analgesic, medical, or surgical treatment
    b. Provide "concrete" diagnostic evidence
    c. Provide legal documentation
    d. Provide "happy faces" for the patient's chart

36. The preemptive scoring system is a:
    a. Visual analog scale
    b. Subjective scoring system
    c. Simple descriptive scale
    d. Numerical rating scale

37. The University of Melbourne Pain Scale is based on:
    a. Hematologic values
    b. Australian regulations
    c. Behavioral and physiologic responses
    d. Physiologic responses

38. The Glasgow Composite Pain Scale is based on specific behavioral signs in which of the following species?
    a. Feline
    b. Ferret
    c. Equine
    d. Canine

39. The Colorado State University Veterinary Medical Center Acute Pain Scale uses which of the following options as an indication of pain?
    a. Number scale
    b. Recorded sounds
    c. Artistic renderings of animals at various levels of pain
    d. Happy to sad faces

40. Which of the following is *not* one of the 3 primary factors included in a quality-of-life scale?
    a. Social factors
    b. Interpersonal factors
    c. Physical factors
    d. Behavioral factors

41. A mental nerve block provides analgesia to the:
    a. Maxilla
    b. Lower lip and incisors on the ipsilateral side
    c. Upper lip and nose
    d. Premolars and molars

42. For which of the following can the lidocaine patch be used to provide analgesia?
    a. Skin abrasions
    b. Lacerations
    c. Hot spots
    d. All of the above

43. In the Pain Buster Soaker catheter, the local anesthetic is delivered by:
    a. Elastomeric reservoir pump
    b. CRI
    c. Syringe pump
    d. IV infusion

44. For which kind of pain would an interpleural block be recommended?
    a. Heart pain
    b. Pancreatic pain
    c. Colon pain
    d. Kidney pain

45. For which of the following would a brachial plexus block provide analgesia?
    a. Thorax
    b. Forefeet
    c. Distal to the elbow
    d. Proximal to the elbow

46. The sciatic nerve block provides analgesia to the:
    a. Medial portion of the thigh, tibia, and tarsus and akinesia of the quadriceps femoris muscle
    b. Caudal muscles of the thigh
    c. Portions distal to the elbow
    d. Lumbosacral space and the first or second intercoccygeal space

47. If a tourniquet is used when injecting a local anesthetic intravenously, the block is referred to as the:
    a. Baer's block
    b. Bayer's block
    c. Byer's block
    d. Bier's block

48. An epidural injection in a dog is injected between:
    a. L7-S1
    b. L4-L5
    c. L5-L6
    d. S1-S2

49. Which of the following statements is *not* true regarding acupuncture?
    a. The points and channels of acupuncture follow neurovascular pathways
    b. Acupuncture treats pain by inducing neuromodulation along peripheral, central, and autonomic pathways
    c. Acupuncture treatments can involve: needling, electroacupuncture, low-level laser, and manual pressure
    d. Acupuncture relies on nonspecific identification of the structures responsible for generating pain

50. Which of the following examples does acupuncture usually involve?
    a. Veterinary manual therapy
    b. The use of herbs for analgesia
    c. The insertion of thin, sterile needles into specific anatomic sites richly supplied with nerve endings
    d. Diluted substances in homeopathic remedies

51. Which of the following are contraindications for acupuncture?
    a. Pregnancy
    b. Sepsis
    c. Severe bleeding abnormalities
    d. All of the above

52. Myofascial pain syndrome entails the palpation of:
    a. Taut bands and trigger points
    b. Swollen segments of muscle
    c. Nodules of infection
    d. Nerve bundles

53. Herbs used for COX inhibition do *not* include:
    a. Ginger
    b. Devils claw
    c. Capsaicin
    d. White willow bark

54. Examples of complementary therapy for pain management include:
    a. Manual therapy
    b. Magnet therapy
    c. Homeopathy
    d. All of the above

55. During cryotherapy, the cold temperature raises the activation threshold of:
    a. Reflex muscles
    b. Blood vessels
    c. Tissue nociceptors
    d. Painful nerves

56. When should cryotherapy be applied for best response?
    a. During the acute inflammatory phase of tissue healing
    b. After exercise to lessen inflammatory response
    c. Immediately following surgery
    d. All of the above

57. Caution should be used with cryotherapy if a patient has:
    a. A large percentage of fat
    b. Localized vascular compromise
    c. Areas of previous frostbite
    d. b and c

58. The primary benefit of cryokinetics is to:
    a. Aid the patient's ability to perform pain-free, low-level exercise
    b. Cool down a body that is overheating
    c. Allow an athlete to compete at the highest levels with no pain
    d. Take the place of local anesthetic injections in advance of athletic stress

59. Cold or white skin after a 20-minute cryotherapy session may indicate:
    a. Circulation is restored and normal
    b. Possible cold-induced tissue damage
    c. The need for external heat creams or rubs
    d. The need for more melanin in the diet

60. Cryotherapy can include:
    a. Ice packs
    b. Cold immersion baths
    c. Ice massage
    d. All of the above

61. Which of the following scenarios is thermotherapy *not* useful for?
    a. Chronic pain
    b. Muscle spasm
    c. Acute inflammation
    d. Stretching to enhance collagen extensibility

62. Treatment for joint mobility includes:
    a. ROM
    b. Stretching exercises
    c. a and b
    d. None of the above

63. Which of the following is *not* true for passive range of motion?
    a. Treatment should be in a quiet, comfortable area
    b. A muzzle should be applied for initial treatments
    c. The patient's limb (of interest) is fully supported
    d. The patient's position is unimportant

64. Which of the following is the target tissue for lengthening a muscle that is contracted?
    a. Joint capsule
    b. Muscle belly
    c. Tendon
    d. Ligament

65. Which of the following is an example of an active range of motion exercise?
    a. Aquatic therapy
    b. Walking in snow or sand
    c. Climbing stairs
    d. All of the above

66. Therapeutic exercises do *not* include:
    a. Pulling or carrying weights
    b. Cavaletti rails
    c. Treadmill walking
    d. Wheelbarrowing

67. Transcutaneous electrical nerve stimulation is a form of:
    a. LLLT
    b. NEMS
    c. EEG
    d. EMG

68. A contraindication for transcutaneous electrical nerve stimulation (TENS) includes:
    a. Cruciate ligament reconstruction
    b. Rehab after orthopedic injury
    c. Animals with pacemakers
    d. Chronic OA

69. When should low-level laser therapy *not* be used?
    a. Over muscle trigger points
    b. Over acupuncture points
    c. With osteoarthritis and muscle spasms
    d. Over areas of malignancy or cancer

70. Massage techniques may include:
    a. Effleurage
    b. Petrissage
    c. Trigger point therapy
    d. All of the above

71. Extracorporeal shock wave treatment (ESWT) could be indicated for:
    a. Pregnancy
    b. Osteoarthritis
    c. Neoplasms
    d. Heart disease

72. Which tool is used to measure passive range of motion in companion animals?
    a. Calipers
    b. Slide rule
    c. Goniometer
    d. Oliometer

73. When should therapeutic ultrasound *not* be used?
    a. When the patient's area of interest has plastic or metal implants
    b. When the ultimate result is to decrease pain
    c. When the goal is to accelerate wound healing
    d. When the patient's ROM should be increased

74. Phototherapy can be used for:
    a. Soft-tissue injuries
    b. Wound healing
    c. Chronic pain
    d. All of the above

75. In cats, aquatic therapy is contraindicated for:
    a. Muscle weakness
    b. OA
    c. Cardiac dysfunction
    d. Geriatric care

76. An example of a proprioception exercise used for cats is:
    a. Jump rope
    b. Swimming
    c. Balance board
    d. Massage

77. What organization requires that pain be included in every veterinary patient assessment regardless of a presenting complaint?
    a. North American Veterinary Technician Association
    b. American College of Veterinary Anesthesia and Analgesia
    c. American Animal Hospital Association
    d. American Veterinary Medical Association

78. How can pain negatively impact the patient?
    a. Treatment costs money so the client will refuse it
    b. Pain promotes inflammation, which delays wound healing
    c. Pain can induce viral diseases
    d. Pain can cause cataracts to form

79. Which pain scale should be used?
    a. Does not matter as long as you like it and it makes you happy
    b. The longest and most complex is always the best
    c. The shortest and simplest is always the best
    d. It is important to choose one system to be used by the entire veterinary team

80. How painful is abscess drainage?
    a. Mild
    b. Moderate
    c. Severe
    d. Extremely severe

81. How painful is a ovariohysterectomy?
    a. Mild
    b. Moderate
    c. Severe
    d. Extremely severe

82. How painful is a thoracotomy?
    a. Mild
    b. Moderate
    c. Severe
    d. Extremely severe

83. What kind of scale is a visual analog scale (VAS)?
    a. Subjective
    b. Objective
    c. a and b
    d. None of the above

84. The Colorado State Canine and Feline Pain Scales fall under which category?
    a. Objective
    b. Subjective
    c. Both a and b
    d. None of the above

85. Which pain scale is considered "state of the art"?
    a. Colorado State Canine and Feline Pain Scales
    b. A scale that you make for yourself
    c. Glasgow Pain Scoring System
    d. Client-specific outcome measures scale

86. How often should a pain score be given to the client?
    a. Never
    b. Every 6 months
    c. Yearly
    d. Every time the pain score is assessed

87. Which of the following parameters do horses most commonly exhibit for various states of pain?
    a. Behavior parameters
    b. Emotional parameters
    c. Physiologic parameters
    d. All of the above

88. Pain that is abnormal and not beneficial for the patient is called:
    a. Adaptive pain
    b. Maladaptive pain
    c. Physiologic pain
    d. Peripheral pain

89. Where can inflammatory pain occur?
    a. Muscles, joints, skin, and periosteum
    b. Thorax
    c. Abdomen
    d. All of the above

90. The most common types of pain experienced by horses are:
    a. Ocular and head pain
    b. Spine and pelvic pain
    c. Orthopedic pain and abdominal/colic pain
    d. Foot and dental pain

91. What pain scoring systems are available for horses?
    a. Obel Laminitis Pain Scale
    b. AAEP lameness grade definition
    c. Horse Grimace Scale
    d. All of the above

92. Which of the following clinical signs might a cow in pain exhibit?
    a. Dull and depressed
    b. Inappetence and grinding teeth
    c. A stance with one foot behind the other
    d. All of the above

93. Goats are intolerant of painful procedures. How do sheep react to a painful procedure?
    a. They refuse to eat
    b. They show subtle signs of pain
    c. They always vocalize when in pain
    d. They develop a fever from pain

94. Squealing is a normal behavior in pigs. When could squealing be considered a result of pain?
    a. When a painful area is palpated
    b. When squealing becomes excessive
    c. When squealing involves a lack of social behavior
    d. All of the above

95. What is a benefit of using local anesthetics?
    a. Local anesthetics produce true analgesia resulting in the complete absence of pain for the duration of the block
    b. Long term (chronic) pain states may be diminished or eliminated
    c. These drugs are nonscheduled agents
    d. All of the above

96. Side effects of local anesthetics can include:
    a. Cardiovascular effects
    b. CNS effects
    c. Allergic reactions
    d. All of the above

97. Which of the following is a local block used for onychectomy procedures?
    a. Leg block
    b. Brachial plexus block
    c. Circumferential ring block
    d. Foot block

98. Of the following listed blocks, which is not a dental nerve block?
    a. Mandibular nerve block
    b. Mental nerve block
    c. Infraorbital nerve block
    d. Retrobulbar nerve block

99. What block can be performed before surgery of the abdominal cavity?
    a. Sacrococcygeal block
    b. Incisional block
    c. Mental nerve block
    d. Bier's block

100. Which bones serve as a landmark for an intercostal block?
    a. Sternum
    b. Thoracic vertebrae
    c. Humerus
    d. Ribs

101. What are the advantages of an interpleural block over the intercostal block?
    a. Ability to redose easily
    b. Ease of administration
    c. Ability to provide analgesia following median sternotomy
    d. All of the above

102. Which block can be used in a castration procedure for companion animals, large animals, and exotic animals?
    a. Intratesticular block
    b. Epidural block
    c. Intra-articular block
    d. Intrapleural block

103. Which of the following is considered an excellent block that can be used for cats with a urinary blockage?
    a. Epidural
    b. Sacrococcygeal block
    c. Pelvic block
    d. Penile block

104. Of the following procedures, which is not an indication for an epidural block?
    a. Cesarean section
    b. Tibial–femoral fractures
    c. TECA procedure
    d. Cruciate ligament repair

105. What type of needle is recommended for an epidural catheter?
    a. Tuohy-type
    b. Butterfly catheter needle
    c. 16-gauge IV catheter needle
    d. Auto-vac needle

106. Which of the following is an indication for an epidural in a horse?
    a. Difficult parturition
    b. Caslick's closure
    c. Urethrostomy
    d. All of the above

107. What can happen to goats if they experience unrelieved pain?
    a. Faint
    b. Death
    c. Goats will roll and vocalize
    d. Goats can suddenly become lame

108. What type of nerve block is used to dehorn cattle?
    a. Cornual nerve block
    b. Epidural nerve block
    c. Facial nerve block
    d. Disbudding nerve block

109. In which ruminant species can an epidural nerve block be performed?
    a. Cattle
    b. Sheep and goats
    c. Camelids
    d. All of the above

110. Which of the following are goals of physical rehabilitation therapy?
    a. Decreased pain and inflammation
    b. Maintained or increased joint ROM and flexibility
    c. Maintained or increased strength
    d. All of the above

111. Benefits of massage include which of the following?
    a. Decreased muscle spasms and increased local blood and lymphatic flow
    b. Help for the patient to reach "nirvana"
    c. No physiological benefits
    d. Cannot be performed on canine species

112. What modalities does thermotherapy encompass?
    a. Heat therapy only
    b. Cold therapy only
    c. Laser therapy
    d. Heat and cold therapy

113. When starting a patient on aquatic swimming therapy, which of the following would be a main recommendation?
    a. Start the patient on a long, difficult program to increase tolerance
    b. Swim several times a day, building in 30-minute increments
    c. Slowly introduce aquatic therapy depending on patient's level
    d. Aquatic therapy swimming is recommended for all patients regardless of incisions

114. Traditional Chinese veterinary medicine (TCVM) includes what five branches?
    a. Diet and food, exercise Qigong, Tui-na, acupuncture, and herbal medicine
    b. Yin-yang, eight principles, zang-fu organs, four levels, and six stages
    c. Wood, fire, earth, metal, and water
    d. Heart, blood, spleen, lung, and kidney

115. Why is electrical stimulation used at select acupuncture points?
    a. To warm acupuncture points
    b. To release endorphins at high frequency
    c. To increase the duration of effect
    d. To cause a permanent effect

116. What is a myofascial trigger point (MTrP)?
    a. A "jump sign"
    b. A hyperirritable spot in skeletal muscle that is associated with a hypersensitive palpable nodule in a taut band
    c. A muscle spasm that causes intense pain
    d. None of the above

117. What is a "jump sign"?
    a. A reaction to pain from MTrPs palpation
    b. When the patient has recovered and can jump high
    c. A behavior exhibited when a patient is startled
    d. A behavior exhibited when the patient receives an injection

118. In chiropractic practice, what is the role of the veterinary technician?
    a. Takes the preliminary history
    b. Conducts the initial examination
    c. Pain assessment
    d. All of the above

119. What is the definition of obesity?
    a. 10% heavier than the optimal weight for the breed in question
    b. 20% heavier than the optimal weight for the breed in question
    c. An increase in fat tissue mass sufficient to contribute to disease
    d. None of the above

120. Negative effects of obesity include:
    a. Specific disease conditions
    b. Reduced life span
    c. Abnormally high body condition scores
    d. All of the above

121. A traumatic cause of OA in dogs includes obesity as a risk factor. What is the most common traumatic cause of OA in dogs?
    a. Ruptured cruciate ligaments
    b. Torn Achilles group
    c. Hip dysplasia
    d. Phalangeal fracture

122. Which of the following statements is false regarding the negative effects of pain?
    a. Pain produces a catabolic state
    b. Pain enhances immune response
    c. Pain promotes inflammation
    d. Pain increases the anesthetic risk

123. What inhibits the aggrecanase enzymes responsible for cartilage degradation in cats?
    a. Docosahexaenoic acid (DHA)
    b. Eicosapentaenoic acid (EPA)
    c. Arachidonic acid (AA)
    d. Methionine

124. What is "porphyrin staining" in rodents?
    a. Hair standing on end
    b. Color of cage litter from urine
    c. Red tears which may encircle the eye
    d. None of the above

125. How is pain typically characterized in rabbits?
    a. Reduction in food and water intake
    b. Bruxism
    c. Closed eyes
    d. Lateral recumbency

126. What is a common cause of pain in ferrets?
    a. Arthritis
    b. Dystocia
    c. Ear mites
    d. Albinism

127. Signs of pain in birds can include:
    a. Weaving in cage
    b. Eating fecal droppings
    c. Self-isolation
    d. Aggressiveness

128. A sign of chronic pain in a reptile includes:
    a. Increased respiratory rate
    b. Restlessness
    c. Immobility
    d. Florid displays

129. Abnormal behavioral signs that could indicate pain in fish could include:
    a. Anorexia, rapid opercular movements, clamped fins
    b. Attempting to attack, eating tank mates, breathing air at surface
    c. Listing, "shimmies," curling
    d. Gasping, hurdling, drifting

130. During the initial onset of pain, all of the following physiologic changes occur, *except:*
    a. Sympathetic tone increases
    b. Vasoconstriction
    c. Increased myocardial work
    d. Decreased oxygen consumption

131. What is meant by the term *noxious stimulus*?
    a. A toxic overdose of a drug
    b. A damaging or potentially damaging tissue stimulus
    c. An nitrous oxide reaction
    d. The changing of the nervous system based on the environment

132. If a painful stimulus is traveling in an afferent direction, what does this mean?
    a. Toward the area of inflammation
    b. Toward the central nervous system
    c. Away from the central nervous system
    d. Not moving at all

133. What is the minimal stimulus required to elicit a transmittable electrical signal from a peripheral sensory receptor?
    a. The action potential
    b. Polymodal nociceptors
    c. Threshold
    d. Secondary modulation

134. What are the two main nerve fiber types associated with transmitting pain sensation information to the central nervous system?
    a. A-delta and C fibers
    b. A-beta and C fibers
    c. A-nociceptors and C nociceptors
    d. Interleukins and substance P

135. Pain known as *first pain*, because it is often the first pain felt after injury, is often described as sharp and short lived. This pain signal is transmitted by what nociceptor?
    a. A-Beta
    b. C fibers
    c. Histamine
    d. A-delta

136. Which of the following correctly lists (in order) the four events involved in the pain pathway?
    a. Transduction, transmission, modulation, perception
    b. Perception, modulation, transmission, transduction
    c. Perception, inhibition, conduction, inflammation
    d. Transduction, modulation, transmission, perception

137. Which of the following terms describes the changing, inhibiting, or amplifying of an impulse within the spinal cord?
    a. Transmission
    b. Perception
    c. Modulation
    d. Inflammation

138. What is the function of the dorsal horn of the spinal cord?
    a. To sense an awareness of pain
    b. To regulate blood pressure
    c. To receive and manage sensory information from the peripheral nerves
    d. To excrete excitatory neurotransmitters

139. Which type of fibers does the "gate control theory" state are responsible for increasing the inhibitory effects of interneurons, thereby reducing transmission of painful stimuli?
    a. C fibers
    b. A-beta
    c. Myelin
    d. A-delta

140. Pain originating from injury to the skin, muscles, joints, and deep tissues is termed:
    a. Somatic pain
    b. Visceral pain
    c. Deep pain
    d. Referred pain

141. Where do the peripheral nerve fibers A-delta and C fibers terminate?
    a. The brain
    b. The hypothalamus
    c. The skin
    d. The dorsal horn of the spinal cord

142. What type of nociceptors respond to the release of endogenous chemicals from damaged cells?
    a. Chemoreceptors
    b. Thermoreceptors
    c. Mechanoreceptors
    d. Beta receptors

143. Which of the following chemicals is *not* considered a major inflammatory mediator of pain?
    a. Histamine
    b. Substance P
    c. Bradykinin
    d. Estrogen

144. What type of nerve fiber is responsible for a diffuse, burning type of pain accompanying tissue damage and inflammation?
    a. A-beta fibers
    b. C fibers
    c. A-delta fibers
    d. Myelinated fibers

145. Which of the following answers represents the three zones of gray matter in the spinal cord?
    a. Dorsal horn, ventral horn, intermediate zone
    b. Dorsal horn, ventral horn, lateral horn
    c. Dorsal horn, intermediate zone, central zone
    d. Ventral horn, lateral horn, white matter

146. What area of the cerebrum is responsible for the higher processing and awareness of pain?
    a. Medulla oblongata
    b. Intermediate zone of the spinal cord
    c. Adrenal glands
    d. Somatosensory cortex

147. Pain arising from the skin and muscles is known as
    _____.
    a. Visceral pain
    b. Somatic pain
    c. Neuropathic pain
    d. Referred pain

148. What type of pain can develop from damage to the peripheral nervous system?
    a. Referred pain
    b. Central sensitization
    c. Visceral pain
    d. Neuropathic pain

149. What type of pain can be felt because of damage to internal organs?
    a. Visceral pain
    b. Neuropathic pain
    c. Referred pain
    d. Somatic pain

150. What type of nerve fibers are responsible for carrying pain signals from the internal organs?
    a. A-delta fibers
    b. C fibers
    c. A-beta fibers
    d. Myelinated fibers

151. What nerve fibers are responsible for conducting harmless signals that provide information such as touch, pressure, vibration, and movement?
    a. A-beta fibers
    b. C fibers
    c. A-delta fibers
    d. None of the above

152. Which of the following painful conditions is *not* an example of chronic pain?
    a. Osteoarthritis
    b. Chronic otitis externa
    c. Incisional pain following castration
    d. Prolonged cancer treatment

153. Which of the following time frames describes chronic pain?
    a. Pain that lasts only 24 hours
    b. Pain that lasts minutes to hours
    c. Pain that is prolonged (days, weeks, months)
    d. The sharp pain that accompanies IV catheter placement

154. What substance normally blocks the NMDA receptor so that it cannot allow ions to pass freely and generate an impulse?
    a. Sodium
    b. Magnesium
    c. Potassium
    d. Calcium

155. Which term describes the ability of neurons to change their structure and function in response to different environmental stimuli?
    a. Central sensitization
    b. Wind-up
    c. Peripheral sensitization
    d. Neuroplasticity

156. What is one strategy the veterinary clinic can use to help decrease a patient's likelihood of developing central sensitization and all of the negative aspects associated with it?
    a. Provide comfortable bedding
    b. Discontinue vaccines
    c. Start IV fluids
    d. Provide preemptive analgesia

157. The high threshold A-delta nerve fiber is covered in an electrically insulating substance called:
    a. Synapse
    b. Neurotransmitter
    c. Myelin
    d. Substance-P

158. What is the function of myelin?
    a. To act as an inflammatory neurotransmitter
    b. To suppress central sensitization
    c. To decrease the rate of nerve impulse transmission
    d. To increase the rate of nerve impulse transmission

159. The inflammatory mediator histamine originates where?
    a. Mast cells
    b. Damaged tissue
    c. C fibers
    d. A-delta fibers

160. An area innervated by a sensory nerve fiber is called what?
    a. Dermatome
    b. Receptive field
    c. C fibers
    d. A-delta fibers

161. What term describes the series of events that occur within the body after a drug has been administered to a patient?
    a. Pharmacodynamics
    b. Pharmacokinetics
    c. Bioavailability
    d. Efficacy

162. Which of the following terms describes the phenomenon of drug metabolism in which the concentration of a drug is greatly reduced before it reaches the systemic circulation?
    a. First-pass effect
    b. Pass-fail effect
    c. Pharmacokinetics
    d. Pharmacodynamics

163. Which of the following does *not* play a role in a drug's rate of absorption?
    a. Route of administration
    b. Solubility of the drug
    c. Temperature of the patient
    d. Brand of syringe used

164. How much of a drug that is absorbed and reaches systemic circulation is termed _____:
    a. Pharmacodynamics
    b. Pharmacokinetics
    c. Bioavailability
    d. Efficacy

165. Which of the following is a representation of how a drug can be *eliminated* from the body?
    a. Urine excretion
    b. Digestion
    c. Biotransformation
    d. Metabolization

166. In what organ are most drugs metabolized (biotransformed)?
    a. Skin
    b. Liver
    c. Eye
    d. Intestines

167. Which of the following words correctly identifies the tendency of a drug to combine with its intended receptor?
    a. Bioavailability
    b. Efficacy
    c. Affinity
    d. Adherence

168. A drug termed an *antagonist* has which characteristics?
    a. Affinity and efficacy are both present
    b. Affinity is present but poor efficacy
    c. No affinity and no efficacy present
    d. Affinity present but no efficacy

169. Which of the following is an example of an opioid agonist?
    a. Morphine
    b. Naloxone
    c. Butorphanol
    d. Nalbuphine

170. Which of the following opioids would be the best choice for moderate to severe pain?
    a. Butorphanol
    b. Propofol
    c. Hydromorphone
    d. Naloxone

171. Which of the following correctly lists the opioid receptor types?
    a. Kappa, beta, gamma
    b. Kappa, mu, gamma
    c. Kappa, mu, delta
    d. Delta, mu, gamma

172. Which of the following routes of administration is *not* commonly used for opioids in veterinary patients?
    a. Intravenous (IV)
    b. Intramuscular (IM)
    c. Subcutaneous (SQ)
    d. Oral administration (PO)

173. Opioids that are considered the most clinically useful analgesics act as agonists at which of the following receptors?
    a. Beta
    b. Mu
    c. Delta
    d. Kappa

174. Which of the following opioid analgesics is often used as a continuous rate infusion because of its short duration of action (approximately 30 minutes)?
    a. Morphine
    b. Ketamine
    c. Buprenorphine
    d. Fentanyl

175. Which of the following mu agonist opioids also has additional affinity for the NMDA receptor making it potentially useful for neuropathic pain?
    a. Morphine
    b. Methadone
    c. Ketamine
    d. Propofol

176. Which of the following opioids has been shown to cause hyperthermia in felines?
    a. Hydromorphone
    b. Butorphanol
    c. Morphine
    d. Methadone

177. Which of the following drugs is classified as an opioid?
    a. Amantadine
    b. Carprofen
    c. Ketamine
    d. Oxymorphone

178. Which of the following can be used to reverse all opioid agonist effects at all receptors?
    a. Butorphanol
    b. Naloxone hydrochloride
    c. Morphine
    d. Hydromorphone

179. Opioid agonist-antagonist drugs such as butorphanol and nalbuphine exert mild analgesic activity by stimulating which receptor?
    a. Mu
    b. Delta
    c. Kappa
    d. Somatic

180. How do nonsteroidal anti-inflammatory drugs exert their analgesic activity?
    a. Blocking sodium channels
    b. Slowing or stopping the conduction of nerve impulses
    c. Inhibition of the enzyme cyclooxygenase (COX)
    d. Nerve cell depolarization

181. Newer NSAIDs that are COX selective have fewer side effects because they only block which isoenzyme?
    a. COX-1
    b. COX-2
    c. Kappa receptors
    d. Arachidonic acid

182. Many NSAIDs have been used for their role in fever reduction. If a drug is shown to be effective in reducing fever, we say it has _____:
    a. Gastrointestinal effects
    b. Antipyretic effects
    c. Renal effects
    d. Cowbell effects

183. Which is *not* a technique the veterinary technician can use to prevent side effects of NSAID use?
    a. Refill the medication as soon as the owner requests
    b. Discuss adverse effects of the medication with the owner
    c. Create a client information sheet for owners that describes the possible side effects
    d. Call owner to follow up on efficacy of the drug and any side effects the pet may be experiencing

184. Side effects of NSAIDs most commonly affect what major organ system?
    a. The gastrointestinal tract
    b. The eye
    c. The dermis
    d. The urinary bladder

185. If a client calls to report that her dog has started vomiting while taking the NSAID carprofen, what is the best course of action?
    a. Tell the client to give hydrogen peroxide to stimulate more vomiting to ensure all of the carprofen is out of the dog's system
    b. Tell the client to give an antacid to help the pet feel better
    c. Do nothing but monitor for further GI problems such as diarrhea
    d. Tell the client to stop using the carprofen and have a veterinarian see the pet

186. What drug class should be avoided when a patient is on NSAIDs because of the likelihood of adverse GI effects occurring from concurrent administration?
    a. Opioids
    b. Corticosteroids
    c. Local anesthetics
    d. Topical flea and tick treatments

187. Which of the following drugs is classified as a nonsteroidal anti-inflammatory drug?
    a. Amantadine
    b. Carprofen
    c. Ketamine
    d. Oxymorphone

188. When a patient is switching from one NSAID to another, what is the best course of action?
    a. The patient should experience a "washout" period of 3–5 days to minimize the risk of concurrent side effects
    b. The patient should experience a "washout" period of 30 days to minimize the risk of concurrent side effects
    c. The patient should start both drugs concurrently to minimize the likelihood of breakthrough pain
    d. The patient should never switch NSAIDs

189. Using which of the following COX-3–inhibiting NSAIDs is contraindicated in cats?
    a. Meloxicam
    b. Carprofen
    c. Acetaminophen
    d. Robenacoxib

190. Which NSAID is labeled for use in horses and cattle, but has extra label uses in other species?
    a. Acetaminophen
    b. Flunixin meglumine
    c. Carprofen
    d. Meloxicam

191. Which of the following NSAIDs has been proven effective in felines as an analgesic on the lower urinary tract associated with cystitis and urethritis?
    a. Aspirin
    b. Acetaminophen
    c. Flunixin meglumine
    d. Piroxicam

192. How do local anesthetic drugs function?
    a. By reducing inflammation
    b. By blocking impulse conduction in nerve fibers
    c. By facilitating the breakdown of arachidonic acid
    d. By acting as an antipyretic

193. Local anesthetics that are applied *topically* provide desensitization and analgesia to which body system?
    a. The internal organs
    b. The skin and mucous membrane surfaces
    c. The muscles
    d. The brain and spinal cord

194. Which of the following drugs is *not* considered a local anesthetic?
    a. Bupivicaine
    b. Lidocaine
    c. Meperidine
    d. Mepivacaine

195. What determines the potency and speed of onset of local anesthetics?
    a. The volume of local anesthetic infused into an area
    b. The lipid solubility of the drug
    c. The temperature of the local anesthetic
    d. The brand of local anesthetic used

196. Which of the following can be an early sign of toxicity associated with local anesthetics in dogs and cats?
    a. Hematuria
    b. Diarrhea
    c. Vomiting
    d. Muscle twitching and convulsing

197. What nerve block is commonly used to desensitize nerves and add additional analgesia to an onychectomy procedure?
    a. Retrobulbar block
    b. Epidural
    c. Circumferential nerve block
    d. Sacrococcygeal block

198. Which of the following terms is used to describe the injection of a local anesthetic into the area around a peripheral nerve to block sensory and/or motor function?
    a. Spinal anesthesia
    b. Regional anesthesia
    c. Topical anesthesia
    d. Subcutaneous injection

199. Which of the following terms describes the technique when a local anesthetic is injected into the cerebrospinal fluid?
    a. Spinal anesthesia
    b. Regional anesthesia
    c. Topical anesthesia
    d. Epidural anesthesia

200. In what types of procedures would a wound diffusion catheter with local anesthetic be useful?
    a. Limb amputations
    b. Radical mastectomies
    c. Tooth extractions
    d. Both a and b

201. To prolong the duration of action because of vasoconstriction, lidocaine is often available in combination with what other drug?
    a. Bupivicaine
    b. Epinephrine
    c. Atropine
    d. Dexmedetomidine

202. For what is EMLA cream most commonly used in veterinary medicine?
    a. As a topical anesthetic to facilitate IV catheter placement
    b. To desensitize the eye before ocular surgery
    c. To desensitize the trachea before intubation
    d. None of the above

203. Which type of nerve block is useful to provide analgesia before or after surgery of the thoracic cavity?
    a. Infraorbital nerve blocks
    b. Retrobulbar nerve blocks
    c. Intercostal nerve blocks
    d. Mental nerve blocks

204. Which of the following is *not* a property associated with the local anesthetic mepivacaine?
    a. Approved for use in dogs and horses
    b. Moderate duration of action
    c. Metabolized by the lungs
    d. Does not sting on injection

205. Which of the following drugs is *not* considered an alpha-2 agonist?
    a. Dexmedetomidine
    b. Medetomidine
    c. Xylazine
    d. Acepromazine

206. What is the name of the drug used to reverse the alpha-2 agonist dexmedetomidine?
    a. Medetomidine
    b. Levomedetomidine
    c. Xylazine
    d. Atipamezole

207. Which of the following is *not* a characteristic of alpha-2 agonists?
    a. Sedation
    b. Increased heart rate
    c. Analgesia
    d. Muscle relaxation

208. Patients given alpha-2 agonists often have pale mucous membranes and cold extremities in the initial phase because of what side effect of the drug?
    a. Peripheral vasoconstriction
    b. Hypothermia
    c. Hypoglycemia
    d. Decreased hepatic blood flow

209. In contrast to alpha-2 receptors, alpha-1 receptors produce which of the following physiological effects?
    a. Sedation and muscle relaxation
    b. Arousal and excitement
    c. Analgesic and antianxiety effects
    d. None of the above

210. Of the veterinary approved alpha-2 agonists, which one produces the most side effects because of its affinity for the alpha-1 receptor as well as the alpha-2 receptor?
    a. Xylazine
    b. Medetomidine
    c. Dexmedetomidine
    d. Atipamezole

211. Which of the following is *not* a route of administration commonly used for alpha-2 agonists?
    a. Transmucosal
    b. Subcutaneous
    c. Transdermal
    d. Intramuscular

212. What arrhythmias can be seen after administration of an alpha-2 agonist?
    a. Ventricular bradycardia
    b. Sinus bradycardia
    c. First- and second-degree AV block
    d. All of the above

213. What side effect of alpha-2 agonists would warrant their cautious use in diabetic patients?
    a. Hyperglycemia
    b. Initial vasoconstriction
    c. Bradycardia
    d. Decreased hepatic blood flow

214. Which drug is commonly used to reverse the effects of the alpha-2 agonist xylazine?
    a. Dexmedetomidine
    b. Levomedetomidine
    c. Yohimbine
    d. Detomidine

215. Which of the following does not function as an NMDA receptor antagonist?
    a. Ketamine
    b. Methadone
    c. Hydromorphone
    d. Amantadine

216. Which of the following is *not* an example of how *ketamine* can be administered as part of a multimodal pain therapy plan?
    a. As a continuous infusion during general anesthesia
    b. As an epidural injection
    c. When mixed with an opioid in the premedication
    d. By mouth in pill form after surgery

217. Ketamine administration would be contraindicated in which of the following disease processes?
    a. Hypertrophic cardiomyopathy
    b. Congestive heart failure
    c. Unstable shock patients
    d. All of the above

218. Which of the following drugs is an antiviral agent in human patients but was recently shown to function as an NMDA receptor antagonist similar to ketamine?
    a. Hydromorphone
    b. Methadone
    c. Amantadine
    d. Oxymorphone

219. Which of the following drugs classes has been shown to be the most efficacious in the management of neuropathic pain?
    a. Opioids
    b. NMDA receptor antagonists
    c. Nonsteroidal anti-inflammatory drugs
    d. Antibiotics

220. Serotonin syndrome can occur after patients are administered tramadol concurrently with what drug class?
    a. Antibiotics
    b. Antidepressants (SSRIs)
    c. Opioids
    d. Anticholinergics

221. Gabapentin is used to help alleviate the symptoms of neuropathic pain. Which of the following characteristics best describes the sensation associated with neuropathic pain?
    a. Burning or lancing pain
    b. Dull pain
    c. Aching pain
    d. Visceral pain

222. Gabapentin has proven useful for patients experiencing osteoarthritis pain, especially when used in combination with what other drug class?
    a. NSAIDs
    b. Anticholinergics
    c. Antibiotics
    d. Inhalant anesthetics

223. Cats with chronic cystitis are often in pain. Which of the following drugs has been shown to provide relief of pain associated with chronic cystitis?
    a. Amoxicillin
    b. Enrofloxacin
    c. Cefazolin
    d. Amitriptyline

224. Which drug is often administered to cats before undergoing limb amputation or declaw surgery to help prevent neuropathic pain and to lessen the chance of chronic pain developing?
    a. Glucose
    b. Gabapentin
    c. Cefazolin
    d. Carprofen

225. Tricyclic antidepressants are contraindicated in which of the following patients?
    a. Senior patients
    b. Osteoarthritis patients
    c. Diabetic patients
    d. Seizure patients

226. Which of the following drugs has been useful in not only reducing opioid-related nausea and vomiting, but also in reducing the MAC of anesthetic gases needed when given preoperatively?
    a. Maropitant
    b. Carprofen
    c. Morphine
    d. Hydromorphone

227. What is another term for an analgesic plan that involves combining different drug classes acting on different pain pathways?
    a. Multimodal analgesia
    b. Constant rate infusion
    c. Soaker catheter
    d. Take-home medications

228. Morphine has a strong tendency to cause physical dependency or addiction in humans. What is the classification of morphine in the United States and Canada?
    a. Schedule I
    b. Schedule II
    c. Schedule III
    d. Not a scheduled drug

229. Which of the following opioids is least likely to cause vomiting in cats?
    a. Morphine
    b. Methadone
    c. Oxymorphone
    d. Hydromorphone

230. Which of the following opioid drugs is commonly administered via a transdermal patch?
    a. Carprofen
    b. Lidocaine
    c. Morphine
    d. Fentanyl

231. What is a common problem with Fentanyl patches if they become overheated?
    a. They become ineffective
    b. They release excessive amounts of fentanyl
    c. They cause excessive sedation
    d. Both b and c

232. Which of the following opioids is most commonly used for epidural analgesia?
    a. Morphine
    b. Buprenorphine
    c. Bupivicaine
    d. Lidocaine

233. Which of the following take-home medications should be reserved for canine patients only?
    a. Acepromazine
    b. Tramadol
    c. Tylenol with codeine
    d. Fentanyl patch

234. What term describes the administration of anesthetic and analgesic agents and adjuncts to calm and prepare the patient for anesthetic induction?
    a. Maintenance
    b. Recovery
    c. Premedication
    d. Induction

235. Which of the following methods is considered the least suitable choice for anesthetic induction in the canine and feline patient?
    a. IV injection of propofol
    b. IV injection of ketamine/diazepam mixture
    c. IM injection of alfaxalone
    d. Chamber induction with isoflurane

236. What term describes the type of pain that will be experienced from any surgery of the reproductive tract that involves manipulations of organs such as the uterus and ovaries?
    a. Somatic pain
    b. Visceral pain
    c. Preemptive pain
    d. Wind-up pain

237. What would be the most appropriate choice of opioid for preemptive analgesia for a patient undergoing surgery for OVH as a treatment for pyometra?
    a. Hydromorphone
    b. Butorphanol
    c. Buprenorphine
    d. Midazolam

238. Which of the following local blocks is considered a part of a multimodal analgesic plan for a castration?
    a. Ovarian ligament blocks
    b. Intratesticular blocks
    c. Infraorbital nerve block
    d. Maxillary nerve blocks

239. If your patient begins responding to surgical stimulation under anesthesia, what should the technician's next step optimally be?
    a. Turn down the % inhalant anesthetic
    b. Turn up the % of inhalant anesthetic
    c. Administer IV analgesics
    d. None of the above

240. If your patient begins responding to surgical stimulation under anesthesia, and you choose to turn up the inhalant %, what next step also needs to be done to ensure your patient receives the % dialed on the vaporizer in a timely manner?
    a. Increase your fresh gas flow rate
    b. Decrease your fresh gas flow rate
    c. Start a constant rate infusion
    d. Perform local blocks

241. Which of the following surgeries would likely involve using a neuromuscular blocking agent?
    a. Ovariohysterectomy
    b. Castration
    c. Cataract removal surgery
    d. Digit amputation

242. What is the standard dose of lidocaine that should be administered as a "loading" dose before starting a lidocaine CRI?
    a. 1 mg/kg IV
    b. 2 mg/kg IV
    c. 0.2 mg/kg IV
    d. No loading dose is needed

243. What analgesic tool can be used to provide ≤72 hours of continuous analgesia for large incisions such as radical mastectomies?
    a. Wound diffusion catheter
    b. Infraorbital nerve block
    c. Intra-articular nerve block
    d. Intercostal nerve block

244. In patients presenting with fractured ribs, what is the benefit to treating pain in advance of thoracotomy?
    a. Improved ventilation
    b. Decreased anxiety
    c. More consistent breathing pattern
    d. All of the above

245. What is the name of the regional anesthesia technique preferred for analgesia in thoracotomy patients?
    a. Intercostal nerve block
    b. Infraorbital nerve block
    c. Maxillary nerve block
    d. Intratesticular block

246. Which of the following is a risk associated with improperly placed retrobulbar nerve blocks?
    a. Hemorrhage
    b. Perforation of the globe
    c. Damage to the optic nerve
    d. All of the above are risks

247. Which of the following drugs is commonly used in the postoperative period for its combined effects of analgesia and sedation?
    a. Dexmedetomidine
    b. Propofol
    c. Diazepam
    d. Midazolam

248. Which of the following is an example of analgesic therapies used in the postoperative period?
    a. Low-level laser therapy
    b. Hydrotherapy
    c. Massage therapy
    d. All of the above

249. Which of the following opioids is the best choice of analgesic for an ER patient for whom vomiting and/or abdominal contractions are contraindicated?
    a. Methadone
    b. Midazolam
    c. Morphine
    d. Hydromorphone

250. Which of the following opioids would be the *best* choice for ER patients who have experienced some sort or head trauma and may need serial neurological exams?
    a. Morphine
    b. Methadone
    c. Fentanyl
    d. Remifentanil

251. Epidurals are contraindicated in which of the following patients?
    a. Patients with hind-limb trauma
    b. Patients undergoing surgery of the urogenital tract
    c. Diabetic patients
    d. Patients with a coagulation disorder such as von Willebrand's

252. For patients that have to be hospitalized long term, what is meant by keeping them in a "physiologic position"?
    a. Left lateral recumbency
    b. Right lateral recumbency
    c. Sternal recumbency with head elevated
    d. Standing

253. Chronic pain is often divided into what two categories?
    a. Nociceptive pain and neuropathic pain
    b. Somatic and visceral pain
    c. Deep pain and superficial pain
    d. Acute pain and chronic pain

254. Which drug class acts by preventing the loss of bone mass by blocking osteoclasts and helping to manage osteosarcoma pain?
    a. Opioids
    b. Bisphosphonates
    c. Gabapentinoids
    d. Neurokinin-1 inhibitors

255. Which of the following analgesic adjuncts is commonly applied topically?
    a. Gabapentin
    b. Amantadine
    c. Capsaicin
    d. Bisphosphonates

256. Which of the following demonstrates a nonpharmacological modality to treat dogs with chronic osteoarthritis?
    a. Weight loss
    b. Extra padding in sleeping areas
    c. Regular low-impact exercise
    d. All of the above

257. Which of the following neurotransmitters plays a role in the process of pain perception as well as in the vomiting reflex?
    a. Substance P
    b. TrpV1
    c. Epinephrine
    d. Norepinephrine

258. Which of the following analgesic adjuncts works to block NK-1 receptors and subsequent activation of substance P?
    a. Gabapentin
    b. Amantadine
    c. Maropitant
    d. Bisphosphonates

259. Of the inhalant anesthetics, which is the only one thought to have analgesic properties?
    a. Nitrous oxide
    b. Isoflurane
    c. Sevoflurane
    d. None of the above

260. Corticosteroids act as powerful agents in chronic pain management when used for their _____ effects.
    a. Opioid
    b. Anti-inflammatory
    c. Anti-nausea
    d. NMDA receptor antagonism

ⓔ *Answers and rationales available on Evolve http://evolve.elsevier.com/Prendergast/QAvettech/*

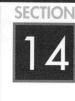
QUESTIONS

1. Which of the following may help decrease dental abrasions in the pet ferret?
   a. Housing the ferret in a wire cage
   b. Offering a raw diet consisting of bones, chicken, and green vegetables
   c. Offering a natural-prey diet or moistening dry kibble
   d. Annual periodontal treatments

2. Which of the following diagnostic tools is *best* used to evaluate real-time GI motility in the ferret?
   a. Magnetic resonance imaging
   b. Computed tomography
   c. Radiography
   d. Fluoroscopy

3. Which of the following are common presenting signs in a ferret with ibuprofen toxicity?
   a. Arrhythmias and vomiting
   b. Generalized neurologic signs
   c. Heart failure
   d. Excessive drooling and tachycardia

4. Which of the listed diseases best fits the statement that follows?
   It is most commonly transmitted by aerosol exposure, but it can also be spread by direct contact with conjunctival and nasal exudates, urine, feces, skin, and sometimes fomites. The incubation period is generally 7 to 10 days in the ferret. The disease spreads by viremia after it is in the body, and it is almost always fatal.
   a. Canine distemper virus
   b. Influenza B
   c. *Pneumocystis carinii*
   d. Cryptococcosis

5. In ferrets, the heart is best auscultated between which of the following ribs?
   a. 5th and 7th
   b. 6th and 8th
   c. 2nd and 4th
   d. 1st and 3rd

6. Ferrets with vestibular signs demonstrate all of the following *except*:
   a. Ataxia
   b. Circling
   c. Left- or right-sided head tilt
   d. Head pressing

7. Which of the following areas contains more than half of all lymphoid tissue in the rabbit?
   a. Nervous system
   b. GI tract
   c. Urinary tract
   d. Heart and lungs

8. Which of the following is a microsporidium obligate intracellular protozoan parasite that causes neurologic disease in rabbits?
   a. *Encephalitozoon cuniculi*
   b. *Baylisascaris procyonis*
   c. *Toxoplasma gondii*
   d. *Pasteurella multocida*

9. Which of the following tools is the most useful option to help diagnose syncope in a rabbit?
   a. Thoracic radiographs
   b. Echocardiogram
   c. Computed tomography of the thorax
   d. Electrocardiogram

10. A lactating doe presents to the clinic for anorexia, depression, lethargy, and fever. What is the most likely the cause of her symptoms?
    a. Septic mastitis
    b. Nonseptic cystic mastitis
    c. GI stasis
    d. Cellulitis

11. Which of the following methods definitively diagnoses *Treponema paraluiscuniculi*?
    a. Complete blood count
    b. Skin biopsy with silver staining
    c. ELISA testing
    d. PCR testing

12. A rabbit presents with a 2-day history of anorexia. You take radiographs and notice an ingesta-filled stomach with large amounts of gas in the intestines and cecum. This is suggestive of what condition in the rabbit?
    a. Acute GI dilation
    b. GI foreign-body obstruction
    c. GI stasis
    d. GI neoplasia

13. Which of the following can be used specifically to diagnose porphyrins in the rabbit's urine?
    a. Wood's lamp
    b. Urine dipstick
    c. Microscopic examination
    d. Urine sedimentation examination

14. In the rabbit, pregnancy toxemia is most likely to occur during which week(s) of gestation?
    a. During the first 2 weeks
    b. During the last week
    c. During the 6th week
    d. During the 5th week

15. Which of the following bacteria are most often associated with antibiotic-associated enterotoxemia in the guinea pig?
    a. *Escherichia coli*
    b. *Pseudomonas aeruginosa*
    c. *Clostridium difficile*
    d. *Salmonella typhimurium*

16. Poor husbandry conditions, along with a humid environment, predispose guinea pigs to which of the following conditions?
    a. *Demodex caviae*
    b. *Trixacarus caviae*
    c. *Gyropus ovalis*
    d. *Bordetella bronchiseptica*

17. A 5-year-old intact male chinchilla presents with a 1-week history of excessive grooming, straining to urinate, repeatedly cleaning the penis, and production of several small spots of urine in the litter box. What is the most likely cause of these signs?
    a. Acute renal failure
    b. Urinary calculi
    c. Penile fur ring
    d. Urinary tract infection

18. What is the most common cause of alopecia and dermatitis in the pet mouse?
    a. Fur mites
    b. Dermatophytes
    c. Contact dermatitis caused by pine shavings
    d. Endoparasites

19. Which of the following factors does *not* contribute to cannibalism of the young by female hamsters?
    a. Lean diet
    b. Increased ambient temperature
    c. Low body weight
    d. Handling the mother and/or the young

20. Hypocalcemia in the sugar glider is primarily caused by an imbalance in which of the following?
    a. Blood calcium, vitamin A, and phosphorus
    b. Dietary calcium, vitamin B, and phosphorus
    c. Blood calcium, vitamin C, and phosphorus
    d. Dietary calcium, vitamin D, and phosphorus

21. An intact male African hedgehog of unknown age presents to the clinic with a 3-day history of lethargy, inappetence, icterus, and diarrhea. Which of the following diseases is most likely to cause these symptoms?
    a. Acute renal failure
    b. Hepatic lipidosis
    c. Bacterial pneumonia
    d. Glomerulosclerosis

22. Which of the following vessels is primarily used for blood collection in the African hedgehog?
    a. Lateral saphenous
    b. Cephalic
    c. Femoral
    d. Jugular

23. An Amazon parrot presents to the hospital with the following clinical signs: blunted choanal papillae, plantar erosions on the planter surfaces of the feet, poor-quality feathering, and poor skin. Diet consists of seeds only. Which of the following diseases is most likely to cause these signs?
    a. Hypovitaminosis C
    b. Hypovitaminosis A
    c. Hypocalcemia
    d. Candidiasis

24. Which of the following values is used to evaluate renal function in the avian patient?
    a. Uric acid
    b. BUN
    c. Creatinine
    d. BUN, creatinine, and uric acid

25. For proper metabolization, ultraviolet lighting is necessary for which of the following?
    a. Vitamin D_3
    b. Magnesium
    c. Calcium and vitamin D_3
    d. Magnesium and calcium

26. Which of the following is not present in the reptilian urinary system?
    a. Loop of Henle
    b. Nephrons
    c. Glomerulus
    d. Ureters

27. Many species of lizards can "drop" or detach their tails if they are grabbed or restrained too tightly. This natural predatory response is referred to as:
    a. Autolysis
    b. Autotomy
    c. Amputation
    d. Dysecdysis

28. Which of the following is most commonly used to obtain a heart rate in a reptilian patient?
    a. Ultrasound
    b. Doppler
    c. Stethoscope
    d. Palpation of pulse

29. Which of the following vessels is most commonly used for blood collection in the lizard?
    a. Cephalic vein
    b. Jugular vein
    c. Ventral abdominal vein
    d. Caudal tail vein

30. Total blood volume in the reptilian patient is approximately what percentage of the body weight?
    a. 5%–8%
    b. 4%–6%
    c. 8%–10%
    d. 10%–12%

31. Total blood volume in the avian patient is approximately what percentage of the body weight?
    a. 5%
    b. 7%
    c. 10%
    d. 12%

32. A snake presents to the clinic for anorexia, striking at the owner, hissing, and a blue-opaque coloring to the eyes and skin. What is likely occurring in this snake?
    a. Contact dermatitis
    b. Fungal dermatoses
    c. Paramyxovirus
    d. It is about to shed its skin

33. Oral examinations are most commonly performed in snakes using which of the following?
    a. Plastic spatula
    b. Gauze strips
    c. Tape strips
    d. Metal specula

34. Which of the following sites are commonly used for venipuncture in the snake?
    a. Heart and ventral abdominal vein
    b. Heart and caudal tail vein
    c. Heart only
    d. Caudal tail vein and ventral abdominal vein

35. The bones of the tortoise shell are covered with structures called scutes. What are scutes made of?
    a. Bone
    b. Epidermis
    c. Dermis
    d. Keratin

36. Which of the following species does not have a diaphragm?
    a. African hedgehog
    b. Sugar glider
    c. Box turtle
    d. Golden hamster

37. Sexing a tortoise is generally easy. The plastron in the male tortoise is usually:
    a. Convex
    b. Concave
    c. Wider and thicker compared to the female
    d. Narrower compared to the female

38. Which of the following is a condition in which uric acid is deposited into the joints and visceral organs and is caused by dehydration, kidney disease, and a high-protein diet?
    a. Hypovitaminosis A
    b. Metabolic bone disease
    c. Gout
    d. Hypocalcemia

39. A female tortoise presents to the clinic with the following clinical signs: straining, lethargy, anorexia, and bloody discharge from the cloaca. What is the most common cause of this presentation?
    a. GI foreign body
    b. Internal parasites
    c. Hypervitaminosis A
    d. Dystocia

40. A complete radiographic series in the turtle and tortoise include which of the following views?
    a. Dorsoventral and lateral
    b. Ventrodorsal and lateral
    c. Anterior-posterior, dorsoventral, and lateral
    d. Anterior-posterior, ventrodorsal, and lateral

41. The normal feces of a parrot contain which of the following?
    a. Primarily Gram-positive organisms
    b. Primarily Gram-negative organisms
    c. An equal mixture of Gram-positive and Gram-negative organisms
    d. The feces are mostly sterile and do not contain bacteria

42. You have been asked to obtain a blood sample for a CBC and chemistry panel from a 100-g cockatiel. Which of the following vessels is most commonly used in this species?
    a. Medial metatarsal vein
    b. Cutaneous ulnar vein
    c. Cephalic vein
    d. Jugular vein

43. A healthy bird can only lose ≤10% of its blood volume safely. You have been asked to draw a blood sample from a 1-kg macaw. What is the maximum amount of blood that can be taken from this patient safely?
    a. 1 mL
    b. 10 mL
    c. 15 mL
    d. 5 mL

44. In the avian patient, into which of the following muscles are intramuscular injections generally administered?
    a. Pectoral
    b. Epaxial
    c. Biceps
    d. Quadriceps

45. A figure-8 bandage is used for immobilization of which of the following bones?
    a. Femur, tibiotarsus, and tarsometatarsus
    b. Femur and tibiotarsus
    c. Ulna, radius, and metacarpals
    d. Humerus, radius, and ulna

46. Which of the following vessels is most commonly used for blood collection in the chinchilla?
    a. Cephalic
    b. Lateral saphenous
    c. Auricular
    d. Jugular

47. Which of the following vessels is most commonly used for intravenous catheterization in a larger lizard such as an iguana?
    a. Femoral
    b. Cephalic
    c. Caudal tail vein
    d. Jugular

48. An iguana presents to the clinic with the following clinical signs: seizures, tremors, anorexia, kyphosis, pliable long bones, and a chronic femoral fracture. The patient has been housed without the proper UV lighting and has been given a diet of dog food, iceberg lettuce, and tofu. From which of the following diseases is this patient likely suffering?
    a. Gout
    b. Metabolic bone disease
    c. Hypercalcemia
    d. Hypervitaminosis A

49. A snake presents to the clinic 12 hours after suspected foreign-body ingestion. Which of the following diagnostics should be performed first?
    a. Computed tomography
    b. Complete blood count
    c. Chemistry panel
    d. Whole-body radiographs

50. Atropine is not suggested for use in which of the following species?
    a. Birds
    b. Snakes
    c. Rabbits
    d. Lizards

51. The hydration status in the avian patient is best evaluated by assessing which of the following?
    a. Capillary refill time
    b. Venous refill time
    c. Mucous membranes for tacky saliva
    d. Quality of the feathers

52. Which of the following bones is pneumatic in the avian patient?
    a. Ulna
    b. Radius
    c. Tibiotarsus
    d. Femur

53. What percentage of body weight can be tube fed at any given time to a bird?
    a. 2%
    b. 5%
    c. 10%
    d. 12%

54. Which of the following are daily maintenance fluid amounts for the avian patient?
    a. 50–60 mL/kg/day
    b. 10–20 mL/kg/day
    c. 75–100 mL/kg/day
    d. 100–150 mg/kg/day

55. Which of the following two metals most commonly cause heavy metal toxicity after ingestion by birds?
    a. Lead and gold
    b. Zinc and copper
    c. Lead and zinc
    d. Cast iron and copper

56. A bird presents to the clinic after chewing on a galvanized wire cage for the previous several days. Clinical signs include weight loss, polyuria, polydipsia, anemia, weakness, and seizures. What are these signs and history indicative of?
    a. Lead toxicity
    b. Zinc toxicity
    c. Iron toxicity
    d. Copper toxicity

57. The pupil in birds and reptiles is made up of which type of muscle?
    a. Smooth muscle
    b. Cardiac muscle
    c. Striated skeletal muscle
    d. A mix of smooth and skeletal muscle

58. The most common cause for penile prolapse in the chinchilla is:
    a. Malnutrition
    b. Fur ring formation
    c. Improper breeding with female
    d. Bacterial infection

59. A hamster presents to the clinic with the following symptoms: diarrhea, matting around the tail, lethargy, and a hunched abdomen. Which of the following diseases is most likely the causative agent?
    a. GI stasis
    b. Cystic calculi
    c. Wet tail
    d. Dental disease

60. Which of the following drugs would likely be contraindicated for use in a rabbit that presented for GI stasis and moderate-to-severe dental pain?
    a. Buprenorphine
    b. Fentanyl
    c. Butorphanol
    d. Oxymorphone

61. An owner calls the clinic regarding her sick guinea pig. She tells you that her pet has not eaten in 16 hours and has been "picky" with her food during the previous few weeks. She has noticed drooling, overgrooming, and small-sized feces. It sounds as if the veterinarian should examine the guinea pig. Although a diagnosis can't be made on the phone, what is the most likely cause of the animal's signs?
    a. Cystic ovaries
    b. Dental disease
    c. *Pasteurella multocida*
    d. Trichobezoar

62. The most common neoplasia in the unspayed female rabbit is:
    a. Uterine adenocarcinoma
    b. Mast cell tumors
    c. Squamous cell carcinoma
    d. Osteosarcoma

63. Which of the following diseases causes upper respiratory tract signs including sinusitis, rhinitis, excessive tearing, snorting, sniffling, and nasal exudate?
    a. *Pasteurella multocida*
    b. Bacterial enteritis
    c. Allergic dermatitis
    d. Pneumonia

64. You have been asked to obtain 10 mL of blood from one ferret for blood donation to another ferret. Which of the following vessels is most likely the best choice for venipuncture?
    a. Cephalic
    b. Lateral saphenous
    c. Auricular
    d. Cranial vena cava

65. In the avian patient, what is the choana?
    a. Part of the urinary system where the ureter connects to the kidney
    b. Opening at the roof of the mouth that connects the trachea to sinuses and the nares
    c. The common holding area for urine, urates, and feces before being excreted from the body
    d. Small metacarpal bone in the distal wing

66. Which of the following bones are considered pneumatic in most avian species?
    a. Humerus and ulna
    b. Femur and tibiotarsus
    c. Tibiotarsus and tarsometatarsus
    d. Humerus and femur

67. Which of the following in *not* considered a potential complication of intraosseous catheterization?
    a. Difficulty maintaining patency
    b. Bone infection
    c. Pain
    d. Hematoma formation

68. Which of the following is the most common and largest space used for subcutaneous fluid administration in the avian patient?
    a. Wing web
    b. Between the shoulder blades
    c. Inguinal area
    d. Over the back, behind the pelvis

69. Moldy peanuts are a common cause of which of the following in the avian patient?
    a. Myotoxicity
    b. *Salmonella*
    c. *Escherichia coli*
    d. *Clostridium difficile*

70. In the bird, air sac cannulas are placed into which of the following?
    a. Cervicocephalic air sac
    b. Clavicular air sac
    c. Caudal thoracic and abdominal air sacs
    d. Cranial thoracic air sac

71. Alopecia at the tail tip, symmetrical alopecia along the trunk of the body, intense pruritus, and enlarged vulva are symptoms in the ferret that indicate what disease?
    a. Green slime disease
    b. Insulinoma
    c. External parasites
    d. Adrenal disease

72. A ferret presents to the emergency clinic for anorexia, vomiting, lethargy, diarrhea, and generalized weakness. The owner stated that these symptoms started 36 hours earlier. A GI foreign body is suspected. Which of the following diagnostics would be used to determine whether a foreign body is present?
    a. Magnetic resonance imaging
    b. Chemistry panel
    c. Radiography
    d. Complete blood count

73. Which of the following is a common cause of upper respiratory disease in the prairie dog?
    a. Odontoma
    b. Mast cell tumor
    c. Adenocarcinoma
    d. Spindle cell sarcoma

74. Which of the following vessels is most commonly used for collection of a complete blood count and chemistry panel in the prairie dog?
    a. Cephalic vein
    b. Lateral saphenous vein
    c. Jugular vein
    d. Caudal tail vein

75. Which of the following vessels are most commonly used for collection of a complete blood count (CBC) and chemistry panel in the sugar glider?
    a. Jugular vein, cranial vena cava, medial tibial artery
    b. Lateral saphenous vein, femoral vein, medial tibial artery
    c. Cranial vena cava, cephalic vein, and lateral saphenous vein
    d. Jugular vein, femoral vein, lateral tail veins

76. Which of the following diseases causes an acute onset of hind limb paresis or paralysis in the captive sugar glider?
    a. Lymphoid neoplasia
    b. Cardiomyopathy
    c. Nutritional osteodystrophy
    d. Obesity

77. Which of the following species is considered arboreal?
    a. Chinchilla
    b. Prairie dog
    c. Guinea pig
    d. Sugar glider

78. Which of the following mammals has a cloaca where the gastrointestinal, urinary, and reproductive tract empty?
    a. Chinchilla
    b. Prairie dog
    c. Guinea pig
    d. Sugar glider

79. The captive diet of sugar gliders includes all of the following *except*:
    a. Chicken
    b. Insects
    c. Fruits
    d. Nectar

80. Pet skunks should be vaccinated against all of the following diseases *except*:
    a. Rabies
    b. Feline panleukopenia
    c. Canine distemper
    d. Canine parvovirus

81. A captive obese pet skunk presents with the following clinical signs: exercise intolerance, weight loss, lethargy, dyspnea, anorexia, coughing, ascites, pale mucous membranes, and cold extremities. What disease process is likely occurring?
    a. Hepatic lipidosis
    b. Dental disease
    c. Cardiomyopathy
    d. Canine distemper virus

82. Hedgehogs are which of the following, requiring a high-protein diet?
    a. Insectivores
    b. Strict carnivores
    c. Herbivores
    d. Nectarivores

83. A hospitalized hedgehog is offered part of a hardboiled egg as a treat. He suddenly becomes stiff and contorted, starts making licking motions with his tongue, and starts heavily salivating. What is occurring?
    a. A seizure
    b. Self-anointing behavior
    c. Anxiety toward caretaker
    d. Wobbling hedgehog syndrome

84. You have been asked to obtain a complete blood count and chemistry panel for a pet hedgehog. What vessels are most commonly used?
    a. Lateral saphenous and jugular
    b. Cephalic and cranial vena cava
    c. Femoral and medial saphenous
    d. Jugular and cranial vena cava

85. Which of the following diseases in the hedgehog is characterized by progressive ataxia, weight loss, paralysis, and eventual death?
    a. Wobbling hedgehog syndrome
    b. Tubulointerstitial nephritis
    c. Hepatic adenocarcinoma
    d. Plasmacytoma

86. Which of the following is the causative agent of Tyzzer's disease?
    a. *Clostridium piliforme*
    b. *Escherichia coli*
    c. *Lawsonia intracellularis*
    d. *Francisella tularensis*

87. Which statement about tularemia in rabbits is true?
    a. Wild rabbits are highly susceptible
    b. Wild rabbits are the cause of most epizootic infections
    c. *Francisella tularensis* is the etiologic agent
    d. All of the above

88. Which is the correct order in the avian gastrointestinal tract descending from the oral cavity?
    a. Crop, gizzard, proventriculus
    b. Proventriculus, gizzard, crop
    c. Gizzard, proventriculus, crop
    d. Crop, proventriculus, gizzard

89. The feathered tracts in birds from which feathers originate are called:
    a. Barbules
    b. Rectrices
    c. Pterylae
    d. Remiges

90. The pectoral muscles in a bird attach to which of the following anatomical structures?
    a. Keel
    b. Pygostyle
    c. Notarium
    d. Synsacrum

91. What is the function of the operculum found in some psittacines?
    a. To prevent the inhalation of foreign bodies
    b. To humidify the air
    c. To absorb saline from the nostrils
    d. To connect the sinuses to the choanal slit

92. Which of the following is responsible for sound generation in the bird?
    a. Infraorbital sinus
    b. Glottis
    c. Syrinx
    d. Larynx

93. Which of the following species lacks an epiglottis?
    a. Amazon parrot
    b. German shepherd
    c. Persian cat
    d. New Zealand white rabbit

94. Which of the following in birds is the final holding area for urine, urates, feces, and eggs before excretion from the body?
    a. Choana
    b. Cloaca
    c. Cecum
    d. Vent

95. Because of a lack of diaphragm in the avian patient, which of the following organs surrounds the apex of the heart?
    a. Pancreas
    b. Cecum
    c. Liver
    d. Kidneys

96. Bird diets that include only seeds are often deficient in which of the following?
    a. Vitamin C
    b. Vitamin D
    c. Vitamin B
    d. Vitamin A

97. Clinical signs in a bird that include loose green feces, green urates, lethargy, inappetence, ascites, abnormal beak and nails, and poor feather quality are often indicative of:
    a. Renal failure
    b. Hepatic disease
    c. Fungal overgrowth
    d. Cardiac disease

98. Most gas exchange in fish takes place in which of the following?
    a. Operculum
    b. Lungs
    c. Bronchi
    d. Gills

99. How many chambers does the fish heart contain?
    a. 4
    b. 2
    c. 3
    d. 5

100. Why is it important to maintain a reptile within its preferred optimal temperature zone (POTZ)?
    a. The POTZ enables animals to metabolize drugs
    b. The POTZ enables animals to digest food properly
    c. The POTZ enables animals to heal after an injury or surgery
    d. All of the above

101. The term *gravid* is used for reptiles that are:
    a. Oviparous
    b. Viviparous
    c. Ovoviviparous
    d. Sterile

102. In the skin of chameleons, which of the following allows for reflectivity of visible light that results in a color change?
    a. Melanocytes
    b. Heterophils
    c. Azurophils
    d. Chromatophores

103. Iguanas have teeth that are replaced many times throughout life. The teeth do not have roots but are attached to the jaw. This type of dentition is called:
    a. Hypsodont
    b. Elodont
    c. Pleurodont
    d. Monophyodont

104. Large femoral pores in the iguana are indicative of:
    a. Male lizard
    b. Systemic infection
    c. Juvenile lizard
    d. Breeding female

105. The reproductive organ in the male lizard consists of:
    a. Single phallus
    b. Paired hemipenes
    c. External testicles
    d. Bilobed phallus

106. Which of the following anatomical structures is located on the dorsal portion of the head and acts as a photoreceptor, helping to regulate hormone production and thermoregulatory behavior in the lizard species?
    a. Thyroid gland
    b. Jacobson's organ
    c. Spectacle
    d. Parietal eye

107. Which of the following species is arboreal?
    a. Leopard gecko
    b. Jackson's chameleon
    c. Bearded dragon
    d. Savannah monitor

108. Which of the following statements is true regarding carnivorous lizards?
    a. They do not require calcium as part of their diets
    b. They do not require vitamin A in their diets
    c. They do not require UV-B lighting
    d. They require live prey

109. Why is UV-B lighting so important for herbivorous, insectivorous, and omnivorous lizards?
    a. UV-B lighting helps to keep these patients warm
    b. UV-B lighting helps with absorption of phosphorus and conversion of vitamin A
    c. UV-B lighting is required for absorption of vitamin C and normal behavior
    d. UV-B lighting is required for absorption of calcium and Vitamin D_3 synthesis

110. Heating a reptile cage safely can be accomplished by all of the following *except*:
    a. Heat rock
    b. Heater under tank
    c. Ceramic radiant heating element outside the cage
    d. Incandescent light bulb placed outside the cage

111. Rostral abrasions in the captive lizard are most commonly caused by:
    a. Fungal infections
    b. Facial impact with terrarium walls
    c. Trauma from cage mates
    d. Trauma from feeding live prey

112. Dysecdysis is the abnormal shedding of skin in a reptile. Which of the following is a common complication resulting from dysecdysis?
    a. Fungal infection of the dermis
    b. Subsequent systemic bacterial infection
    c. Extremity necrosis, especially of the toes or tail tip
    d. Constipation caused by eating the shed skin

113. Cloacal prolapse in the lizard is caused by all of the following *except*:
    a. Egg laying
    b. Foreign-body impaction
    c. Straining to defecate
    d. Septicemia

114. Diets high in purines cause which of the following diseases?
    a. Gout
    b. Heart failure
    c. Salmonellosis
    d. Liver failure

115. Ferrets are vaccinated annually for which of the following diseases?
    a. Rabies and feline panleukopenia
    b. Rabies and canine distemper
    c. Rabies and canine parvovirus
    d. Rabies and canine corona virus

116. The normal lifespan of a domestic ferret is:
    a. 2–4 years
    b. 7–10 years
    c. 10–12 years
    d. 5–7 years

117. You have been asked to place an intraosseous catheter in a very critical ferret. Which bone is most commonly used?
    a. Radius
    b. Ulna
    c. Fibula
    d. Femur

118. Which of the following white blood cells are predominant in the rabbit?
    a. Monocytes and neutrophils
    b. Lymphocytes and heterophils
    c. Metamyelocytes and azurophils
    d. Eosinophils and bands

119. What percentage of body weight is composed of bone in the rabbit?
    a. 13%
    b. 20%
    c. 8%
    d. 5%

120. Night feces in the rabbit are also referred to as:
    a. Cecotrophs
    b. Cecumliths
    c. Fusustrophs
    d. Colonoliths

121. Why is hay an important part of the rabbit diet?
    a. High in calories and vitamin C
    b. High in digestible fiber and helps wear the teeth
    c. Contains indigestible fiber that helps with weight management, dental disease, and gut health
    d. Helps maintain gut motility and is high in vitamins A, D, and E

122. Oblique skull radiographs are used to evaluate which of the following in a rabbit?
    a. Incisors
    b. Lower dental arcade only
    c. Upper dental arcade only
    d. Tooth roots

123. Pain in the rabbit is often exhibited by all of the following *except*:
    a. Moaning
    b. Bruxism
    c. Anorexia
    d. Reduced grooming and activity

124. The female rabbit is referred to as:
    a. Jill
    b. Bitch
    c. Doe
    d. Hobb

125. Male rabbits are referred to as:
    a. Bucks
    b. Hobbs
    c. Toms
    d. Colts

126. What is the range of the gestational period in a rabbit?
    a. 30–35 days
    b. 34–38 days
    c. 31–32 days
    d. 28–30 days

127. What is the normal rectal temperature range in the rabbit?
    a. 101° F–104° F
    b. 99.5° F–102.5° F
    c. 100° F–103° F
    d. 98.5° F–100.5° F

128. What percentage is the normal range for packed cell volume (PCV) in the rabbit?
    a. 25%–35%
    b. 33%–45%
    c. 44%–50%
    d. 50%–57%

129. Which of the following animals does *not* have molars that grow continuously throughout life?
    a. Rats
    b. Rabbits
    c. Chinchillas
    d. Guinea pigs

130. To keep the skin and coat healthy, a chinchilla should be offered a daily:
    a. Multivitamin
    b. Dust bath
    c. Vitamin C tablet
    d. Handful of dried papaya

131. Suitable bedding for the chinchilla includes all of the following *except*:
    a. Newspaper
    b. Recycled newspaper products
    c. Aspen shavings
    d. Pine shavings

132. Chinchillas are prone to all of the following diseases *except*:
    a. Dental disease
    b. Heat stroke
    c. Back fractures
    d. Choke

133. The average weight of an adult chinchilla ranges between:
    a. 400 g–600 g
    b. 200 g–400 g
    c. 600 g–900 g
    d. 800 g–1200 g

134. The female guinea pig is referred to as a:
    a. Hen
    b. Sow
    c. Queen
    d. Doe

135. A guinea pig presents with hind leg lameness. Physical examination findings include obesity, plantar thinning, and mild ulceration. These findings are indicative of which of the following diseases?
    a. Gout
    b. Vitamin C deficiency
    c. Pododermatitis
    d. *Streptobacillus spp.* infection

136. Scruffing is not recommended in chinchillas because of which of the following potential issues:
    a. It is painful for them
    b. Fur slip
    c. Scruffing is actually fine in chinchillas
    d. Chinchillas do not have enough skin around the neck region to scruff them properly

137. Which of the following is not a sign of dental disease in chinchillas, rabbits, and guinea pigs?
    a. Discharge from the ears
    b. Drooling
    c. Anorexia
    d. Overgrooming

138. Which of the following diets is most appropriate for a ferret?
    a. Oxbow Herbivore Care
    b. Oxbow Carnivore Care
    c. Ground alfalfa pellets
    d. Sweet potato baby food

139. Which of the following species has a duplex uterus and two cervices?
    a. Ferret
    b. Guinea pig
    c. Rat
    d. Rabbit

140. The proper diet in a ferret contains:
    a. 30%–40% protein and 15%–30% fat
    b. 50%–60% protein and 15%–30% fat
    c. 40%–50% protein and 15%–30% carbohydrates
    d. 25%–30% protein and 50% carbohydrates

141. Which of the following feathers are trimmed as part of the avian wing trim?
    a. Primary feathers
    b. Secondary feathers
    c. Tertiary feathers
    d. Tail feathers

142. Which of the following does *not* contribute to pododermatitis in the avian patient?
    a. Obesity
    b. Hypovitaminosis A
    c. Improper perch surfaces
    d. Psittacine beak and feather virus

143. A blue-and-gold macaw presents to the clinic with the following signs: depression, lethargy, anorexia, dyspnea, nasal and ocular discharge, conjunctivitis, and biliverdinuria (green urates). What disease should be at the top of the differential diagnosis list?
    a. Papillomatosis
    b. Psittacine beak and feather disease
    c. Proventricular dilation disease
    d. Avian chlamydophila

144. Which of the following leukocytes are usually the most numerous cells in avian blood?
    a. Eosinophils
    b. Heterophils
    c. Basophils
    d. Lymphocytes

145. Azurophils are leukocytes that are only found in what group of animals?
    a. Amphibians
    b. Mammals
    c. Birds
    d. Reptiles

146. Clinical signs of dystocia in the chelonian include all of the following *except*:
    a. Anorexia
    b. Lethargy
    c. Straining
    d. Seizures

147. The upper and lower shells of a turtle are referred to as:
    a. Plastron and carapace
    b. Anterior shell and posterior shell
    c. Epiplastral and endoplastral
    d. Hypoplastral and xiphiplastral

148. Where is the heart located in the snake?
    a. In the middle of the body, similar to a monitor lizard
    b. About 25% down the length of the body from the nares
    c. Just below the base of the skull
    d. About 2 inches below the skull

149. Which of the following statements is correct regarding the snake respiratory tract?
    a. Snakes have air sacs similar to those in birds
    b. Snakes have complete cartilaginous tracheal rings
    c. Most species have a single right lung and a nonfunctioning left lung
    d. The lungs run the entire length of the snake's body

150. Which of the following is *not* considered an appropriate bedding substrate for a snake?
    a. Indoor/outdoor carpet
    b. Newspaper
    c. Gravel/corncob bedding
    d. Cypress mulch

ⓔ *Answers and rationales available on Evolve*
http://evolve.elsevier.com/Prendergast/QAvettech/

Answer Key

SECTION 1

1. d	50. d	100. d	150. b
2. a	51. d	101. c	151. a
3. c	52. a	102. b	152. c
4. c	53. c	103. a	153. b
5. d	54. c	104. b	154. c
6. b	55. a	105. d	155. d
7. b	56. d	106. d	156. a
8. a	57. d	107. b	157. c
9. c	58. d	108. b	158. d
10. d	59. b	109. d	159. b
11. c	60. c	110. b	160. a
12. a	61. d	111. c	161. d
13. c	62. a	112. a	162. c
14. c	63. b	113. d	163. d
15. a	64. a	114. d	164. b
16. d	65. c	115. b	165. c
17. b	66. b	116. b	166. a
18. d	67. a	117. b	167. b
19. a	68. a	118. c	168. b
20. d	69. a	119. b	169. d
21. b	70. b	120. b	170. a
22. c	71. c	121. a	171. a
23. a	72. c	122. a	172. d
24. d	73. b	123. d	173. c
25. c	74. d	124. c	174. d
26. b	75. c	125. d	175. c
27. a	76. a	126. c	176. a
28. a	77. a	127. d	177. d
29. a	78. d	128. b	178. d
30. c	79. a	129. d	179. a
31. a	80. b	130. b	180. b
32. a	81. a	131. a	181. d
33. b	82. c	132. c	182. d
34. a	83. c	133. a	183. d
35. d	84. b	134. b	184. d
36. a	85. b	135. d	185. a
37. a	86. b	136. c	186. d
38. d	87. a	137. d	187. c
39. a	88. a	138. b	188. b
40. a	89. b	139. d	189. b
41. d	90. a	140. c	190. a
42. c	91. b	141. b	191. c
43. b	92. b	142. b	192. b
44. c	93. c	143. a	193. a
45. a	94. b	144. c	194. a
46. d	95. b	145. a	195. d
47. d	96. c	146. c	196. d
48. a	97. c	147. b	197. d
49. c	98. a	148. a	198. d
	99. a	149. b	199. c

200. d	257. d	314. b	371. d
201. b	258. c	315. b	372. d
202. c	259. d	316. b	373. d
203. a	260. d	317. d	374. a
204. b	261. b	318. b	375. b
205. b	262. c	319. b	376. d
206. d	263. b	320. a	377. b
207. a	264. c	321. c	378. a
208. d	265. c	322. b	379. d
209. c	266. a	323. a	380. c
210. d	267. d	324. c	381. c
211. b	268. a	325. d	382. d
212. b	269. c	326. d	383. b
213. d	270. b	327. a	384. c
214. b	271. c	328. c	385. d
215. a	272. b	329. b	386. b
216. a	273. b	330. d	387. c
217. c	274. d	331. a	388. b
218. b	275. d	332. b	389. d
219. d	276. d	333. b	390. b
220. b	277. d	334. b	391. b
221. c	278. b	335. b	392. b
222. b	279. c	336. b	393. d
223. b	280. b	337. a	394. b
224. a	281. c	338. a	395. b
225. a	282. d	339. b	396. c
226. c	283. d	340. d	397. b
227. c	284. a	341. d	398. d
228. b	285. a	342. d	399. d
229. d	286. b	343. b	400. b
230. a	287. a	344. d	401. b
231. b	288. c	345. c	402. b
232. c	289. a	346. b	403. c
233. c	290. b	347. a	404. d
234. c	291. b	348. d	405. b
235. b	292. a	349. c	406. c
236. a	293. c	350. e	407. b
237. a	294. c	351. c	408. c
238. d	295. b	352. d	409. b
239. c	296. d	353. d	410. b
240. c	297. a	354. a	411. c
241. b	298. c	355. c	412. e
242. c	299. d	356. d	413. b
243. c	300. d	357. b	414. a
244. a	301. c	358. b	415. c
245. b	302. a	359. d	416. b
246. d	303. b	360. b	417. b
247. d	304. b	361. a	418. d
248. b	305. a	362. d	419. b
249. c	306. b	363. a	420. d
250. b	307. a	364. c	421. a
251. b	308. c	365. b	422. c
252. b	309. d	366. c	423. b
253. d	310. b	367. d	424. d
254. a	311. d	368. b	425. a
255. c	312. c	369. b	426. a
256. d	313. a	370. a	427. b

428. b	485. c	542. a	599. b
429. b	486. a	543. c	600. c
430. c	487. d	544. c	601. a
431. d	488. d	545. b	602. b
432. b	489. d	546. b	603. d
433. b	490. a	547. b	604. c
434. c	491. a	548. b	605. d
435. a	492. b	549. d	606. a
436. b	493. c	550. d	607. c
437. c	494. b	551. d	608. a
438. a	495. a	552. c	609. d
439. c	496. b	553. b	610. c
440. a	497. c	554. d	611. b
441. d	498. d	555. b	612. b
442. c	499. c	556. a	613. b
443. c	500. c	557. a	614. b
444. d	501. c	558. d	615. d
445. a	502. d	559. c	616. d
446. c	503. c	560. e	617. a
447. b	504. a	561. d	618. c
448. c	505. d	562. d	619. c
449. b	506. d	563. b	620. b
450. c	507. d	564. d	621. b
451. a	508. b	565. b	622. b
452. b	509. b	566. b	623. c
453. b	510. b	567. b	624. d
454. b	511. d	568. c	625. a
455. c	512. c	569. c	626. b
456. c	513. b	570. d	627. c
457. d	514. d	571. d	628. b
458. a	515. c	572. b	629. d
459. c	516. b	573. c	630. c
460. b	517. b	574. d	631. b
461. a	518. b	575. a	632. b
462. c	519. b	576. d	633. c
463. d	520. a	577. c	634. a
464. b	521. c	578. c	635. c
465. d	522. b	579. a	636. b
466. d	523. c	580. b	637. d
467. b	524. b	581. d	638. a
468. d	525. d	582. d	639. a
469. b	526. b	583. a	640. b
470. b	527. b	584. b	641. c
471. c	528. c	585. d	642. a
472. b	529. b	586. c	643. c
473. b	530. a	587. b	644. e
474. a	531. c	588. a	645. b
475. c	532. d	589. b	646. c
476. d	533. b	590. d	647. a
477. b	534. b	591. a	648. c
478. b	535. c	592. a	649. a
479. c	536. c	593. c	650. b
480. d	537. c	594. c	651. d
481. b	538. b	595. d	652. b
482. b	539. a	596. d	653. b
483. d	540. c	597. c	654. b
484. a	541. b	598. d	655. c

656. c	11. a	68. c	6. c
657. c	12. b	69. a	7. c
658. b	13. a	70. b	8. b
659. d	14. b	71. a	9. a
660. d	15. c	72. d	10. a
661. d	16. c	73. b	11. c
662. a	17. e	74. c	12. d
663. b	18. c	75. d	13. b
664. d	19. b	76. b	14. b
665. b	20. d	77. b	15. d
666. b	21. d	78. b	16. d
667. c	22. c	79. a	17. c
668. b	23. d	80. d	18. d
669. b	24. d	81. d	19. d
670. c	25. c	82. b	20. d
671. b	26. d	83. d	21. c
672. d	27. d	84. c	22. b
673. b	28. b	85. c	23. c
674. c	29. a	86. c	24. c
675. c	30. b	87. c	25. b
676. c	31. b	88. b	26. c
677. a	32. d	89. b	27. a
678. b	33. b	90. a	28. b
679. c	34. d	91. c	29. c
680. d	35. b	92. d	30. a
681. b	36. b	93. c	31. b
682. a	37. a	94. b	32. a
683. b	38. c	95. a	33. d
684. b	39. d	96. c	34. d
685. a	40. d	97. c	35. d
686. c	41. d	98. d	36. c
687. b	42. d	99. b	37. a
688. d	43. a	100. b	38. c
689. a	44. e	101. a	39. c
690. a	45. d	102. d	40. a
691. b	46. b	103. d	41. b
692. b	47. a	104. c	42. d
693. d	48. c	105. d	43. b
694. d	49. d	106. b	44. d
695. a	50. b	107. c	45. d
696. b	51. b	108. c	46. c
697. d	52. d	109. c	47. a
698. a	53. d	110. a	48. b
699. c	54. b	111. c	49. a
700. b	55. c	112. d	50. c
	56. a	113. a	51. d
SECTION 2	57. d	114. b	52. b
1. c	58. c	115. d	53. b
2. a	59. c	116. b	54. b
3. d	60. d	117. d	55. c
4. b	61. d		56. c
5. b	62. c	**SECTION 3**	57. b
6. b	63. c	1. b	58. a
7. d	64. b	2. c	59. b
8. d	65. c	3. b	60. b
9. b	66. b	4. a	61. a
10. b	67. b	5. c	62. b

63. a
64. d
65. c
66. d
67. b
68. c
69. d
70. a
71. d
72. b
73. b
74. c
75. b
76. d
77. c
78. c
79. c
80. b
81. b
82. b
83. c
84. c
85. d
86. c
87. d
88. d
89. a
90. c
91. d
92. a
93. c
94. b
95. d
96. c
97. b
98. a
99. b
100. d
101. a
102. b
103. c
104. b
105. d
106. d
107. b
108. a
109. a
110. b
111. a
112. c
113. b
114. b
115. c
116. b
117. d
118. a
119. c

120. c
121. b
122. c
123. c
124. d
125. a
126. c
127. b
128. b
129. b
130. a
131. a
132. d
133. b
134. c
135. b
136. b
137. c
138. c
139. d
140. d
141. c
142. a
143. c
144. c
145. c
146. b
147. c
148. c
149. a
150. a
151. c
152. c
153. b
154. b
155. d
156. d
157. d
158. b
159. a
160. d
161. b
162. d
163. b
164. d
165. d
166. b
167. c
168. b
169. c
170. c
171. d
172. a
173. b
174. c
175. d
176. a

177. c
178. c
179. b
180. d
181. c
182. c
183. d
184. c
185. b
186. b
187. a
188. a
189. b
190. a
191. b
192. b
193. b
194. b
195. a
196. b
197. c
198. d
199. d
200. c
201. c
202. d
203. c
204. d
205. d
206. c
207. a
208. a
209. d
210. a
211. d
212. a
213. b
214. a
215. d
216. b
217. a
218. a
219. c
220. c
221. d
222. d

SECTION 4

1. b
2. b
3. b
4. a
5. c
6. d
7. d
8. c
9. c

10. b
11. d
12. a
13. c
14. b
15. d
16. c
17. b
18. b
19. b
20. a
21. d
22. b
23. b
24. a
25. b
26. c
27. b
28. a
29. b
30. b
31. a
32. c
33. a
34. a
35. b
36. b
37. c
38. b
39. c
40. d
41. b
42. a
43. d
44. c
45. b
46. b
47. b
48. c
49. b
50. b
51. b
52. b
53. a
54. c
55. b
56. b
57. b
58. b
59. a
60. b
61. b
62. a
63. a
64. c
65. c
66. b

67. a	124. a	181. b	6. c
68. b	125. d	182. b	7. b
69. d	126. b	183. d	8. c
70. a	127. b	184. a	9. b
71. c	128. b	185. b	10. d
72. b	129. b	186. b	11. c
73. a	130. c	187. a	12. c
74. b	131. a	188. c	13. b
75. c	132. b	189. b	14. c
76. b	133. b	190. b	15. d
77. b	134. c	191. a	16. c
78. c	135. a	192. c	17. d
79. c	136. a	193. b	18. c
80. c	137. b	194. c	19. c
81. b	138. c	195. c	20. d
82. c	139. b	196. b	21. d
83. a	140. d	197. c	22. c
84. a	141. b	198. d	23. b
85. b	142. a	199. c	24. c
86. c	143. b	200. d	25. c
87. a	144. a	201. c	26. c
88. a	145. a	202. b	27. d
89. b	146. b	203. b	28. b
90. c	147. d	204. d	29. a
91. c	148. b	205. d	30. c
92. a	149. a	206. c	31. c
93. d	150. d	207. b	32. d
94. b	151. a	208. a	33. d
95. b	152. c	209. c	34. a
96. a	153. d	210. d	35. c
97. c	154. a	211. b	36. c
98. b	155. a	212. c	37. c
99. d	156. d	213. b	38. d
100. b	157. b	214. b	39. d
101. b	158. d	215. c	40. c
102. a	159. a	216. b	41. d
103. b	160. b	217. b	42. d
104. c	161. d	218. c	43. b
105. b	162. a	219. b	44. a
106. b	163. b	220. c	45. b
107. b	164. c	221. d	46. a
108. b	165. d	222. b	47. b
109. d	166. b	223. a	48. d
110. a	167. c	224. c	49. d
111. c	168. b	225. c	50. a
112. c	169. b	226. b	51. a
113. b	170. b	227. b	52. c
114. a	171. a	228. b	53. b
115. b	172. d	229. c	54. d
116. b	173. c	230. c	55. b
117. b	174. b		56. a
118. d	175. c	**SECTION 5**	57. b
119. a	176. d	1. d	58. a
120. b	177. c	2. b	59. d
121. b	178. b	3. d	60. d
122. c	179. c	4. d	61. b
123. d	180. a	5. d	62. a

63. b	120. a	177. b	234. c
64. d	121. a	178. a	235. b
65. a	122. d	179. d	236. b
66. d	123. d	180. a	237. d
67. b	124. c	181. c	238. c
68. c	125. a	182. b	239. b
69. a	126. d	183. c	240. a
70. d	127. b	184. d	241. c
71. a	128. c	185. c	242. d
72. b	129. b	186. a	243. a
73. c	130. c	187. a	244. a
74. a	131. a	188. d	245. d
75. c	132. c	189. a	246. b
76. a	133. c	190. d	247. b
77. b	134. d	191. a	248. c
78. d	135. b	192. d	249. c
79. a	136. b	193. b	250. d
80. d	137. a	194. a	251. d
81. a	138. a	195. a	252. b
82. a	139. a	196. a	253. d
83. d	140. c	197. c	254. b
84. b	141. c	198. d	255. a
85. b	142. b	199. c	256. b
86. c	143. c	200. c	257. c
87. d	144. a	201. d	258. b
88. a	145. d	202. d	259. b
89. b	146. c	203. a	260. c
90. c	147. a	204. c	261. d
91. a	148. c	205. a	262. c
92. d	149. c	206. b	263. c
93. a	150. a	207. d	264. d
94. b	151. d	208. b	265. a
95. b	152. b	209. b	266. c
96. a	153. b	210. b	267. c
97. b	154. a	211. b	268. c
98. d	155. c	212. a	269. d
99. d	156. d	213. b	270. b
100. a	157. d	214. b	271. a
101. c	158. a	215. c	272. b
102. c	159. c	216. d	273. a
103. a	160. c	217. c	274. c
104. c	161. a	218. b	275. c
105. a	162. a	219. a	276. a
106. b	163. c	220. a	277. b
107. a	164. b	221. c	278. a
108. b	165. a	222. c	279. b
109. b	166. b	223. b	280. d
110. d	167. b	224. b	281. b
111. c	168. b	225. d	282. b
112. d	169. c	226. a	283. c
113. c	170. d	227. b	284. d
114. d	171. d	228. b	285. b
115. a	172. c	229. b	286. c
116. c	173. a	230. b	287. d
117. a	174. a	231. c	288. b
118. d	175. c	232. c	289. c
119. c	176. d	233. d	290. c

291. b	348. b	405. c	8. a
292. a	349. d	406. d	9. a
293. b	350. a	407. c	10. c
294. b	351. c	408. d	11. d
295. c	352. b	409. b	12. a
296. b	353. c	410. a	13. d
297. b	354. c	411. b	14. a
298. d	355. c	412. c	15. a
299. d	356. d	413. b	16. b
300. b	357. d	414. a	17. a
301. d	358. c	415. d	18. b
302. b	359. d	416. a	19. a
303. c	360. c	417. c	20. c
304. c	361. a	418. d	21. c
305. b	362. b	419. a	22. d
306. d	363. a	420. c	23. d
307. b	364. c	421. a	24. b
308. a	365. d	422. d	25. c
309. d	366. b	423. c	26. c
310. c	367. b	424. a	27. b
311. b	368. a	425. b	28. d
312. a	369. d	426. a	29. d
313. a	370. b	427. b	30. c
314. a	371. d	428. c	31. d
315. b	372. b	429. c	32. b
316. b	373. a	430. b	33. c
317. b	374. d	431. b	34. d
318. b	375. b	432. b	35. a
319. d	376. a	433. c	36. c
320. d	377. b	434. b	37. a
321. b	378. d	435. c	38. d
322. a	379. b	436. c	39. c
323. c	380. a	437. b	40. d
324. a	381. d	438. d	41. a
325. c	382. d	439. d	42. b
326. d	383. b	440. a	43. a
327. c	384. c	441. c	44. c
328. a	385. d	442. d	45. b
329. d	386. b	443. c	46. c
330. a	387. b	444. a	47. a
331. b	388. c	445. b	48. c
332. a	389. b	446. c	49. c
333. b	390. a	447. c	50. a
334. c	391. b	448. b	51. d
335. a	392. c	449. d	52. a
336. c	393. a	450. c	53. c
337. a	394. c	451. b	54. d
338. c	395. b	452. c	55. c
339. b	396. d		56. a
340. b	397. c	**SECTION 6**	57. c
341. b	398. b	1. b	58. b
342. d	399. d	2. d	59. b
343. d	400. a	3. b	60. a
344. c	401. b	4. a	61. b
345. c	402. a	5. d	62. d
346. a	403. d	6. d	63. a
347. d	404. b	7. c	64. c

65. a	122. d	179. b	236. a
66. a	123. b	180. a	237. d
67. a	124. d	181. b	238. b
68. b	125. a	182. d	239. d
69. a	126. a	183. c	240. c
70. d	127. b	184. d	241. d
71. d	128. b	185. a	242. d
72. d	129. a	186. c	243. b
73. a	130. d	187. c	244. a
74. d	131. d	188. b	245. c
75. b	132. d	189. c	246. a
76. d	133. a	190. a	247. b
77. a	134. d	191. d	248. a
78. a	135. d	192. c	249. d
79. b	136. b	193. b	250. d
80. c	137. c	194. d	251. d
81. d	138. a	195. a	252. d
82. d	139. c	196. c	253. c
83. b	140. c	197. b	254. b
84. a	141. b	198. c	255. d
85. d	142. d	199. b	256. b
86. a	143. a	200. c	257. d
87. c	144. c	201. a	258. d
88. c	145. a	202. c	259. d
89. a	146. d	203. a	260. d
90. a	147. d	204. d	261. c
91. a	148. b	205. d	262. c
92. c	149. c	206. c	263. b
93. d	150. d	207. b	264. a
94. a	151. c	208. a	265. c
95. a	152. b	209. d	266. d
96. a	153. a	210. d	267. b
97. d	154. c	211. d	268. d
98. c	155. c	212. b	269. b
99. a	156. c	213. d	270. b
100. c	157. b	214. b	271. d
101. b	158. a	215. b	272. b
102. d	159. b	216. d	273. c
103. c	160. c	217. d	274. d
104. a	161. b	218. a	275. c
105. a	162. d	219. d	276. c
106. c	163. a	220. a	277. a
107. b	164. b	221. a	278. b
108. c	165. c	222. c	279. c
109. d	166. a	223. a	280. b
110. d	167. c	224. b	281. c
111. c	168. c	225. d	282. c
112. b	169. a	226. d	283. c
113. d	170. c	227. d	284. c
114. d	171. a	228. b	285. b
115. b	172. c	229. a	286. a
116. a	173. b	230. d	287. b
117. d	174. b	231. b	288. b
118. a	175. b	232. c	289. c
119. a	176. d	233. b	290. d
120. c	177. c	234. a	291. c
121. d	178. a	235. b	292. d

293. c	350. d	407. d	51. d
294. c	351. c	408. d	52. b
295. c	352. c	409. b	53. c
296. c	353. c	410. a	54. a
297. b	354. b	411. b	55. d
298. d	355. b		56. a
299. b	356. b	**SECTION 7**	57. a
300. b	357. b	1. a	58. a
301. d	358. d	2. c	59. d
302. d	359. a	3. c	60. a
303. c	360. b	4. a	61. b
304. d	361. c	5. d	62. c
305. c	362. b	6. d	63. c
306. c	363. c	7. b	64. a
307. c	364. a	8. b	65. a
308. d	365. d	9. a	66. c
309. b	366. a	10. b	67. c
310. a	367. b	11. d	68. b
311. b	368. a	12. c	69. c
312. c	369. b	13. d	70. a
313. d	370. b	14. c	71. b
314. b	371. a	15. b	72. a
315. c	372. d	16. c	73. b
316. a	373. b	17. a	74. a
317. c	374. c	18. c	75. d
318. a	375. b	19. d	76. d
319. b	376. a	20. a	77. b
320. a	377. b	21. b	78. c
321. b	378. b	22. b	79. b
322. b	379. b	23. b	80. d
323. b	380. b	24. c	81. a
324. d	381. c	25. d	82. a
325. c	382. a	26. c	83. a
326. b	383. c	27. b	84. c
327. c	384. b	28. b	85. a
328. b	385. d	29. c	86. b
329. a	386. c	30. a	87. c
330. b	387. c	31. b	88. a
331. a	388. c	32. d	89. a
332. b	389. b	33. d	90. b
333. b	390. c	34. d	91. c
334. d	391. b	35. c	92. b
335. c	392. d	36. a	93. c
336. b	393. b	37. c	94. b
337. b	394. a	38. d	95. d
338. b	395. a	39. b	96. c
339. d	396. c	40. c	97. b
340. c	397. a	41. c	98. b
341. b	398. d	42. a	99. d
342. b	399. b	43. c	100. a
343. d	400. c	44. c	101. a
344. c	401. d	45. b	102. b
345. c	402. a	46. d	103. d
346. b	403. d	47. c	104. a
347. a	404. d	48. c	105. b
348. c	405. b	49. b	106. a
349. b	406. a	50. a	107. d

108. d
109. c
110. a
111. b
112. c
113. d
114. d
115. c
116. d
117. a
118. b
119. b
120. a
121. c
122. b
123. d
124. b
125. c
126. b
127. c
128. b
129. d
130. a
131. b
132. d
133. d
134. b
135. a
136. c
137. b
138. a
139. b
140. d
141. b
142. b
143. a
144. b
145. b
146. c
147. c
148. b
149. b
150. b
151. a
152. c
153. a
154. a
155. c
156. b
157. b
158. c
159. a
160. c
161. c
162. a
163. a
164. b

165. c
166. d
167. a
168. c
169. b
170. d
171. a
172. b
173. d
174. c
175. a
176. d
177. a
178. c
179. a
180. b
181. a
182. a
183. c
184. a
185. d
186. b
187. b
188. c
189. b
190. c
191. a
192. b
193. b
194. c
195. d
196. d
197. a
198. b
199. d
200. c
201. c
202. b
203. b
204. a
205. c
206. a
207. b
208. c
209. d
210. b
211. c
212. c
213. c
214. b
215. b
216. d
217. b
218. c
219. d
220. b
221. d

222. b
223. a
224. d
225. d
226. a
227. a
228. d
229. c
230. c
231. a
232. d
233. a
234. c
235. c
236. d
237. c
238. a
239. b
240. d
241. b
242. b
243. a
244. c
245. c
246. d
247. c
248. a
249. d
250. a
251. d
252. b
253. a
254. c
255. a

SECTION 8

1. a
2. a
3. a
4. d
5. a
6. a
7. a
8. d
9. b
10. a
11. b
12. b
13. b
14. c
15. d
16. b
17. b
18. b
19. a
20. d
21. c

22. b
23. c
24. a
25. b
26. a
27. a
28. c
29. a
30. a
31. d
32. a
33. d
34. c
35. b
36. a
37. b
38. d
39. d
40. c
41. d
42. d
43. a
44. b
45. d
46. d
47. c
48. a
49. c
50. d
51. b
52. c
53. d
54. c
55. a
56. d
57. c
58. c
59. c
60. a
61. a
62. c
63. d
64. a
65. c
66. d
67. c
68. c
69. a
70. c
71. b
72. c
73. a
74. c
75. d
76. b
77. b
78. c

79. c	136. a	193. b	250. d
80. c	137. c	194. c	251. a
81. c	138. d	195. a	252. b
82. a	139. a	196. b	253. a
83. b	140. a	197. c	254. a
84. c	141. c	198. a	255. c
85. c	142. a	199. b	256. d
86. d	143. c	200. d	257. b
87. a	144. d	201. c	258. d
88. a	145. d	202. b	259. d
89. a	146. a	203. a	260. b
90. d	147. d	204. b	261. a
91. c	148. b	205. d	262. a
92. b	149. a	206. c	263. b
93. d	150. c	207. a	264. a
94. c	151. a	208. d	265. b
95. c	152. c	209. a	266. b
96. d	153. d	210. d	267. a
97. b	154. b	211. c	268. c
98. d	155. c	212. a	269. a
99. c	156. d	213. b	270. b
100. b	157. d	214. c	271. b
101. d	158. a	215. a	272. b
102. c	159. c	216. d	273. b
103. d	160. d	217. b	274. b
104. a	161. d	218. c	275. d
105. c	162. b	219. d	276. b
106. d	163. a	220. a	277. a
107. d	164. d	221. c	278. c
108. c	165. a	222. b	279. d
109. b	166. c	223. c	280. a
110. b	167. b	224. c	281. d
111. a	168. c	225. b	282. b
112. b	169. a	226. b	283. d
113. c	170. c	227. b	284. a
114. c	171. b	228. d	285. b
115. c	172. a	229. b	286. c
116. d	173. b	230. a	287. a
117. b	174. d	231. a	288. c
118. b	175. b	232. b	289. b
119. c	176. c	233. c	290. a
120. b	177. c	234. d	291. d
121. c	178. a	235. a	292. b
122. c	179. c	236. b	293. c
123. c	180. c	237. d	294. d
124. d	181. d	238. b	295. a
125. a	182. b	239. c	296. c
126. c	183. b	240. a	297. a
127. a	184. c	241. b	298. c
128. b	185. b	242. c	299. c
129. d	186. c	243. c	300. b
130. d	187. d	244. b	301. a
131. c	188. b	245. d	302. d
132. b	189. c	246. c	303. b
133. c	190. a	247. b	304. c
134. a	191. c	248. d	305. a
135. a	192. a	249. a	306. c

307. d	364. b	421. d	29. d
308. c	365. b	422. c	30. c
309. a	366. c	423. d	31. a
310. b	367. b	424. b	32. c
311. a	368. d	425. c	33. a
312. c	369. d	426. b	34. c
313. b	370. b	427. d	35. b
314. d	371. d	428. c	36. d
315. d	372. d	429. a	37. a
316. c	373. d	430. b	38. a
317. d	374. b	431. c	39. b
318. d	375. d	432. a	40. c
319. a	376. d	433. b	41. a
320. c	377. a	434. b	42. d
321. c	378. b	435. c	43. d
322. b	379. c	436. a	44. b
323. b	380. d	437. c	45. a
324. a	381. a	438. b	46. a
325. d	382. a	439. c	47. d
326. a	383. b	440. a	48. a
327. d	384. c	441. d	49. b
328. b	385. d	442. b	50. d
329. b	386. a	443. a	51. a
330. a	387. d	444. a	52. c
331. b	388. c	445. a	53. c
332. c	389. b	446. d	54. a
333. c	390. d	447. d	55. a
334. a	391. c		56. b
335. c	392. a	**SECTION 9**	57. a
336. a	393. b	1. a	58. a
337. b	394. b	2. c	59. b
338. b	395. a	3. a	60. a
339. c	396. d	4. c	61. a
340. b	397. a	5. a	62. b
341. a	398. d	6. d	63. b
342. d	399. a	7. d	64. b
343. a	400. c	8. a	65. c
344. b	401. d	9. c	66. a
345. d	402. d	10. b	67. b
346. c	403. a	11. d	68. b
347. b	404. b	12. b	69. a
348. c	405. c	13. a	70. b
349. d	406. b	14. d	71. a
350. d	407. d	15. b	72. a
351. d	408. d	16. b	73. b
352. b	409. b	17. b	74. d
353. c	410. b	18. a	75. b
354. c	411. b	19. b	76. b
355. b	412. b	20. c	77. c
356. b	413. a	21. b	78. c
357. d	414. d	22. c	79. c
358. a	415. c	23. d	80. b
359. c	416. b	24. d	81. b
360. b	417. a	25. a	82. d
361. b	418. b	26. b	83. b
362. d	419. a	27. c	84. a
363. c	420. b	28. a	85. c

86. c	143. c	200. a	257. b
87. a	144. a	201. d	258. a
88. a	145. c	202. b	259. b
89. c	146. c	203. c	260. b
90. a	147. a	204. c	261. b
91. a	148. c	205. a	262. a
92. d	149. b	206. b	263. d
93. c	150. a	207. c	264. b
94. b	151. a	208. a	265. c
95. b	152. b	209. d	266. d
96. b	153. c	210. c	267. a
97. d	154. c	211. d	268. a
98. c	155. d	212. c	269. a
99. a	156. d	213. b	270. c
100. d	157. a	214. a	271. d
101. d	158. c	215. b	272. d
102. c	159. a	216. b	273. b
103. c	160. d	217. d	274. d
104. a	161. d	218. b	275. b
105. c	162. d	219. b	276. b
106. c	163. d	220. d	277. b
107. d	164. c	221. b	278. b
108. c	165. c	222. a	279. a
109. d	166. a	223. c	280. c
110. b	167. c	224. d	281. b
111. c	168. d	225. d	282. d
112. d	169. b	226. c	283. b
113. c	170. b	227. b	284. b
114. b	171. c	228. b	285. b
115. b	172. b	229. b	286. c
116. c	173. b	230. c	287. d
117. a	174. a	231. a	288. a
118. d	175. c	232. d	289. b
119. b	176. a	233. b	290. a
120. b	177. a	234. a	291. c
121. a	178. a	235. c	292. b
122. c	179. d	236. b	293. d
123. b	180. d	237. d	294. c
124. b	181. a	238. c	295. a
125. a	182. d	239. b	296. a
126. a	183. b	240. d	297. b
127. c	184. c	241. c	298. b
128. b	185. b	242. b	299. d
129. d	186. d	243. d	300. d
130. c	187. a	244. c	301. d
131. b	188. b	245. d	302. c
132. c	189. b	246. c	303. c
133. d	190. d	247. b	304. d
134. b	191. b	248. b	305. b
135. a	192. b	249. a	306. a
136. c	193. b	250. c	307. a
137. c	194. b	251. c	308. d
138. c	195. c	252. a	309. a
139. a	196. c	253. d	310. d
140. d	197. d	254. d	311. b
141. a	198. b	255. c	312. b
142. d	199. d	256. c	313. c

314. a	371. b	428. a	485. b
315. c	372. c	429. d	486. a
316. c	373. c	430. a	487. a
317. a	374. b	431. b	488. b
318. c	375. b	432. d	489. a
319. b	376. c	433. a	490. d
320. b	377. a	434. c	491. b
321. b	378. c	435. c	492. d
322. d	379. b	436. d	493. c
323. c	380. c	437. c	494. a
324. d	381. c	438. a	495. d
325. d	382. b	439. b	496. a
326. a	383. b	440. c	497. d
327. a	384. d	441. c	498. c
328. b	385. d	442. d	499. b
329. c	386. d	443. c	500. d
330. c	387. a	444. c	501. c
331. c	388. b	445. d	502. b
332. d	389. b	446. d	503. c
333. c	390. b	447. a	504. c
334. b	391. d	448. c	505. c
335. b	392. a	449. d	506. a
336. b	393. c	450. a	507. b
337. a	394. a	451. c	508. a
338. b	395. c	452. c	509. a
339. b	396. b	453. c	510. b
340. b	397. c	454. a	511. a
341. b	398. a	455. d	512. a
342. c	399. d	456. d	513. c
343. c	400. b	457. d	514. a
344. a	401. b	458. a	515. a
345. c	402. b	459. c	516. b
346. c	403. c	460. d	517. a
347. b	404. b	461. c	518. d
348. a	405. c	462. b	519. b
349. b	406. c	463. a	520. c
350. d	407. c	464. c	521. d
351. b	408. a	465. c	522. c
352. c	409. d	466. d	523. a
353. a	410. d	467. c	524. b
354. b	411. d	468. d	525. c
355. a	412. b	469. c	526. a
356. b	413. b	470. b	527. d
357. c	414. b	471. c	528. b
358. b	415. b	472. a	529. a
359. d	416. a	473. b	530. b
360. a	417. d	474. a	531. c
361. c	418. c	475. d	532. a
362. c	419. d	476. d	533. c
363. a	420. d	477. b	534. c
364. a	421. c	478. d	535. c
365. a	422. d	479. a	536. c
366. c	423. a	480. d	537. a
367. c	424. c	481. d	538. d
368. a	425. b	482. d	539. a
369. c	426. c	483. c	540. c
370. d	427. c	484. a	541. a

542. b	598. d	654. a	33. a
543. a	599. b	655. c	34. b
544. c	600. d	656. b	35. d
545. d	601. c	657. d	36. c
546. d	602. b	658. c	37. a
547. b	603. a	659. b	38. b
548. d	604. d	660. b	39. b
549. d	605. d	661. c	40. a
550. a	606. a	662. b	41. c
551. a	607. d	663. c	42. a
552. b	608. a	664. a	43. b
553. b	609. d	665. b	44. d
554. c	610. b	666. c	45. b
555. a	611. d	667. a	46. b
556. d	612. a	668. c	47. a
557. a	613. b	669. c	48. c
558. a	614. c	670. b	49. b
559. b	615. a	671. d	50. d
560. d	616. d	672. c	51. e
561. c	617. a	673. d	52. c
562. b	618. c	674. d	53. c
563. c	619. b	675. c	54. b
564. a	620. b		55. a
565. a	621. a	**SECTION 10**	56. d
566. a	622. b	1. b	57. d
567. c	623. c	2. d	58. b
568. b	624. b	3. b	59. c
569. c	625. a	4. d	60. b
570. d	626. d	5. b	61. a
571. d	627. b	6. b	62. a
572. d	628. c	7. c	63. c
573. a	629. d	8. c	64. a
574. a	630. d	9. b	65. b
575. a	631. d	10. d	66. c
576. a	632. a	11. a	67. d
577. c	633. c	12. d	68. a
578. b	634. b	13. a	69. a
579. c	635. b	14. d	70. d
580. d	636. b	15. a	71. d
581. b	637. c	16. b	72. d
582. b	638. c	17. c	73. c
583. b	639. a	18. a	74. b
584. c	640. b	19. b	75. a
585. d	641. a	20. c	76. b
586. a	642. b	21. a	77. d
587. d	643. d	22. a	78. c
588. d	644. a	23. c	79. d
589. b	645. c	24. b	80. d
590. b	646. d	25. c	81. d
591. d	647. b	26. a	82. b
592. b	648. b	27. a	83. c
593. a	649. b	28. a	84. b
594. b	650. c	29. b	85. a
595. a	651. d	30. d	86. b
596. c	652. c	31. c	87. a
597. b	653. d	32. b	88. c

89. c	145. d	201. c	257. a
90. b	146. a	202. d	258. b
91. b	147. c	203. b	259. c
92. a	148. b	204. c	260. c
93. b	149. b	205. b	261. d
94. d	150. c	206. d	
95. c	151. d	207. b	**SECTION 11**
96. e	152. d	208. a	1. a
97. b	153. a	209. d	2. b
98. c	154. d	210. a	3. b
99. b	155. c	211. b	4. d
100. c	156. b	212. a	5. a
101. b	157. c	213. a	6. b
102. b	158. c	214. c	7. d
103. a	159. d	215. a	8. d
104. b	160. d	216. b	9. b
105. b	161. c	217. a	10. a
106. b	162. d	218. d	11. a
107. d	163. c	219. b	12. c
108. d	164. d	220. d	13. c
109. a	165. c	221. c	14. c
110. b	166. a	222. b	15. b
111. b	167. d	223. b	16. c
112. b	168. a	224. d	17. c
113. a	169. b	225. c	18. a
114. c	170. c	226. b	19. b
115. c	171. d	227. b	20. a
116. b	172. d	228. d	21. d
117. a	173. b	229. b	22. a
118. b	174. c	230. d	23. c
119. a	175. b	231. c	24. d
120. c	176. b	232. a	25. c
121. a	177. b	233. b	26. d
122. b	178. a	234. c	27. c
123. b	179. d	235. b	28. a
124. c	180. b	236. c	29. c
125. b	181. b	237. a	30. d
126. a	182. b	238. c	31. d
127. e	183. a	239. a	32. d
128. c	184. d	240. c	33. b
129. c	185. d	241. c	34. b
130. a	186. d	242. b	35. a
131. a	187. b	243. c	36. b
132. c	188. a	244. d	37. b
133. b	189. d	245. b	38. c
134. c	190. b	246. d	39. d
135. b	191. c	247. b	40. d
136. c	192. c	248. a	41. a
137. d	193. c	249. b	42. a
138. c	194. b	250. e	43. c
139. b	195. a	251. c	44. a
140. b	196. b	252. a	45. a
141. a	197. d	253. c	46. a
142. b	198. b	254. b	47. c
143. c	199. b	255. a	48. d
144. b	200. b	256. c	49. d

50. b	107. d	164. c	221. b
51. b	108. d	165. c	222. d
52. d	109. d	166. c	223. c
53. a	110. d	167. a	224. b
54. a	111. a	168. c	225. b
55. c	112. a	169. a	226. b
56. c	113. c	170. b	227. d
57. c	114. a	171. b	228. a
58. b	115. b	172. c	229. c
59. b	116. b	173. b	230. a
60. d	117. d	174. d	231. c
61. a	118. b	175. d	232. d
62. b	119. d	176. a	233. c
63. c	120. d	177. b	234. c
64. c	121. c	178. b	235. b
65. b	122. a	179. d	236. b
66. a	123. b	180. a	237. c
67. c	124. c	181. d	238. b
68. a	125. b	182. d	239. c
69. b	126. b	183. c	240. b
70. c	127. b	184. c	241. b
71. b	128. a	185. b	242. c
72. c	129. a	186. c	243. c
73. b	130. d	187. a	244. a
74. b	131. a	188. c	245. e
75. a	132. c	189. a	246. d
76. c	133. a	190. c	247. c
77. a	134. c	191. d	248. b
78. b	135. b	192. b	249. c
79. c	136. b	193. d	250. a
80. c	137. c	194. a	251. a
81. a	138. d	195. a	252. b
82. b	139. b	196. d	253. c
83. d	140. b	197. b	254. b
84. c	141. a	198. a	255. a
85. d	142. d	199. c	256. a
86. c	143. b	200. b	257. c
87. c	144. d	201. c	258. b
88. c	145. c	202. b	259. d
89. c	146. b	203. a	260. a
90. c	147. a	204. b	261. d
91. a	148. c	205. c	262. a
92. d	149. b	206. a	263. a
93. a	150. d	207. b	264. a
94. a	151. a	208. b	265. c
95. d	152. b	209. a	266. d
96. c	153. b	210. d	267. d
97. a	154. a	211. a	268. a
98. c	155. b	212. b	269. b
99. b	156. b	213. a	270. a
100. d	157. b	214. d	271. d
101. d	158. b	215. d	272. c
102. b	159. a	216. b	273. b
103. a	160. d	217. b	274. c
104. b	161. b	218. a	275. a
105. d	162. d	219. a	276. b
106. a	163. a	220. c	277. c

278. d	335. b	392. c	449. d
279. d	336. a	393. a	450. c
280. b	337. c	394. b	451. c
281. a	338. d	395. c	452. b
282. d	339. c	396. d	453. c
283. b	340. a	397. a	454. b
284. b	341. d	398. b	455. d
285. a	342. b	399. a	456. b
286. c	343. c	400. c	457. a
287. d	344. d	401. b	458. d
288. b	345. c	402. c	459. a
289. b	346. a	403. b	460. d
290. d	347. c	404. d	461. a
291. c	348. d	405. b	462. d
292. a	349. d	406. c	463. d
293. c	350. a	407. a	464. c
294. a	351. b	408. d	465. b
295. d	352. c	409. d	466. a
296. a	353. a	410. d	467. b
297. c	354. b	411. b	468. d
298. b	355. d	412. b	469. d
299. a	356. a	413. d	470. a
300. b	357. b	414. d	471. d
301. d	358. a	415. b	472. b
302. b	359. b	416. b	473. c
303. c	360. b	417. c	474. b
304. d	361. c	418. a	475. b
305. c	362. c	419. b	476. c
306. c	363. d	420. c	477. d
307. a	364. c	421. b	478. d
308. b	365. c	422. d	479. c
309. b	366. d	423. b	480. b
310. b	367. a	424. a	481. a
311. a	368. d	425. b	482. b
312. d	369. d	426. c	483. b
313. b	370. b	427. a	484. a
314. a	371. a	428. c	485. c
315. d	372. d	429. a	486. d
316. c	373. c	430. d	487. d
317. b	374. b	431. c	488. d
318. b	375. c	432. a	489. d
319. b	376. c	433. c	490. b
320. c	377. d	434. b	491. b
321. c	378. b	435. d	492. a
322. b	379. b	436. a	493. b
323. b	380. a	437. b	494. d
324. a	381. b	438. b	495. d
325. c	382. a	439. c	496. d
326. c	383. a	440. a	497. c
327. a	384. b	441. a	498. b
328. a	385. b	442. d	499. a
329. a	386. b	443. b	500. b
330. c	387. d	444. b	501. c
331. d	388. b	445. d	502. b
332. c	389. c	446. d	503. a
333. b	390. a	447. a	504. d
334. d	391. d	448. b	505. d

506. b	563. a	21. d	78. b
507. b	564. d	22. d	79. a
508. d	565. c	23. a	80. a
509. c	566. d	24. a	81. b
510. a	567. d	25. b	82. c
511. b	568. b	26. a	83. b
512. d	569. a	27. c	84. d
513. b	570. b	28. d	85. c
514. c	571. a	29. d	86. b
515. a	572. d	30. c	87. c
516. c	573. c	31. c	88. c
517. b	574. b	32. d	89. d
518. d	575. c	33. c	90. c
519. c	576. b	34. b	91. d
520. c	577. b	35. c	92. c
521. c	578. a	36. b	93. a
522. c	579. c	37. b	94. c
523. a	580. d	38. d	95. b
524. b	581. b	39. b	96. a
525. c	582. a	40. b	97. a
526. c	583. d	41. b	98. c
527. b	584. c	42. d	99. c
528. a	585. c	43. c	100. a
529. c	586. b	44. a	101. a
530. b	587. b	45. b	102. d
531. d	588. b	46. b	103. d
532. a	589. b	47. d	104. c
533. a	590. b	48. d	105. a
534. c	591. c	49. d	106. b
535. d	592. b	50. a	107. d
536. a	593. d	51. c	108. a
537. c	594. a	52. d	109. c
538. d	595. b	53. d	110. c
539. a	596. a	54. a	111. b
540. a	597. d	55. c	112. b
541. c		56. c	113. d
542. c	**SECTION 12**	57. c	114. c
543. c		58. b	115. a
544. a	1. a	59. d	116. d
545. d	2. a	60. c	117. a
546. a	3. c	61. d	119. c
547. b	4. b	62. c	120. d
548. d	5. b	63. b	121. b
549. a	6. c	64. d	122. b
550. c	7. a	65. c	123. c
551. d	8. d	66. b	124. d
552. c	9. a	67. a	125. b
553. a	10. c	68. d	126. c
554. b	11. c	69. d	127. d
555. d	12. c	70. b	128. a
556. b	13. c	71. c	129. a
557. c	14. b	72. d	130. b
558. d	15. c	73. a	131. b
559. d	16. b	74. a	132. a
560. a	17. a	75. a	133. a
561. c	18. b	76. b	134. c
562. b	19. a	77. c	135. a
	20. d		

136. d	193. b	23. a	80. a
137. c	194. d	24. d	81. b
138. c	195. d	25. c	82. c
139. b	196. b	26. c	83. a
140. d	197. b	27. c	84. b
141. d	198. b	28. c	85. c
142. d	199. a	29. c	86. d
143. a	200. b	30. a	87. d
144. c	201. d	31. d	88. b
145. c	202. d	32. d	89. d
146. a	203. a	33. b	90. c
147. b	204. c	34. d	91. d
148. c	205. a	35. a	92. d
149. b	206. c	36. b	93. b
150. b	207. b	37. c	94. d
151. a	208. d	38. d	95. d
152. a	209. c	39. c	96. d
153. d	210. b	40. b	97. c
154. c	211. c	41. b	98. d
155. c	212. c	42. d	99. b
156. d	213. c	43. a	100. d
157. c	214. a	44. b	101. d
158. c	215. b	45. c	102. a
159. c	216. a	46. b	103. b
160. a	217. a	47. d	104. c
161. c	218. a	48. a	105. a
162. a	219. b	49. d	106. d
163. a	220. c	50. c	107. b
164. c	221. a	51. d	108. a
165. b	222. d	52. a	109. d
166. b	223. c	53. c	110. d
167. a	224. b	54. d	111. a
168. b	225. a	55. c	112. d
169. d		56. d	113. c
170. a	**SECTION 13**	57. d	114. a
171. b	1. c	58. a	115. c
172. c	2. b	59. b	116. b
173. a	3. a	60. d	117. a
174. c	4. b	61. c	118. d
175. d	5. c	62. c	119. c
176. b	6. a	63. d	120. d
177. c	7. a	64. b	121. a
178. b	8. d	65. d	122. b
179. b	9. c	66. a	123. a
180. c	10. d	67. b	124. c
181. b	11. a	68. c	125. a
182. d	12. c	69. d	126. a
183. c	13. b	70. d	127. c
184. b	14. b	71. b	128. c
185. c	15. d	72. c	129. a
186. a	16. a	73. a	130. d
187. c	17. b	74. d	131. b
188. c	18. c	75. c	132. b
189. d	19. d	76. c	133. c
190. d	20. b	77. c	134. a
191. a	21. c	78. b	135. d
192. a	22. b	79. d	136. a

137. c
138. c
139. b
140. a
141. d
142. a
143. d
144. b
145. a
146. d
147. b
148. d
149. a
150. b
151. a
152. c
153. c
154. b
155. d
156. d
157. c
158. d
159. a
160. b
161. b
162. a
163. d
164. c
165. a
166. b
167. c
168. d
169. a
170. c
171. c
172. d
173. b
174. d
175. b
176. a
177. d
178. b
179. c
180. c
181. b
182. b
183. a
184. a
185. d
186. b
187. b
188. a
189. c
190. b
191. d
192. b
193. b

194. c
195. b
196. d
197. c
198. b
199. a
200. d
201. b
202. a
203. c
204. c
205. d
206. d
207. b
208. a
209. b
210. a
211. c
212. d
213. a
214. c
215. c
216. d
217. d
218. c
219. b
220. b
221. a
222. a
223. d
224. b
225. d
226. a
227. a
228. b
229. b
230. d
231. d
232. a
233. c
234. c
235. d
236. b
237. a
238. b
239. c
240. a
241. c
242. b
243. a
244. d
245. a
246. d
247. a
248. d
249. a
250. d

251. d
252. c
253. a
254. b
255. c
256. d
257. a
258. c
259. a
260. b

SECTION 14

1. c
2. d
3. b
4. a
5. b
6. d
7. b
8. a
9. d
10. a
11. b
12. c
13. a
14. b
15. c
16. d
17. c
18. a
19. b
20. d
21. b
22. d
23. b
24. a
25. c
26. a
27. b
28. b
29. d
30. a
31. c
32. d
33. a
34. b
35. d
36. c
37. b
38. c
39. d
40. c
41. a
42. d
43. b
44. a
45. c

46. d
47. c
48. b
49. d
50. c
51. b
52. d
53. b
54. a
55. c
56. b
57. c
58. b
59. c
60. c
61. b
62. a
63. a
64. d
65. b
66. d
67. d
68. c
69. a
70. c
71. d
72. c
73. a
74. c
75. a
76. c
77. d
78. d
79. a
80. d
81. c
82. a
83. b
84. d
85. a
86. a
87. d
88. d
89. c
90. a
91. a
92. c
93. a
94. b
95. c
96. d
97. b
98. d
99. b
100. d
101. a
102. d

103. c	**115.** b	**127.** a	**139.** d
104. a	**116.** d	**128.** b	**140.** a
105. b	**117.** d	**129.** a	**141.** a
106. d	**118.** b	**130.** b	**142.** d
107. b	**119.** c	**131.** d	**143.** d
108. c	**120.** a	**132.** c	**144.** b
109. d	**121.** a	**133.** a	**145.** d
110. a	**122.** d	**134.** b	**146.** d
111. b	**123.** a	**135.** c	**147.** a
112. c	**124.** c	**136.** b	**148.** b
113. d	**125.** a	**137.** a	**149.** c
114. a	**126.** c	**138.** b	**150.** c